BS60
50
0

UNDERWATER MEDICINE

Underwater Medicine

STANLEY MILES

C.B., M.D., M.Sc., D.T.M. & H., F.R.C.P., F.R.C.S.,
Surgeon Rear-Admiral;
Dean of Postgraduate Medical Studies, University of Manchester;
formerly Director of Medical Research,
Royal Naval Medical School, Alverstoke, Hants

THIRD EDITION

STAPLES PRESS LONDON

Granada Publishing Limited
First published in Great Britain 1962 by Staples Press
3 Upper James Street London WIR 4BP
Second edition 1966
Third edition 1969, reprinted 1972

ISBN 0 286 62723 X

Printed in Great Britain by
Ebenezer Baylis & Son Limited
Worcester and London

CONTENTS

FOREWORD

IT IS with considerable pleasure that I write a few words to introduce Surgeon Captain Miles's book on Underwater Medicine. New books usually present an apologia for their appearance. None is necessary here. The wide and active public interest in diving and the underwater world has made this book a real necessity. More and more ordinary and extraordinary citizens are taking up independent underwater swimming as a hobby and recreation. Any medical man may find himself responsible for advising such people. He now has available to him an integrated account of physical principles, physiological risks, medical problems and all the related hazards.

It is fitting that a member of the Royal Navy should write this book. While in no way detracting from the great pioneer work of other nations, the British contribution to our knowledge of diving and the physical and physiological problems involved is not widely appreciated even by the British themselves.

The first real practical dive in which a man wore a leather suit and a brass helmet and had compressed air pumped through his helmet took place off the Needles in 1754 and was described by Dr Richard Pococke in his *Travels in England*. Fullerton, a naval surgeon, suggested in 1805 that divers should be free and carry a reservoir charged with air, highly condensed. August Siebe introduced the first safe air diving apparatus for general use in 1819. Sir Robert Davis, who later succeeded him, worked with Dr J. S. Haldane and Sir Leonard Hill and these great pioneers contributed to almost all aspects of diving and submarine escape. In 1905 J. S. Haldane and Captain Damant produced the famous decompression tables which largely defeated the grave risks of decompression sickness. In 1930 British naval air divers descended to 300 ft. in the open sea and encountered nitrogen narcosis for the first time. On reading the original accounts of these dives one senses a strong undercurrent of indignation that not all these intrepid men could behave with absolute parade ground correctness under these conditions. This mystery was illuminated shortly afterwards by the brilliant work of Behnke, Thomson and Shaw of the United States Navy. The British diver is peculiarly resistant to this narcosis as judged by reports from other countries. It has been suggested that this is due to exposure to the daily tot of rum and disciplined behaviour in front of the officer of the watch after evenings ashore in Portsmouth.

7

In 1933 two Royal Naval officers, Captain Damant and Surgeon Lieutenant Commander Phillips breathed oxygen at four atmospheres absolute. Both experienced acute oxygen poisoning and Phillips convulsed; the first definite record of acute oxygen poisoning.

In 1878 H. A. Fleuss designed the earliest form of self-contained breathing apparatus with a cylinder of compressed gases, a counter-lung and a canister containing tow impregnated with potash. He tested the apparatus alone, personally, in the Thames.

During the Second World War the Royal Navy, stimulated by the remarkable Italian success in disabling the battleships in Alexandria harbour, developed a highly efficient organization to cope with all aspects of underwater warfare and the attendant physiological and diving problems. Human torpedoes (charioteers), frogmen, beach reconnaissance groups, baby submarine divers, harbour clearance teams and varying types of underwater commandos and saboteurs were developed in large numbers. In 1945 Great Britain led the world in these types of activities from both the operational and scientific aspects. However, since these days the diving authorities in this country have had little to do with the world-wide publicity of the underwater advances which have popularized independent diving as a sport and recreation. The attitude of the Royal Navy, perhaps unfortunately, remains strictly professional and practical. The contrasting names for nitrogen narcosis in France (rapture of the deep) and in Britain (the 'narks') mentioned by the author are a delightful example of this.

The discussions of submarine escape in this book are well worth reading as they are an excellent exercise concerning almost all physical and physiological principles and problems in underwater survival.

Finally the author, although a great enthusiast and optimist, has rightly included sections dealing with drowning and resuscitation. The sea remains dangerous and unpredictable and those who go down under the sea should study her with the same devotion and respect as those who go down to the sea in ships.

K. W. Donald, D.S.C., M.A., M.D., D.SC., F.R.C.P.,
Professor of Medicine, University of Edinburgh,
Scientific Consultant to the Royal Navy,
Consulting Physician to the Navy in Scotland

PREFACE

Wherever there is water, salt or fresh, warm or cold, in the open sea or in underground inland caves there will be men who will wish to explore and exploit it. Improved breathing apparatus and protective clothing is enabling man to remain in water longer and to venture deeper with the result that, today, in addition to the naval requirements of underwater-warfare, there is increasing application to commercial development and recreational activity.

Throughout the world are many groups of men who spend much of their time in and under water. They include, not only naval divers and frogmen, but commercial divers working on salvage, seeking underwater supplies of oil and coal, examining wrecks and gathering pearls. Many more are there for pleasure and interest such as the 'Skin' Divers, Spear Fishermen, Sub-Aqua Club members, Underwater Research Groups, Marine Biologists, Archaeologists, Underwater Cave Explorers and Photographers. Whatever the interest or profession there is no doubt that more and more men and women are going in and under water. All are entering a new environment in which as they extend their activities, common problems of adaptation are faced and new hazards met.

This book is an attempt to review and bring together current work and knowledge of the medical problems of the underwater environment, to consider the dangers and their avoidance and to look at the potential man has before him.

The first hope therefore is that what is written may contribute in some way to the lessening of the risk to life and health of those whose work or play brings them into intimate contact with the seas or inland waters. Secondly it will be apparent that, in spite of what is already known, there are vast areas of uncertainty, the challenge of which must stimulate further thought and effort.

Underwater Medicine, as such, is a relatively new field in which, though there is a good foundation of factual knowledge, much is still speculation. The reader should have no difficulty in separating fact from fantasy. Dreaming must always be the fore-runner of discovery and the author asks that, on the occasions when he trespasses into the realm of fancy, he may be forgiven in the belief that, where there are gaps in knowledge they may as well be temporarily filled with ideas until the truth is established. In Underwater Medicine there are many such gaps.

9

Finally the author would like sincerely to acknowledge his deep gratitude to many friends in this and other countries for help and encouragement and in particular to his colleagues at the Royal Naval Physiological Laboratory and the Admiralty Experimental Diving Unit. These include Professor K. W. Donald for continued encouragement and his kindness in writing a foreword. Dr H. J. Taylor for allowing reproduction of pictures of the R.N. Physiological Laboratory of which he is Superintendent, Margaret Trimboy and John Davis for help with many of the drawings and Sir Robert Davis for allowing reproductions of illustrations from his own book on Deep Diving. Most valuable help with, and criticism of, the various chapters has been generously given by Commander John Carr, Superintendent of Diving, Surgeon Lieutenant Commander Eric Mackay, Surgeon Lieutenant Peter Barnard and Messrs H. V. Hempleman and P. B. Bennett. To them all—many thanks. There are many others too, Doctors, Divers, Draughtsmen, who in their various ways have made most useful and welcome contributions. Finally the permission of the Medical Director General of the Navy, Surgeon Vice-Admiral W. R. S. Panckridge, to publish this work is greatly appreciated.

Hill Head: 1st June 1961

PREFACE TO SECOND EDITION

IN THE past three years there has been a marked increase in interest in underwater activities in naval, commercial, academic and recreational fields. Much publicity has been given to the underwater exploits of Cousteau, Link and Bond whose success in maintaining men in underwater compartments has inspired the imagination of all.

Two very important international conferences have been held. In November, 1962 the British Sub-Aqua Club were hosts to the World Underwater Federation at a conference on Underwater Activities in London. This has been reported in a publication 'The Undersea Challenge' produced by the Palantype Organization. More recently the National Academy of Sciences in America held a Second Symposium on Underwater Physiology, the proceedings of which were published in 1963. In addition there has been a growing interest by the medical profession in the uses of high pressure oxygen in the treatment of certain accidents and illnesses, the success of which depends on a sound knowledge of pressure physiology.

The changes which have been made in this edition reflect some of these recent advances but, by and large, the basic physics and physiology must remain unchanged. New references have been added where these are appropriate.

Hill Head: 1st September 1964

PREFACE TO THIRD EDITION

THE IMPETUS which underwater development has received in the last five years has been remarkable particularly in the extension of both time and depth of man's underwater capability.

Man himself has not changed but the ways and means of increasing his underwater activity have introduced new stresses and techniques. This is largely due to growing naval and commercial interests. It has therefore been necessary to re-write much of the text and add a new Chapter on 'Saturation Diving'.

The growing complexity of equipment, underwater vehicles and submarines makes it all the more important that man himself, the crucial unit in the effort, is at all times given careful consideration for his health and well being. This cannot be too strongly emphasized.

Hill Head: 1st March 1969

UNDERWATER MEDICINE

PART I

The Environment

CHAPTER I

The Challenge

IT IS most important, right at the outset, to realize that the problems of man's adaptation to a watery environment are primarily those of temperament. True all manner of physical adjustments are necessary and the study of these must occupy the bulk of subsequent chapters but time and time again in the practice of underwater medicine one is brought up against some psychological impasse. Why this is so may become apparent if thought is given to the reasons why, amongst all the possible outlets for man's exploring instincts, the urge to investigate the depths of the oceans is quite low down on the list.

The history of man's achievement in exploration covers first the land and surface of the seas and then the air. He could explore the land on foot even to the tops of the highest mountains. To voyage over the seas he needed boats which over the years have increased in efficiency and to conquer the atmosphere, an achievement of a relatively few decades, the aeroplane has been developed to an astounding degree. Today he has reached beyond the atmosphere into space where, though formidable obstacles confront him, there is every reason to believe that, with the aid of modern science, he will enlarge his already considerable accomplishments. In short man has, since he inhabited the earth, extended his sphere of activity to include its surface, its atmosphere and beyond. Always into the unknown.

It is indeed strange that the urge to explore and conquer has not caused man to investigate more fully the depths of the oceans. Indeed there are many physical barriers in the change of medium, the absence of respirable air and the great pressures to be encountered but these can be no more formidable than those which face the potential space traveller. No one quite knows what will be the rewards of the conquest of the outer space but there is no doubt that the seas and sea-bed hold a great source of wealth.

To find the reason why undersea exploration has not kept pace with extra-territorial adventuring it is necessary to look beyond the physical barriers. Instinctively man distrusts the sea. In his development from primitive life he has escaped from it. In his pre-natal life he recapitulates the struggle of the human race to establish itself as land dwelling. To him, subconsciously perhaps, the sea is the primitive womb of all living things. He has no wish to return. To trek across deserts, through jungles

2

or over ice fields, to climb great mountains and to soar through the air is to advance, to return beneath the sea is to retreat. He is afraid of its storms and appalled at the enveloping darkness of the deeps. To drown is quite the worst form of death he can imagine.

It is against such a background of inherent suspicion that man is at last seriously coming to accept the great underseas challenge and before he attempts to overcome the physical barriers it is necessary for him to come to terms with the new environment, an achievement needing both courage and understanding.

It is against this background too, that the science and art of underwater medicine must be considered. To the man in the street the promise of a climb up a high mountain or a flight in a modern aircraft may be accepted with anticipation of an exhilarating experience but few would accept with anything but alarm the offer of a descent in a diving bell or even a trip in a submarine.

THE GROWING AWARENESS

It is difficult to know just what has stimulated the present growing awareness of the potential of underwater development but there is no doubt that more and more people are becoming actively interested. Probably the biggest single factor is the development, in recent years, of the self-contained breathing apparatus, the 'aqua lung' or its equivalent, which has made underwater exploration available to all. This has been glamorized by such enthusiasts as Jacques Cousteau and Hans Hass whose writings and television programmes have done much to foster interest in what goes on beneath the waves.

Before this however, in the warm coastal waters of Japan and Korea, women—the Diving Amas—had been, for over 2,000 years, harvesting shell fish, seaweed, sponges and even pearls from the sea-bed. They still continue, their methods little changed, being still dependent on their ability of breath holding. This limits them to a range not exceeding 100 ft. in depth. Recent physiological studies of these remarkable women have contributed much to the understanding of man's adaptation underwater (Rahn 1965).

The extensive use of 'Frogmen' in the Second World War has produced a series of dramatic anecdotes of man's adaptation to the underwater environment in a specialized and individual form of conflict which cannot fail to stimulate an appreciation of what may be achieved by similar application in times of peace.

The conventional diver connected to the surface by means of his air pipe and body line has done little, in spite of a splendid record of salvage to his credit, to inspire all but a devoted few. When in a Norwegian Fjord in 1956 a British Naval Diver, Lieutenant George Wookey, established a world record dive of 600 ft. there was little publicity though this was in every way an achievement as important as the first four-minute mile. Though unspectacular it is the experience gained by this type of diving which has provided the basis of modern diving of every kind. It showed the limitations of Standard Diving even with mixture breathing. Wookey's dive with a five minute bottom time and many hours of uncomfortable decompression was undoubtedly the limit for this form of diving and showed that alternative techniques would be necessary for further achievement.

Speaking to a gathering of members of the British Sub-Aqua Club in Brighton early in 1960, Sir Alistair Hardy, an eminent zoologist, drew attention to the importance of the underwater environment. He propounded an interesting theory that man's far distant ancestors, finding food on land becoming scarce, ventured into shallow coastal waters to supplement their diet with sea food. In so doing, he suggested they learnt to swim and lost their hair. Far more important was his suggestion that once more, man, faced with a population growing more rapidly than the resources of food on land, might again turn to the sea to augment supplies. This did not mean an improvement of conventional fishing techniques but that man would find the means to work below the sea and to domesticate the marine creatures. In fact to develop organized underwater farming.

This Brighton meeting has been repeated annually with ever increasing enthusiasm. It is basically a scientific conference which has attracted the world's top workers in underwater problems. At the same time it has encouraged underwater photography, with competitive exhibitions.

The most important conferences however for the underwater medical workers have been the series of International Symposia on Underwater Physiology organized in Washington by the National Academy of Science and the United States Navy. They have been held in 1955, 1963 and 1966. It is proposed to maintain this three year interval and future conferences might well be held in other interested countries. These meetings led in 1968 to the formation of an Undersea Medical Association to ensure adequate exchange of knowledge and international cooperation.

Also in 1960 Cousteau, on a lecture tour of the United States was telling his listeners of his plans, then well on the way to success, to build an underwater farm in the Mediterranean. He envisaged, in his

underwater farm yard, sea creatures herded and penned and referred
to an 'underwater pig farm'. If his dreams come true 'salt pork' might
be available 'fresh'!

Cousteau and his divers wasted no time in following up his proposals
with active trials and in 1962 maintained 2 men at 35 ft. for 7 days
(Conshelf 1). This was followed by the 'Conshelf 2' and 'Conshelf 3'
projects. In the former, in 1963, 5 men spent 1 month at 33 ft. and 2
men, 7 days at 85 ft. In Conshelf 3 in 1965, 6 men spent 22 days at 330 ft.
This remarkable achievement was well documented and studied
particularly with regard to the more personal problems of habitability.
(See Chapter XII.)

Meanwhile Ed Link in 1962 had kept one man at 200 ft. for 24 hours
and later in 1964, 2 men at 432 ft. for 49 hours.

This was exciting progress only to be matched by the U.S. Navy's
'Sealab' projects which established 'Sealab I' in 1964 a fairly crude
pressurized cylinder in which 4 men lived for 11 days at 192 feet. This
was followed the next year by 'Sealab II' in which 28 men lived and
worked at 205 feet for 15–30 days. In 1969 'Sealab III' is underway in
which, if all goes well, five diving teams of eight men will occupy the
underwater station for periods of 12 days at a depth of 600 ft. From
such bases it should be possible to make sorties to even greater depths.
(Bond 1967, 1968.)

'The Navy', the official publication of 'The Navy League', in
November, 1960, published a group of articles on 'The Underseas and
their Importance to the Service', 'Deep Sea Exploration', 'Offshore Oil
Production in the Middle East' and 'Questing for Coal Beneath the Sea'.
These articles left no possible doubt of the growing importance of their
common subject, as did a paper by Tom Gaskell in 1963 to the Royal
Society of Arts.

It may well be that the year 1960 was a most significant one for
'Underwater Medicine'. Not only did many articles, including those
listed above, appear in scientific and popular publications but International Conferences on underwater problems were held in Barcelona and
Cannes. Also in Sydney, Australia, the first International Conference
on Life-Saving techniques devoted much of its time to the study of the
causes and treatment of drowning and paid serious attention to other
allied problems.

Thus at last it seems man is beginning to realize that to accept the
underwater challenge may well secure for him rich and material rewards.
The military aspects must of course remain of vital importance, for
control under the sea may well become of greater importance than

control above. For this reason it is likely that the world's navies will continue to be the pioneers of underwater development and make an important contribution to this growing enterprise.

THE APPROACH

The challenge accepted, the means must be studied. It is immediately obvious that man without artificial aids is very limited in his aquatic activity.

Unassisted, man may swim on the surface but only experts attain speeds exceeding 2 m.p.h. and with intense training some long-distance swimmers may keep going for 12 hours or more. Underwater the earliest achievements are best seen in the pearl-diver where the need to breathe must confine a dive to a few minutes and physiological factors limit the depth to about 100 ft.

Historians quote cases of military operations where men seeking concealment have hidden or moved completely submerged underwater breathing through reeds or short tubes. The modern version of this is the 'Schnorkel tube'. This, enabling the user to relax, or move slowly with almost the whole body submerged, is very sparing of effort and allows continuous underwater observation from the surface. For diving the depth and duration is as restricted as that of the pearl-diver.

Conventional diving in which air is pumped down under adequate pressure to a diver wearing a flexible suit and rigid helmet is still the most usual form of commercial diving, employed extensively in salvage and underwater construction. The mobility of the diver is greatly restricted and the apparatus and organization required precludes its use for recreational purposes. For practical purposes it is rarely used below 200 ft. though 600 ft. has been reached. The diver cannot move very far on the sea-bed and must take care in negotiating objects lest his air supply and life-line become entangled. He is however usually under the care of his surface attendants whose efficiency is unaffected by the environmental changes below.

The self-contained diver, carrying on his back cylinders of air or other breathing mixture, is however able to move at will through the water or along the bottom. He need not be attached to a surface vessel and is by and large entirely responsible for his own safety. He must therefore be disciplined to appreciate and avoid the hazards which depth may present. This form of underwater activity shows the greatest promise and there is no doubt that, with time, the depth and duration will be increased. Mobility may be increased by wearing fins or by towing through the water with mechanical aids. Methods by which this form of diving may be extended will be discussed in subsequent chapters. Ultimately it is believed that he will be able to work from a pressurize underwater base spending long periods, even weeks, on the sea-bed.

In the methods so far described the diver is moving freely in intimate contact with the environment, a facility which is essential if he is to take full advantage of his surroundings.

Much that has been learnt about the world below the waves however has been achieved by direct inspection from the submersible observation chamber of the bathyscaphe. The stories of deep-sea exploration in Piccard's Bathyscaphe Trieste make stirring reading. This work will continue and play a vital part in man's accumulation of knowledge of the ocean deeps; the 'abyss' as it is frequently called. In it however the observers take with them their natural atmosphere and are not subject to the physiological stresses with which this book is primarily concerned.

Similarly mention must be made of the true submarine. The underwater boat in which men maintain, by artificial means, a natural environment which, with the introduction of nuclear power, may be maintained for weeks or even months. This again protects the occupants from the hazards of prolonged high pressure.

At present the activities of divers are far removed from those of submariners but it seems inevitable that the two should be drawn together and men may descend in a pressurized submarine and dive from such a base already deeply submerged. This is still a hope for the future but that it is by no means improbable will be made clear in the following pages.

The approach to the conquest of the vast reaches below the sea is just becoming apparent. That these reaches are indeed vast will be realized if it is remembered that almost two-thirds of the earth's surface is sea and its volume is over three hundred million cubic miles.

THE PRIZE

The ultimate prize may be summarized as the complete freedom of the seas and the sea-bed. At the moment complete conquest would seem physically and physiologically impossible. There are however large areas where the depth is less than 1,000 ft. This includes wide expanses of the sea-floor, extensive continental shelves and peaks of ocean-bed mountain ranges, many of which are shallower than 500 ft. and offers a very wide scope for man's endeavour. These areas must be the proving ground and already progress is being made.

Vast supplies of valuable animal food are there waiting to be controlled and protected from their natural enemies. Marine vegetation
may be a further source of nutriment or raw material. Coal and oil are
known to be present in the sea-floor and scattered deposits of many
minerals have been shown to be available. Much, too, still remains to be
salvaged from sunken ships and for the marine biologist, and the
archaeologist, there are great opportunities for study and research.

That this is no idle dream may be appreciated if the present-day
activity of man in and under water is tabulated.

(i) *Free Swimming.* Swimming and diving play an important part in
recreation and from the ranks of those already at home in the water,
may be recruited the best 'skin'-divers. Much can be learnt from studying the physiological reactions of swimmers, both sprinters and long
distance, which will be of value in assessing man's general adaptability
to the aquatic environment as a whole.

(ii) *Standard or Helmet Diving.* This, the basis of present knowledge,
still continues in commercial diving in harbour construction work,
salvage, mining, cable-laying, bridge building and many other important
activities.

(iii) *Skin-diving.* With a simple Schnorkel tube this gives pleasure to
many and an early glimpse at the wonders below the sea. Spear-fishermen
are thrilled by the three-dimensional chase in the quarry's own realm.

(iv) *Self-contained Diving (Scuba or Aqualung diving).* With self-
contained breathing apparatus new worlds are opened up. Photographers have facilities in colour and motion unparalleled on land.
Archaeologists explore forgotten cities. Marine biologists can study
their subjects under natural conditions. In dark inland caverns, water-
filled tunnels hitherto inaccessible, are probed by intrepid divers. Pearl-
gatherers by these newer methods are increasing their harvest.

Under a shield of military security frogmen are increasing their
efficiency in defence and attack.

(v) *Surface Demand Diving.* This is a compromise between scuba and
standard diving in which air or a mixture of breathing gases is supplied
to the diver from the surface or from reservoirs in a submersible
decompression chamber or sea-bed complex. The breathing supply pipe
also acts as a safety line and the diver wears a light-weight suit and swim
fins to give maximum mobility.

(vi) *Saturation Diving.* Taking advantage of the fact that in time
tissues saturate with breathing gases at any particular depth a prolonged
stay can be accomplished for the same decompression routine once
saturation is reached. This means residence under pressure either in

sea-bed or ship born chambers with working sorties into the sea without pressure change. Prolonged final decompression only is needed.

(vii) *Caisson Work*. Many engineering constructional projects, especially the building of tunnels below great waterways, necessitate men working in compressed air for long periods. In this work they face many of the hazards met under water. To increase their potential needs the same research as that of the diver and from their experience much is learnt which is applicable to underwater problems.

(viii) *The Submarine*. Though at present an instrument of war there are aspects of submarine service where familiarity with the undersea environment is of the utmost importance. The development of current methods of submarine escape has been possible only with the understanding of high-pressure physiology and man's behaviour in water. The adaptation of the submarine for commercial purposes and deep-sea research will bring closer together the activity of the submariner and the diver.

(ix) *Pressure Medicine*. The experience of diving physiologists is being used by physicians and surgeons in the treatment of many conditions where tissue oxygen supply is impaired by exposing patients to high pressure oxygen. A number of larger hospitals are installing pressure chambers as additional therapeutic facilities.

An attempt has been made in this chapter to show the wideness of the underwater environment as it primarily affects man. For the student of underwater medicine the problem is essentially one of man's adaptation to an entirely strange environment. Without the help of complicated breathing apparatus, and a wide appreciation of the hazards little adaptation can be achieved. With carefully constructed equipment and appreciation of the problems safe progress will be made. There are many pitfalls for the unwary and there is no other field in which a little knowledge may be so dangerous.

READING AND REFERENCES

Bond, G. F. (1967). *Medical Problems of Multiday Saturation Diving in Open Water*. Proc. 3rd Symposium on Underwater Physiology, Ed. Lambertson—Williams and Wilkins Co., Baltimore.

—(1968). *Medical Aspects of Life Underwater*. Second Naval Medical Scientific Symposium. Naval Medical Institute and Christian-Albrechts University, Kiel, Germany.

Carson, R. L. (1956). *The Sea Around Us*. Staples Press, London.

Cousteau, J. Y. (1953). *The Silent World*. Hamish Hamilton Ltd., London.

—(1960). *Farm Under the Sea*. Report in the *Sun Herald*, Sydney, Australia. 13 March, 1960.

Dietz, R. S. (1958). 'Deep Sea Research in the Bathyscaphe Trieste'. *The New Scientist*, Vol. 3, No. 74 (17 April, 1958).

Dugan, J. (1960). *Man Explores the Sea*. Penguin Books Ltd., London.

Gaskell, T. F. (1963). 'Man Explores the Sea'. *J. Roy. Soc. Arts*, 111, 784.

Hardy, A. (1960). 'Now Subaquatic Man'. Report by Peter Collins in the *Sunday Times*, London. 6 March, 1960.

McKee, A. (1967). *Farming the Sea*. Souvenir Press, London.

'The Navy'. 'Section on Oceanography'—various authors. *The Navy*. November, 1960.

Piccard, A. (1956). *In Baloon and Bathyscaphe* (Translation). Cassell and Co. Ltd., London.

Rahn, H. (1965). *Breath hold Diving and the Ama of Japan*. National Academy of Sciences, Washington.

Tailliez, P. (1954). *To Hidden Depths*. Wm. Kimber, London.

CHAPTER II

The Physical Approach

BEFORE studying man in water consideration should be given to important physical characteristics of the medium. These include pressure, specific gravity, viscosity, temperature and changes in the conduction of light and sound waves. Of these pressure is by far the most important factor.

The problem is further complicated by the fact that man, as a land animal must, even when submerged in water, still obtain supplies of oxygen and lose carbon dioxide by gaseous interchange in the lung alveoli. He cannot utilize the oxygen dissolved in the water as do fishes and the entry of water into the respiratory passages may result in drowning. Thus to maintain his existence under water oxygen must be supplied and carbon dioxide removed by artificial means. In other words the respiratory system must be insulated from the medium and be kept in continuous association with some respirable atmosphere.

PRESSURE

Man on land is adapted to exist within the normal range of atmospheric pressure though on the highest mountains this pressure may be so low as to prejudice his oxygen supply.

At or near sea-level the atmospheric, or barometric pressure is usually a little above 760 mm.Hg. The small fluctuations associated with meteorological variations can, as far as pressure in the water is concerned, be neglected.

To be more precise the atmospheric pressure is said to be STANDARD when at a temperature of $0°$ C. the height of the column in a mercury barometer is 760 mm. This 'Standard Atmospheric Pressure', i.e. 760 mm.Hg, is the unit of pressure used in underwater practice and is called ONE ATMOSPHERE.

For compactness the conventional barometer consists of an inverted mercury-filled tube with a vacuum above the mercury. It could, however, be made with water in which case standard atmospheric pressure would support a column of fresh water 34 ft. high or sea water 33 ft. high.

Alternatively the pressure could be signified in units of weight per unit of area, i.e. in pounds per square inch or grammes per square centimetre.

Thus in table form:

760 mm. mercury (Hg)
≡ 29·9 inch mercury (Hg)
≡ 34 ft. fresh water
≡ 33 ft. salt water
≡ 14·7 lb. per sq. inch.
≡ 1033·3 grammes per sq. cm.
≡ 1 ATMOSPHERE.

(Meteorologists use the 'millibar' as a unit of barometric pressure where 1,000 millibars are equivalent to approximately 750 mm.Hg under standard conditions.)

As most of the significant changes due to pressure on man in water occur in the sea it is customary to use the pressure of 33 ft. water as being that of 1 atmosphere.

Owing to the pressure of the atmosphere at the water surface a man (or other object) entering the water is already under this pressure of 1 atmosphere.

If the man is taken to a depth of 33 ft. he is subjected to a pressure caused by the water above him (33 ft. = 1 atmosphere) plus the atmospheric pressure, i.e. a total of 2 atmospheres. For every further 33 ft. he descends an additional atmosphere of pressure is added, so that at 99 ft., for example, he would be under a total pressure of 4 atmospheres (3 of water plus 1 of atmospheric pressure).

It is well, at this stage, to clarify a small point which may occasionally lead to misunderstanding. Where, in underwater operations, depth pressure gauges are being used it is usual for these to be constructed to give a 'zero' reading at the surface. At 99 ft. a gauge would register an equivalent pressure of 3 atmospheres, not the true or absolute pressure of 4 atmospheres. To avoid confusion therefore it is important that when gauge pressure is quoted the word 'gauge' should be emphasized and similarly it is correct and safe when referring to total pressure to describe this as 'absolute' pressure.

Thus a man at 99 ft. below the surface is subject to a pressure of 4 atmospheres *absolute* or 3 atmospheres *gauge*.

In this book, however, the common practice will be followed in that any unqualified reference to pressure will refer to absolute pressure. Where gauge pressure is used it will be referred to as such.

THE CHANGE FROM AIR TO WATER

It is impossible in underwater medicine to divorce air or gas pressure from water pressure as air or other breathing mixture must be supplied. Consideration must also be given to changes affecting the air spaces in the body, the lungs and respiratory passages, middle ear and sinuses and the gastro-intestinal gases.

The fundamental laws governing the behaviour of both gases and liquid must therefore be known.

Water is virtually incompressible, air and other gases can be compressed.

The earth's atmosphere at sea-level is more tightly packed or denser whereas at the peak of Everest it is rarefied and exerts a pressure of about 0·3 of an atmosphere. On land, except for the highest mountain ranges or in high-altitude flying, pressure changes are rarely effective but on entering water there is an abrupt change in the pressure distance ratio.

Altitude in feet	Pressure in atmospheres absolute
30,000	0·30
20,000	0·46
10,000	0·69
5,000	0·83
SEA-LEVEL	1·00
Depth in feet	
100	4·00
250	8·55
500	16·15
1,000	31·30

It is apparent from this table that, as compared with changes in altitude on land or in the air, changes in depth in water involve very much greater changes in pressure.

It has already been stated that water is incompressible and air compressible. What about man? The soft tissues behave as a fluid and therefore together with the body fluids and bony skeleton are incompressible. The laws which apply to liquids can therefore be applied to human tissues immersed in water. Such laws are—

(i) If a pressure is applied to the surface of a fluid it is transmitted to all parts of that fluid.

(ii) The pressure at any point in a fluid is the same in all directions if the fluid is at rest.

(iii) In a homogeneous liquid the pressure at all points in the same horizontal plane is equal.

It is often very difficult to understand why the tissues of man are not distorted when subjected to underwater pressure. Archimedes, about 250 B.C., most certainly was aware of this. It is not easy however to appreciate that, for example, a diver in a flexible suit at 600 ft. though each square inch of his body is under a pressure of almost 2½ cwt., is himself quite unaware of this. The heart beats normally, a blood-pressure reading if taken would be much the same as on the surface, and superficial vessels pulse unhindered. In fact the organs of the body function normally without restriction.

A glance at Figure 1 may help. In 1a a body is immersed in water and is subject to the pressures from all directions as indicated by the arrows. If the body is removed it will be seen that the space it occupied is now filled with water (Fig. 1b). This volume of water is no more restricted than the surrounding water and it exerts equal and opposite pressures

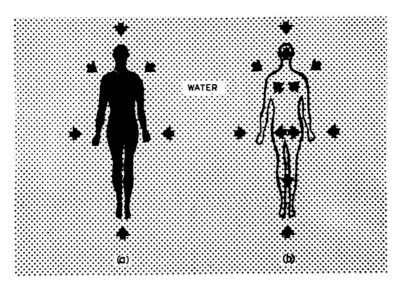

WATER

(a)   (b)

FIG. 1. Man in water

in all directions. So would the tissues of man in the same position. The vascular pulses and activity of the muscular organs would continue their functioning being only concerned with producing local pressure differences quite independent of the overall environmental pressure.

THE HUMAN AIR CAVITIES AND THE GAS LAWS

It is impossible to consider the effects of pressure on man without taking into account the effect of that pressure on the air contained in the lungs, respiratory passages, middle ears, sinuses and viscera. Under water this air is isolated but as depth and pressure increase the incompressible tissues take up the pressure of the surrounding water and are undistorted. However, this state can only be upheld if the pressure of the enclosed air is also increased to that of the enclosing tissues. This can be achieved artificially by supplying compressed air at a pressure equivalent to the water pressure at the depths of the individual. If this is not done one of two things may happen. If the surrounding tissues will allow it the enclosed air may contract to meet the increasing pressure. Failing this, if the volume cannot be reduced the pressure will be unchanged and a pressure difference be built up between the air and the surrounding tissues, the result of which may be disastrous.

Air or other gases must always obey the 'gas laws' and of these Boyle's Law is of fundamental importance in underwater physiology.

BOYLE'S LAW

'The pressure of a given quantity of gas whose temperature remains unchanged varies inversely as its volume.'

$PV = K$. When P = pressure, V = volume and K = constant.

This simply means that if the pressure of a given amount of gas is doubled it must be compressed to half its volume. An enclosed volume of gas cannot be subjected to increased pressure unless it occupies a smaller space.

The importance of this under water is well illustrated in Figure 2, which represents the changes taking place if an inverted bell, or bucket, containing air is pushed under water.

The changes illustrated form the basis of underwater medicine and their understanding is of paramount importance. It is worth while therefore at this stage mastering the important implications, especially as the inverted bell can, to all intents and purposes, be taken as representing the air contained in the lungs of a man who goes under water.

At the surface the bell contains a given mass of air which occupies the volume of the bell and exerts a pressure of 1 atmosphere.

If the bell is now lowered 33 ft. through the water its lower end, being open, is subjected to the increased water pressure, i.e. a pressure of the atmosphere plus that of 33 ft. of water, a total of 2 atmospheres. The pressure on the air in the bell has in fact been doubled and therefore it must contract to half its volume. This is achieved by the water level rising half way up the bell. At 33 ft. therefore the volume of air in the bell is halved and its pressure doubled though its mass (the number of molecules present) is unchanged. (It should be pointed out that no account is being taken of slight variations which may occur as a result of changes in the amount of air dissolving in the water.)

If the bell is now lowered a further 33 ft. to a depth of 66 ft. a further

BOYLE'S LAW AND DIVING
PV = K

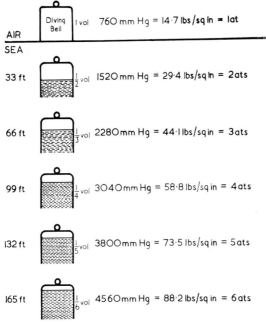

FIG. 2

33 foot's-worth of water pressure is added giving now a total of 3 atmospheres of pressure on the confined air which must therefore be compressed to $\frac{1}{3}$ of its original volume by water rising $\frac{2}{3}$ the way up.

Similarly if the bell is lowered to 99 ft. the air would be compressed to
$\frac{1}{4}$ of the original volume, at 132 ft. to $\frac{1}{5}$ of the volume and so on until at
627 ft., for example, it would be reduced to $\frac{1}{20}$ of the original volume
when the pressure of the water and the air at that depth would be 20
atmospheres. This is of course a pressure of 20 atmospheres 'absolute'
i.e. it includes the one atmosphere of the air at sea-level. A pressure
gauge at this depth would read only 19 atmospheres 'gauge'.

It may however, in practice, be necessary to maintain air under water
at a constant volume, i.e. occupying an unchanging space. How can this
be done?

Two methods are available. The first and simplest (Fig. 3A) is to contain the air in a rigid case, i.e. in the present example to seal off the bottom of the bell. In this case both pressure and volume of the air are

unchanged but as depth increases the container is subjected to an increasing external pressure. At 627 ft., for example, with only one atmosphere of pressure inside, the case would need to be strong enough to withstand a pressure of 19 atmospheres, i.e. about 280 lb. per sq. inch. It would be essential, therefore, to construct the chamber of material of sufficient strength to withstand the pressure difference of the proposed

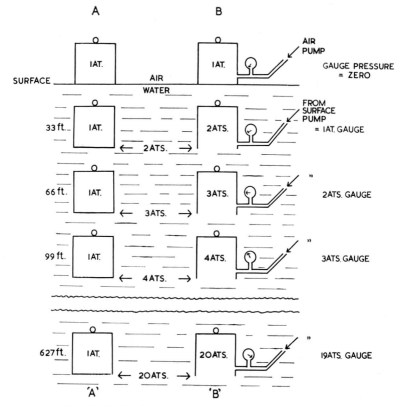

FIG. 3. Maintaining constant gas volume under water

operating depth. This principle is in fact used in the construction of the submarine whose hull must therefore be of the optimal shape and strength to withstand the pressure difference at its maximum cruising depth. The depth, therefore, to which a submarine may dive must be limited by the strength of its hull for the air it contains remains at atmospheric pressure and constant volume whilst the external pressure increases with depth.

The second method of maintaining a constant volume of air under the increasing pressure of depth is to keep pumping in more air to maintain the pressure at that of the surrounding water pressure (Fig. 3B). In the case of the diving bell the bottom may be left open provided a pipe from an air pump is attached to supply air at the required pressure. To keep the bell full of air at 33 ft. it would have to be pumped up to a pressure of 2 atmospheres. (1 atmosphere on the pump gauge.) At 99 ft. an air pressure of 4 atmospheres would be needed and at 627 ft. 20 atmospheres. (The pump gauge reading in each case 3 atmospheres and 19 atmospheres, respectively.) In practice a pressure a little above those given would cause bubbles of air to escape from the edges of the bell and give an assurance to those working the pump that an adequate supply was being provided to maintain the volume. This method is indeed that used to supply air to the diver who being in a flexible suit needs air at the pressure of his surroundings. The supply may be obtained from a source of compressed air on the surface or gas cylinders carried by the diver himself.

RELATIVE VOLUME CHANGES

To return to the simple inverted bell (Fig. 2) where with increasing pressure the volume of trapped air decreases a further important observation may be made.

As the bell descends through the water the volume of the air within it decreases so that at 33 ft. it is half what it was on the surface, at 66 ft. a third and at 99 ft. a quarter. As it gets deeper, therefore, for each additional atmosphere of pressure the relative change in volume becomes less. In the first 33 ft. it is halved (a 50% reduction). From 66 ft. to 99 ft. it changes only from $\frac{1}{3}$ to $\frac{1}{4}$ of the original volume, i.e. a 25% reduction. At greater depths the reduction in volume for each additional atmosphere of pressure becomes less. Indeed when dropping from 627 ft. to 660 ft. the volume decreases from $\frac{1}{20}$ to $\frac{1}{21}$ of the original, a reduction of only 4·8% for the additional atmosphere of pressure.

It will be seen later that this is of the utmost importance to man in water. Changes of depth near the surface are likely in certain circumstances to involve much greater volume changes in enclosed air than similar changes at much greater depths. A diver dropping uncontrolled through the water may do himself severe injury if near the surface and yet if already deep may escape unharmed from a similar fall.

CHANGES IN AIR DENSITY

Once more studying the simple bell as it descends in the water, it will be realized that changes in density of the air also occur. On the surface

3

the volume of air had a specific mass. When halved by being taken down to 33 ft. this same mass was concentrated in half the volume. Thus its density was doubled. At 99 ft. the density would be four times as great and at 627 ft. it would be twenty times as great. In other words the air is becoming 'thicker'. This increasing air density is a major problem in underwater medicine. In the study of respiration and in the design of breathing apparatus density is a factor to be considered with problems of air movement and resistance and is an important limiting factor to human efficiency under water.

SOLUBILITY AND PARTIAL PRESSURES

Not only must the physical effects of changes in pressure and volume be considered but also the influences these changes have on the passage in and out of solution of the constituents of air or other breathing mixtures.

On land under normal atmospheric pressures there is an equilibrium between the gases in the lung alveoli and the quantities of them dissolved in the blood stream and tissues. The lungs are designed to produce a large surface area where liquid (blood) and gases can be brought into intimate contact to enable oxygen to be taken up by the blood and carbon dioxide to be liberated into the air. Changes in pressure of the gases within the lung must upset this equilibrium.

Furthermore because air is a mixture of gases, mostly nitrogen and oxygen, these gases must be considered quite separately for their effects on the human body depend upon their individual or 'partial' pressures.

These effects can best be studied by reference to two further 'gas laws' which are:

(i) *Dalton's Law* which states that—'in a mixture of gases the pressure exerted by one of those gases is the same as it would exert if it alone occupied the same volume.'

and (ii) *Henry's Law* which states that—'at a constant temperature, the amount of a gas which dissolves in a liquid, with which it is in contact, is proportional to the partial pressure of that gas.'

It is first necessary to be quite clear on what is meant by partial pressure and air at atmospheric pressure will serve as a good example. Air is a mixture of—

NITROGEN = 79%

OXYGEN = 21% approximately

(The small quantity of carbon dioxide, 0·04% and other trace elements can be disregarded at this stage.)

At one atmosphere this mixture exerts a pressure of 760 mm. mercury

(Hg). This pressure is shared by the nitrogen and oxygen in proportion to their presence, i.e. the pressure of

NITROGEN $= 79\%$ of $760 = 600$ mm.Hg
and of OXYGEN $\quad = 21\%$ of $760 = 160$ mm.Hg

$\overline{}$

760 mm.Hg

$\overline{}$

These values are the 'PARTIAL PRESSURES' of the two gases. If, in a given volume where air was exerting a pressure of 760 mm.Hg the oxygen could be totally removed without there being any change in volume, then the pressure exerted by the remaining nitrogen would be 600 mm.Hg, i.e. its partial pressure. This is Dalton's Law.

When gases are in contact with a fluid in which they will dissolve an equilibrium is set up between the amounts of the gases in solution and the partial pressures of the gases in contact with the solution. This depends upon the temperature of the liquid and the coefficient of solubility of the gas.

If pure nitrogen is in contact with water, at $0°$ C., equilibrium is reached when the water contains 2·35ml. of dissolved nitrogen per 100 ml. water. With pure oxygen the figure would be 4·89 ml. oxygen per 100 ml. From this information and a knowledge of the partial pressure of nitrogen and oxygen can be calculated the amounts of these gases dissolved in water when air is in contact at $0°$ C., viz.:

NITROGEN, if p.p. is 760 mm.Hg

then 2·35 ml. is dissolved in 100 ml.

if p.p. is 600 then $\dfrac{600 \times 2\cdot35}{760} = 1\cdot85$ ml. is dissolved in

100 ml.

Similarly—

OXYGEN, if p.p. is 160 then—

$$\frac{160 \times 4\cdot89}{760} = 1\cdot03 \text{ ml. is dissolved in 100 ml.}$$

Thus when air at a pressure of 760 mm.Hg (one atmosphere) is in contact with water at $0°$ C. that water will contain in every 100 ml., in solution 1·85 ml. nitrogen and 1·03 ml. oxygen. This is based on Henry's Law.

If the partial pressures of gases in contact with fluids, or for that matter living tissue, are known and also the temperature and co-efficients of solubility for the gases in the fluid or tissues, then the amount of each gas dissolved can be calculated. Time must of course be allowed for equilibrium to be reached.

It must now be very obvious that, when man is under water and breathing air or a mixture of other appropriate gases, which must be at increased pressure, then profound and far-reaching physiological effects due to varying amounts of these gases diffusing through and dissolving in body fluids and tissues will be inevitable. Though this situation will be discussed time and time again in subsequent chapters, one example may now suffice.

Study the partial pressures in the inverted bell of Figure 3 as it is pushed under water. The results can be tabulated thus:

Depth	TOTAL PRESSURE		PARTIAL PRESSURES	
			Nitrogen	Oxygen
ft.	atmospheres	mm.Hg	mm.Hg	mm.Hg
0 (Surface)	1	760	600	160
33	2	1520	1200	320
66	3	2280	1800	480
99	4	3040	2400	640
132	5	3800	3000	800

It becomes obvious from these greatly increasing values of partial pressures that the amount of the gases dissolving in contact fluids will be proportionally increased.

A more interesting observation from the above figures is, however, that somewhere between 99 ft. and 132 ft. the oxygen partial pressure would be 760 mm.Hg. Actually the depth is 124 ft. and it follows that if a man were breathing air at this depth he would respond to the oxygen in it as if he were breathing pure oxygen at the surface.

This simple fact illustrates the importance, in considering problems of underwater respiration, of thinking in terms of partial pressures of gases involved in relation to their solution in body fluids and tissues. Attention must also be paid in similar terms to the partial pressures of carbon dioxide, water vapour or any other gas present.

SPECIFIC GRAVITY

The specific gravity of pure fresh water at 4° C. is taken as the standard 1·0. This is the ratio of weight to volume, i.e. 1 g. of water occupies 1 ml. More commonly the ratio is given in grammes per litre, i.e. 1000.

The specific gravity of sea water depends largely on its salinity but varies to some extent with temperature and depth. The range is from 1020 to 1030 being high in such salty areas as the Red Sea and low in the North Atlantic.

The effect of temperature on the density of water is interesting. At

4° C. a given mass of water occupies its smallest volume and therefore is most dense. Heat it above this and it expands becoming less dense. Cool it further and it again expands with decreasing density.

It has been stated that water is incompressible. This is not strictly true for it is indeed slightly compressed in the great ocean depths due to very large pressures above and in consequence there will be a corresponding increase in density. This slight compressibility is, however, insignificant in its relationship with man in water and need not be further mentioned or considered.

The importance of the specific gravity of water as it affects man is concerned with his BUOYANCY. Most men, in fresh water, will if they take a full breath, remain on the surface with just a little of the scalp above water, i.e. be positively buoyant. About 10%—the so-called 'negatively buoyant' will actually sink. In sea water the figure is smaller, possibly 2%. Thus man in water displaces just about his own weight of water and therefore needs very little effort to support himself. It is not difficult for a diver to make himself neutrally buoyant so that he would neither sink nor rise. This fact is physiologically significant in that being more or less supported in water he loses his sense of position. The force of gravity is neutralized and proprioceptive sense is ineffective. Men have been blindfolded, supplied with air and lightly suspended under water. They very soon lose their sense of position and frequently undergo disconcerting sensations of rolling over even to the extent of complete emotional breakdown. The condition is not unlike the 'breakaway' phenomenon described in very high flying and it has been used in studies of man's reaction to weightlessness. It is a reaction worthy of further investigation.

Another effect of this relative weightlessness in water is that no longer is there a need for maintenance of postural tone. If the water temperature is close to that of the body, relaxation can be very complete, more so than being at rest in bed, with a minimal tidal volume and oxygen consumption. This fact is of course used in the various techniques of hydrotherapy.

LIGHT AND SOUND WAVES

Man in water must also adjust himself to alterations in the pattern of light and sound. Under water he invariably protects his eyes with a face mask or goggles containing air and as the refractive index of light is different in water, rays passing from water to air are bent with the result that the underwater visual field is reduced and objects appear distorted and nearer than they actually are.

The velocity of sound in water is about 4,700 ft. per sec. as compared with that in air of 1,090 ft. per sec. The effect is briefly to make it difficult or impossible for a man in water to determine the direction from which a sound is reaching him.

Both underwater vision and sound will be considered in greater detail later.

DECOMPRESSION

To appreciate the results of decompression the gases which with increased partial pressure dissolve in excess in the blood must be followed further. From the lungs blood carries the excess dissolved gases to the tissues where further transfers take place. At atmospheric pressure there is an equilibrium between, for example, the partial pressure of atmospheric nitrogen and that dissolved in the blood. Between the blood and the tissues it serves there is a similar equilibrium between the nitrogen in the blood and that in the tissue. The amount of nitrogen in unit volume will depend on the solubility of the nitrogen in the blood or tissue, there being more in a fatty tissue. When the pressure is constant an equilibrium exists with the tissues saturated for that pressure but if the pressure is increased say to four atmospheres the blood will take up four times the amount of dissolved gases until all are saturated for the new pressure. In establishing the new equilibrium not only the solubility of the gases in the tissue must be considered but also the rate at which they diffuse into the tissue. Thus some tissues will saturate very quickly and others quite slowly.

The only way in which the excess respiratory gas can reach the tissues when pressure is raised is from the lungs and via the circulation.

If the pressure is now reduced back to one atmosphere the equilibrium will be upset in the opposite direction. Nitrogen, for example, will now escape from the blood in the lungs and leave the tissues to enter the blood until the former equilibrium at atmospheric pressure is re-established. Provided the reduction of pressure is slow this return to normal may proceed without complication.

It is a well-known physical fact that if a gas is dissolved in a liquid and saturation is reached, sudden reduction in pressure will cause the gas to come out of solution and in fact bubbles will form. This can indeed also happen with tissues in the human body when suddenly decompressed after exposure to certain conditions of pressure. There is, however, a threshold for bubble formation which is a factor of pressure and time of exposure. The whole problem of decompression revolves round the rates at which various tissues tend to saturate and the solubility of gases concerned. With increase in pressure the build-up is at first very rapid, slowing down as saturation is approached. The elimination following decompression is not quite the same pattern in reverse.

The different solubility coefficients which the various tissues of the body exhibit only add to the complexity of the problem. When the time comes to study decompression in more practical detail the difficulty in applying basic physical data to a complex ever-changing organism will be apparent and reliance will be placed on a combination of theoretical compromise and trial and error.

SUMMARY

From what has been said so far, when man's reactions to the aquatic environment are being studied, special attention must be paid to the following conditions:

(i)   Increased pressure.
(ii) Increased density.
(iii) Increased nitrogen partial pressure.
(iv) Increased oxygen partial pressure.
(v)   Changes in vision, hearing and other senses.
(vi) The effects of decompression.

Man is not equipped for complete and total existence under water and must maintain respiratory contact with the atmosphere either directly or artificially from gas cylinders. In the medium he has the advantages of three-dimensional activity but the situation is grossly complicated by his respiratory needs so that the fluid and gaseous environments can never be truly separated.

An understanding of respiratory physiology is the key to underwater medicine and in the next chapter some of the recent advances in this subject will be used to illustrate the way in which the problem may best be approached.

READING AND REFERENCES

Davis, R. H. (1955). *Deep Diving and Submarine Operations.* Siebe Gorman & Co. Ltd., London.
The Royal Naval Diving Manual (1964). B.R. 155C. Admiralty, London.
National Academy of Sciences (U.S.A.). *Handbook of Respiration.* W. B. Saunders, Co., Philadelphia and London.

CHAPTER III

The Physiological Approach

THE study of man in water is the study of man in a new environment. As in the sister sciences of Aviation Medicine, Atomic Medicine, Space Medicine, Climatic Medicine and even Clinical Medicine a common approach is used. The functioning of the human body within its natural environment must be known, the limits of the environment within which the body will function without loss of efficiency must be established and an accurate assessment of the stresses produced by the new environment made.

The basic approach is one of environmental physiology. In underwater medicine the stresses of the environment can be accurately forecast and many of the requirements to adapt man to them may be anticipated. Success depends on careful compromise, for man unaided in water has but a brief and limited usefulness. Artificial means must be provided to assist him and great care is needed to ensure that these aids do not impair his efficiency or prejudice his safety.

Whatever methods are used to extend man's activity under water the aim must always be to provide the various systems of the body with that range of environment in which they may work with maximum efficiency. Many occasions will arise where efficiency is sacrificed for expediency but this must never be accepted as the final compromise.

Physiologists of today have a wide variety of techniques, some simple, some involving complicated apparatus. Many of these have already been adapted for use in water and under pressure and are producing important information. Indeed it is now possible to simulate the underwater environment under laboratory conditions. A familiar pattern of research is used. Man, wholly and system by system, is studied firstly in his normal environment with special attention to those systems likely to be most affected. Secondly he is observed in the artificially produced underwater and pressurized condition and finally he is observed working in the natural underwater environment. This routine is of course supplemented by much theoretical reasoning and a good deal of animal experimentation.

Of the systems of the body most involved, that of respiration is far and away the most important. It is therefore well worth while reviewing current work on this subject with special reference to its application to the underwater situation.

THE RESPIRATORY SYSTEM

THE MECHANICS OF RESPIRATION

Three important structures are involved in the mechanics of respiration, the lungs, the chest wall and the respiratory muscles. Their interrelation can best be appreciated if they are studied first separately and then together.

The chest cage has a well-known springiness (chest elasticity) for which there is a position of rest. Compress the chest cage and on release it returns to this position. Extend it and again on release it does likewise. This position of rest for the 'empty' chest cage is such that if it occupied this position in the living body the lungs would contain about 60% of a maximal inspiration, i.e. 60% of the 'vital capacity'.

Similarly the lungs themselves have an elasticity (lung elasticity) which in this case is tending to collapse them, i.e. to drive the air out. This force therefore, when the lungs are in the chest cage, will tend to reduce the volume of the latter and set up a new elastic equilibrium. This new equilibrium is such that in the living body, when the respiratory muscles are paralysed or inactive, the lungs contain about 40% of the vital capacity. It is from this base line, this balance between chest elasticity and lung elasticity, that, with the help of the respiratory muscles, normal respiration is initiated. The importance of the base line will be further studied when reference is made to methods of artificial respiration. Such methods may involve compression or expansion away from this line.

In normal respiration only two groups of muscles are primarily involved, the diaphragm which increases chest volume downwards and the intercostal muscles which expand the chest cage upwards and outwards. These are essentially muscles of inspiration and their function in increasing chest volume is to displace the elastic equilibrium from the resting position. This is inspiration. When the muscles relax the balance of the elastic forces is re-established at the resting level producing expiration. In short, inspiration results from muscular effort, expiration is the elastic recoil.

Much useful information on the activity of the muscles of respiration has been obtained by electromyography, a technique which enables careful following of electrical activity in selected muscle groups by introducing electrodes and amplifying and recording potential differences. Campbell (1958), using this method, concludes that in breathing up to 50 litres per minute, only the diaphragm and intercostals are active. Above this figure the accessory muscles, e.g. the sterno-mastoids and extensor muscles of the spine, may come into action. He finds no evidence that intercostal muscles play any part in expiration and indeed in forceful expiration the only muscles actively employed are those of the abdominal wall. There is some evidence, however, that intercostals may be active during the early part of expiration. This is most likely a breaking effect on the elastic recoil without which expiration might be quite violent as when a stretched piece of elastic is released.

It is helpful to express this pattern of respiratory mechanics diagrammatically and Figure 4 is an attempt to show the various forces in relation to lung volume.

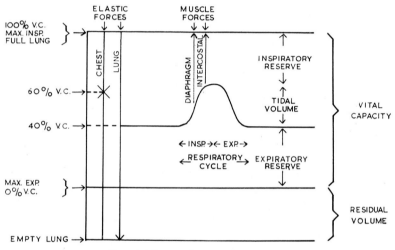

FIG. 4. The mechanics of breathing

From this Figure it is possible to obtain definitions of common terms used in respiratory physiology, viz.:

Vital Capacity—the maximum volume of air which can be inhaled following complete exhalation.

Residual Volume—that volume of air which remains in the lungs after complete exhalation.

Tidal Volume—the volume of air passing in and out of the lungs with each natural inspiration and expiration. This is of course, unlike vital capacity and residual volume, a very variable amount being low when the subject is at rest and high when he is active.

Inspiratory Reserve—(sometimes called 'complemental' air) is that volume which may still be inhaled at the completion of a normal tidal inspiration.

Expiratory Reserve—(sometimes called 'supplemental' air) is that volume of air which may be further exhaled at the completion of a normal tidal expiration. These reserve volumes, of course, decrease as the tidal volume increases.

Figures can be put to these volumes and it is useful to have some knowledge of what to expect in the average man, though individual variations may be very great. Convenient figures are:

	Vital Capacity	*Residual Volume*
	litres	*litres*
AVERAGE MAN	4·5	1·5
SMALL MAN	3·0	1·0
LARGE MAN	6·0	2·0

As respiration is a continuous process it is usual to introduce a time scale to give further useful information. With this, two well-known terms are used:

(i) *Respiratory Rate*—the number of complete respiratory cycles taking place per minute.

(ii) *Minute Volume*—the total volume of air passing in and out of the lungs in one minute. This is of course the multiple of the respiratory rate and the mean tidal volume.

Minute Volume is frequently used as an indication of respiratory requirement for a given effort, but in underwater medicine it may be misleading. Suppose, for example, that a certain task produced a minute volume of 60 litres. If this task were to be performed using a breathing apparatus, to supply air in a steady flow of 60 litres per minute would be quite inadequate. Also, if it was necessary to introduce into the circuit a carbon dioxide canister to remove CO_2 from expired air when the minute volume was 60 litres, it would be quite unreal to use one which was only capable of removing the CO_2 from a steady stream of expired air flowing at 60 litres per minute. Calculations of the resistances involved based on a steady flow rate of 60 litres per minute would also be completely false.

The minute volume is very much a 'mean' figure and does not take into account the variations in rate of flow during the respiratory cycle. For practical purposes therefore, it is essential that the FLOW RATE is known.

RESPIRATORY FLOW RATE

If the flow rate was, in its simplest form, one such that air moved into the lungs at a constant rate throughout inspiration, and similarly out of the lungs during expiration and the times taken for inspiration and expiration were equal, then, for a minute volume of 60 litres, flow rates of 120 litres per minute would be produced during each phase. Human breathing is not as simple as this.

Flow rates have been measured continuously during respiration (Proctor and Hardy, 1949), and it can be shown that the pattern follows very closely a 'sine' curve (Fig. 5). This example is one of moderate respiration and would represent a minute volume of about 30 litres. It will be seen, however, that to achieve this a peak flow rate of 100 litres per minute is reached during inspiration and is almost as great during expiration. If it was necessary to provide this subject with an adequate

RESPIRATORY FLOW PATTERN

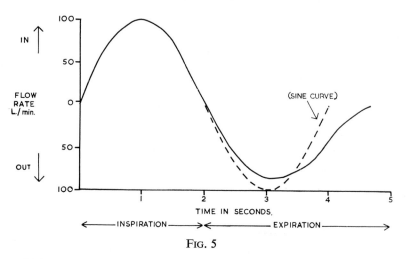

Fig. 5

artificial supply of air, facilities would be needed to ensure the peak flow being met, and if a carbon dioxide absorbing canister were needed then this should be effective for the peak expiratory flows approaching 100 litres per minute. If the question of resistance in the apparatus was involved flows of 100 litres per minute would also have to be reckoned with and not just the mean minute volume of 30 litres.

It has been stated that the respiratory flow rate follows a sine curve. This is only really so for the inspiratory phase; the expiratory phase curve being somewhat flattened and prolonged. The reason for the tapering off of the end of expiration lies in the nature of the elastic forces which, as the chest volume returns to its base or resting level, become much less powerful.

Many methods of measuring chest movement and respiratory flow rates are available and these include:

(i) *The Simple Pneumograph* or *Stethograph* which is a corrugated rubber tube round the chest or abdomen leading to a tambour and recording drum.

(ii) *The Hot Wire Anemometer* which consists of an electrically heated wire held before the mouth and nose. Air flow cools the wire according to the flow rate, and variation in its electric resistance can be recorded.

(iii) *Pressure Recording.* Various forms of delicate manometers attached to air ways can be calibrated to record flow rates.

Reference should be made to recent books and papers on respiratory

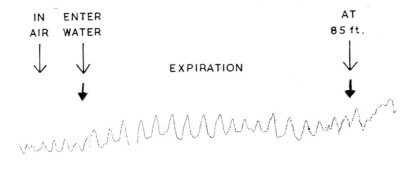

IN   ENTER   AT
AIR   WATER   85 ft.

                    EXPIRATION

INSPIRATION

CHEST MOVEMENT OF ENTERING WATER AND
BEING LOWERED TO 85 FEET

FIG. 6

physiology for details of these and other methods, some of which are listed at the end of the chapter.

Special adaptations are required for work under pressure and under water, and because pressure will alter the internal volume of any air-containing apparatus the simple pneumograph cannot be used.

A simple technique developed at the Royal Naval Physiological Laboratory consists of a length of bicycle valve-rubber tubing supported in a light-weight elastic rubber band. The rubber tubing is filled with mercury and doubled, the length of the loop being sufficient almost to encircle the chest or abdomen. The open ends are sealed with wire electrodes which lead through a long insulated cable to a galvanometer. The band containing the mercury-filled loop is secured slightly stretched around the chest or abdomen. (A pair can be used to record chest and abdominal movements simultaneously.) The wires lead to a galvano-meter, amplifier, stabilizer and pen recorder. Chest or abdominal move-ment alters the resistance of the mercury-filled tube and is reflected on the pen recording. Figure 6 shows such a recording of chest movement in a man descending in a diving bell, with only his head out of water, to a depth of 85 ft. ote the moving away from the base line of the respiratory pattern.

This method gives a picture of chest or abdominal movement but with care it can be calibrated against a spirometer to record volume changes.

In many physiological laboratories more delicate and elegant methods are used. Minute flow recorders are available which measure accurately pressure differences across a tiny diaphragm set in parallel with the inspiratory and expiratory sides of the mouthpiece of a conventional breathing apparatus. With such equipment it should be possible to assess respiratory flow patterns for all types of underwater breathing apparatus.

RESISTANCE TO BREATHING

It is inevitable that when an artificial means of supplying air or respi-ratory gases to the man under water is introduced, additional resistance to flow of air must result. Every attempt should be made to reduce this to a minimum. Resistance to breathing means work by the respiratory muscles and even in natural breathing the work of moving air in and out of the lungs must be considered. An ill-designed breathing apparatus may add to this an unacceptable load.

The work of breathing is essentially the effort required in moving air through a system of tubes and may be considered as such. The work or force required to move a gas through a tube is affected by such things as the rate of flow, the diameter and length of the tube, the influence of gravity and either the viscosity or density of the gas. The requirements of respiration demand variation in flow rate and whether or not appara-tus is used the other conditions do not vary significantly.

The mechanics of air movement in tubes, however, is such that for a given set of conditions the nature of the flow itself may vary with changes in the volume of air being moved in unit time.

In a gentle low-velocity flow through a straight tube the flow is streamlined or 'laminar'. The moving molecules retain an orderly forma-tion in their movement but those in the centre move more rapidly than those at the periphery which are slowed down by the friction between the gas and the inside of the tube (Fig. 7). The pressure required of maintain such a flow is dependent on the peripheral resistance which is proportional to the viscosity of the gas.

If now the flow rate is increased, or the tube narrowed, the peripheral drag is so effective as to cause eddying and distortion of the stream. Only the centre may retain the laminar flow. Finally the whole stream

AIR FLOW IN A TUBE

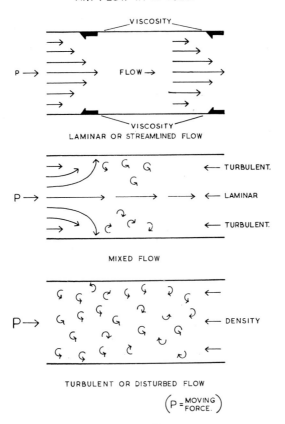

FIG. 7

may become completely disturbed or TURBULENT. In this case the molecules moving in all directions relative to one another do not remain in continuous contact with the tube wall and the viscosity ceases to resist the driving force. However, the turbulence completely destroys any streamlined momentum and the weight of the molecules becomes the resisting force to the flow pressure. In other words whereas in a laminar flow the driving force is proportional to the viscosity, in the turbulent flow it is proportional to the density of the gas.

The conditions under which a laminar flow is converted into a turbulent one can be obtained by the application of Reynolds Number, a factor which takes into account the radius of the tube, the linear velocity of the flow and the density and viscosity of the gas.

$$\text{Reynolds number} = \frac{v\,r\,D}{V} \text{ where } \left. \begin{array}{l} v = \text{velocity} \\ r = \text{radius} \\ D = \text{density} \\ V = \text{viscosity} \end{array} \right\} \begin{array}{l} \text{in C.G.S.} \\ \text{units} \end{array}$$

If less than 1000 the flow is wholly laminar, if more than 1500 it is wholly turbulent.

From the human respiratory system it can be estimated that flow rates below about 20 litres per minute are largely laminar while those of 40 litres per minute and above are largely turbulent. Between these figures the flow is mixed. In simple terms it may be said that in quiet breathing the flow is streamlined and with exercise or breathing against resistance it becomes turbulent.

This aspect of respiratory mechanics is of very great importance in underwater medicine. With the laminar flow, when this is to and fro, it will be observed that air in mid-stream will move further in and out than that of the periphery, an important factor in the consideration of DEAD SPACE. That density should increase the work of turbulent breathing is seen to be important when it is remembered that as depth under water increases so does the density of the air breathed.

All factors which increase the resistance to breathing must be considered, and where possible measured, account being taken of man's natural respiratory resistance as well as that of any apparatus he may use to the flow of the gases involved. Under water both these resistances must increase.

THE RESPIRATORY DEAD SPACE

With every inhalation the last of the inspired breath is contained in the nose, mouth, pharynx, trachea, bronchi and bronchioli. This, in fact, includes all the air except that which enters the actual alveoli, i.e. that which does not come into close contact with the pulmonary capillary bed and which is, as far as respiratory gas exchange is concerned, inactive. The simplest conception of 'dead space' is the total volume of the respiratory passages from the nose and mouth to the entrances of all the alveoli.

This is known as the ANATOMICAL DEAD SPACE and in the average man is about 180 ml. When a breathing apparatus is used which incorporates a mask or mouth-piece with inspiratory and expiratory valves the volume of air between the valves and the mouth and nose, or mouth if the nose is clipped, must be added to the anatomical dead space in any calculation of dead space effect. For every complete respiratory cycle the air occupying the dead space is ineffective in ventilation, i.e. of each breath, about 180 c.c. is wasted. It follows, therefore, that a man breathing rapidly and shallowly must waste very much more dead space air than one who for the same minute volume is breathing slowly and deeply. The latter pattern is therefore more acceptable where economy of supply is important.

The anatomical dead space, however, does not give a true picture of the practical significance of this volume. In certain pathological lung conditions alveoli, which lack an efficient blood supply or large bullæ, may be ventilated with very little gaseous exchange. In such cases the functional dead space is increased. On the other hand, particularly with quiet breathing and where the flow is laminar, the air in mid-stream flowing more rapidly may pass through the slower peripheral stream so that there is a relatively smaller dead space than the actual anatomical volume. At complete rest the tidal volume may approach that of the anatomical dead space and yet oxygenation remains adequate. This has been illustrated by Fowler (1950) who carried out two simple experiments. In the first a volume of pure oxygen equal to the anatomical dead space was inhaled. On exhalation of this volume only 40–50 ml. was pure oxygen. In the second case a subject inhaled a mixture of 80 ml. helium and 20 ml. oxygen (100 ml. in all). On subsequent exhalation, even when as much as 700 ml. had been exhaled, helium was still present. When allowance is made for these changes, reference is usually made to the PHYSIOLOGICAL DEAD SPACE. Techniques for measuring the two dead space volumes are described in standard books on respiratory physiology, but for practical purposes in the healthy subject not at rest physiological and anatomical dead space may be taken as much the same. More important in underwater medicine is to take into account and, wherever possible, reduce any additional dead space which may be introduced by the use of breathing apparatus.

Added dead space results in an increase in tidal volume to maintain the oxygen supply. As the added dead space is increased the compensation may lag behind producing some carbon dioxide retention. It is obvious, therefore, that added dead space, as well as being wasteful of respiratory gas, involves extra and profitless expenditure of energy by

4

the respiratory muscles with, in extreme cases, some loss of efficiency from carbon dioxide retention. This wastage can be ill-afforded under water where increased density already makes breathing more difficult and pressure increases the equivalent volume of air wasted, e.g. a litre lost at 100 ft. is equivalent to a loss of 4 litres at the surface pressure.

MAXIMUM BREATHING CAPACITY

A useful measurement in respiratory physiology is that of maximum breathing capacity. This simply indicates the maximum volume of air which can be moved in and out of the lungs and is usually recorded in litres per minute although the maximum effort can rarely be maintained for more than about 20 seconds. The term maximum breathing capacity (M.B.C.) is not favoured by respiratory physiologists as it involves the combination of two variables, rate and depth of respiration. It is customary therefore, to choose a fixed respiratory rate, usually one which is known to be within the optimal range for most individuals. The subject practises breathing at this rate with the aid of a metronome and when ready attempts over a period of 10 seconds to blow the maximum volume through a gas meter. The highest volume of several tries is taken as the result and recorded in litres per minute. When such a method is used the term applied is MAXIMUM VOLUNTARY VENTILATION (MVV). It is usual also to state the chosen respiratory rate which is indicated by a small figure after the symbol. This measurement will be referred to again but because 'Maximum Breathing Capacity' has a more familiar application this term will be retained in preference to 'Maximum Voluntary Ventilation'. In experiments to be described a rate of 72 breaths per minute is used, which would be symbolized as MVV_{72}.

Breathing air of increased density results in a profound reduction of maximum breathing capacity.

HYPERVENTILATION

More than any other system in the body, respiration is sensitive to emotional influence. The gasping inspiration of sudden fright, the rapid breathing of anxiety, the breath holding of concentration, the hot breath of passion and the cold breath of scorn are but a few examples of this relationship to which reference is made time and time again in all forms of literature. To the physiologist, however, the important irregularity is that of hyperventilation, an increase in rate and/or depth of respiration over and above that required to meet the body's respiratory requirement. If prolonged it may produce an excessive washout of carbon dioxide with disturbance of the blood's acid-base balance resulting in finger tingling and tetany or even loss of consciousness. It may occur voluntarily or involuntarily, the latter being a very common accompaniment of anxiety.

In underwater practice hyperventilation is extremely important. It may be used voluntarily to prolong breath-holding time but is frequently the result of anxiety for there are indeed many anxious moments for the underwater swimmer, especially the inexperienced. In many cases too, the very act of putting into place a mouth-piece and nose clip will promote it. Figure 8 is a typical example of this and shows chest movement before, during and after wearing a mouth-piece and nose clip. Note the drop in minute volume after removal to allow the blood carbon dioxide tension to rise to normal once more.

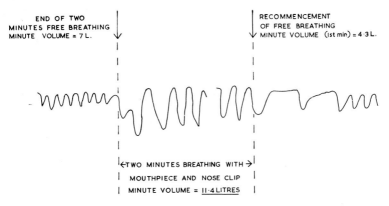

END OF TWO
MINUTES FREE BREATHING
MINUTE VOLUME = 7 L.

RECOMMENCEMENT
OF FREE BREATHING
MINUTE VOLUME (1st min) = 4·3 L.

←TWO MINUTES BREATHING WITH →
MOUTHPIECE AND NOSE CLIP
MINUTE VOLUME = 11·4 LITRES

EFFECT OF MOUTH PIECE AND NOSE CLIP ON BREATHING PATTERN

FIG. 8

THE CONTROL OF RESPIRATION

The respiratory centre, situated at the brain stem, exerts a direct control on the muscles of respiration but is itself very susceptible to influences from elsewhere. The pneumotaxic centre in the upper part of the pons ensures the maintenance of an even rhythm but this is readily disturbed by higher centres. The respiratory rhythm is profoundly influenced by emotion and may be varied within a wide range by conscious effort.

To meet the varying requirements of oxygen for changes in activity of the many systems of the body, especially the muscles, the main control is through the chemo-receptors in the aortic arch and carotid bodies. Through these an increase in the carbon dioxide tension of the blood or a decrease in oxygen tension will result in a stimulation of the centre and increased ventilation. Decrease in carbon dioxide will depress the centre and reduce ventilation but increase in oxygen does not have this effect. Response also occurs to changes in blood pH, acidity increasing respiration.

The centre is directly stimulated by increase in temperature of the blood, a mechanism which, in addition to the carbon dioxide stimulus, ensures an adequate ventilatory response to muscular exercise. Oxygen lack, as well as its stimulating effect on the peripheral chemo-receptors, has a direct local anoxic effect on the centre which may cause depression of activity.

Another factor to remember is the Hering-Breuer reflex. This is generally regarded as a regulator of the respiratory cycle in that inflation and stretching of the lungs reflexly depresses the centre and terminates inspiration. Recent work however (Marshall and Widdicombe, 1958) has suggested that in man this reflex may be weak or absent.

In the underwater environment the controlling mechanism of respiration may be subjected to variations in stimuli not normally encountered. Carbon dioxide may on occasions be difficult to eliminate due to faulty apparatus, increased oxygen tensions retarding the reduction of oxyhaemoglobin in the blood or its damming back by increases in respiratory resistance. Oxygen partial pressures may be reduced without corresponding increases in carbon dioxide tension. Extensive decreases in pressure may cause expansion of intra-pulmonary gases when a weak Hering-Breuer reflex is little or no protection against mechanical lung damage.

DIFFUSION

Attention is usually focused on the diffusion of oxygen through the alveolar membrane, interstitial fluid and capillary membrane to the plasma, where some dissolves, and the red blood cell (through its membrane) where it unites with the haemoglobin. In the healthy lung this is a rapid and short route. In the tissues where oxygen is required, the diffusion is much the same but in the other direction. The driving forces behind the diffusion are the differences between the partial pressures of the gas in the alveoli, and the tensions in the blood and tissues. In life at atmospheric pressure, these pressure differences are adjusted to the relatively constant intra-pulmonary pressure, oxygen flowing in and carbon dioxide flowing out to meet the tissues' fluctuating requirements, complicated only in health by accidental pollutions of the inspired air, and the continuous addition from the respiratory tract lining of water vapour.

When, however, the ambient pressures of the respiratory gases are subject to gross changes or when a wide range of gas mixture replaces the air (mixtures of oxygen with nitrogen or helium and even hydrogen or argon in experimental trials), the process of diffusion becomes a growing threat to orderly metabolism. Even the oxygen dissolving in increasing quantities in plasma may meet tissue requirements from solution, leaving the combined oxygen useless within the red cell, and denying the carbon dioxide the vehicle of reduced haemoglobin for its escape.

Nitrogen, hitherto ignored and apparently inert, assumes a new significance. Increasing pressure drives it in excess into solution. Widely distributed in the circulation, it diffuses into and through the tissues—fast through some, slow through others—until in all new levels of saturation are reached. Being five times more soluble in oil than water the fatty tissues hoard it. Having saturated widespread tissues with increasing pressure it is trapped and may, when pressures fall again, be unable freely to return to the lungs and escape, and must perforce form bubbles on the spot. These bubbles, like intra-parenteral poltergeists, potential emboli, may cause the fleeting havoc of decompression sickness. Still more, this nitrogen, infiltrating the tissues of the brain, exerts narcotic power striking the divers with the 'madness of the deeps'. So much for nitrogen the Inert!

The other gases, too, which may be used in practice, the light helium or in experiments the heavy argon, as they diffuse into tissues, bring with them their special problems, though helium may in many ways, except for its costliness, be called the diver's friend.

JUSTIFICATION?

The reader may be puzzled that this chapter, a rather untidy patchwork of respiratory tenets, some elementary, some controversial, should be here at all. Much of what is written will be referred to again in proper context when the relevant underwater problems are discussed. Other systems, too, might well have been included for few escape the influence of the new environment.

Without doubt, however, respiratory physiology is of such fundamental importance that any who would become specialists in underwater medicine should first serve an apprenticeship in this field. Though the justification for this possibly academic diversion at this stage may not yet be fully appreciated, it is confidently believed that any one who studies the following chapters will ultimately agree that it serves a useful purpose.

READING AND REFERENCES

Campbell, E. J. M. (1958). *The Respiratory Muscles and the Mechanics of Breathing.* Lloyd Luke Ltd., London.

Comroe, J. H. Jr., R. E. Forster, A. B. Dubois, W. A. Briscoe and E. Carlsen. (1959). *The Lung, Clinical Physiology and Pulmonary Function Tests.* The Year Book Publishers Inc., Chicago, U.S.A.

Consolazio, C. F., R. E. Johnson and E. Marck (1951). *Metabolic Methods.* C. V. Mosby Co., St. Louis, U.S.A.

Cooper, E. A. (1955). 'Aerodynamic Principles and their application to Closed Circuit Respiratory Apparatus.' National Coal Board, Physiology Panel Report. Ph.P/P (55) 4.

Fowler, W. S. (1950). 'Lung Function Studies.' *J. Clin. Invest. 29,* 1439.

Haldane, J. S. and J. G. Priestley (1935). *Respiration.* Clarendon Press, Oxford.

Liljestrand, A. (1958). 'The Neural Control of Respiration.' *Physiol. Rev. 38,* 691.

Marshall, R. and J. G. Widdicombe (1958). 'The Weakness of the Hering-Breuer Reflex in Man.' *J. Physiol. 140,* 36P.

Pitts, R. F. (1941). 'Organization of the Respiratory Centre.' *Physiol. Rev. 26,* 609.

Proctor, D. F. and J. B. Hardy (1949). 'Studies in Respiratory Air Flow.' *Bull. J. Hopkins Hosp. 85,* 253.

CHAPTER IV

Underwater Research Facilities

THE burden of underwater medical research has largely fallen upon the shoulders of the navies of the world. Man under water, however, is so completely dependent upon the aid of breathing apparatus, protective clothing and other artificial aids that running parallel to any physiological research programme must be an equally active developmental organization capable of producing apparatus to meet growing demands.

In this country from the start of the twentieth century there has been a close and profitable liaison between the Diving Schools of the Royal Navy and commercial firms such as Siebe Gorman and Heinke. Sir Robert Davis, an inspired chairman of the former, was the author of *Deep Diving and Submarine Operations*, a volume which remains today a valuable, comprehensive and practical text-book. Amongst naval divers who have made outstanding contributions by their experience in the pioneering days should be mentioned Captains Damant and Shelford, and coupled with them on the medical side must be Professors Haldane and Donald. These men have left a legacy in underwater development which inspires their present-day successors whose continuing efforts have provided much of the material for this book.

The pattern of underwater research is emerging on a world-wide scale. Though urgent military demands have necessitated the major developments being primarily a naval responsibility, the extension of diving to peaceful uses has fostered the fruitful co-operation between all the many organizations whose interests extend below the waves. In naval practice, divers and submariners tend to work as separate branches, but the common environment and general development on both sides is slowly bringing them together. In the United States of America this amalgamation has so far advanced that the term 'Submarine Medicine' is used to cover the medical problems of both the submarine and diving.

The Admiralty has wisely directed that in underwater medicine every help and encouragement should be given to civilian organizations interested in this field. The result is that whereas much basic research and development is carried out in Naval Establishments, effective liaison exists with private and commercial enterprises and much progress is made in all directions.

Underwater medicine is dependent primarily on the results of research in general physiology and as the last chapter emphasized, respiratory

physiology in particular. To extend the basic research into the underwater environment, elaborate equipment and special laboratories are
needed. The training of divers and submariners is, of course, the foremost responsibility of a fighting service, but this, too, needs special
facilities which can at the same time be adapted for research. Research
is complementary to training since its ultimate aim is to extend the field
of operation of those who are trained. Research will not only extend the
sphere of activity but will improve methods of training and the selection
of men for training.

The behaviour of man in water can only be finally assessed by observing him at work under water, carrying out his allotted task in the sea
or inland waters. It is possible, however, to simulate very closely under
laboratory conditions the final environment. Having studied man in his
natural environment on land his progress to underwater efficiency may
be examined in the following stages.

  (i)   In water.
 (ii)   Under pressure.
(iii)   In water under pressure.
(iv)   Under the sea or other natural water.

MAN IN WATER

Much valuable information can be obtained from a study of man in
water using such facilities as swimming baths and the tanks which are
found in many research establishments or even open water. Such information includes the metabolic cost and speeds of various forms of
swimming, resistance to immersion, the value of protective clothing and
changes in respiratory pattern. Breathing apparatus can also first be
tested on the surface.

An ideal arrangement is to have a tank in which movement of surface
water can be controlled in order that a subject may remain stationary,
so facilitating recording while swimming through water at a controlled
rate. In fact what is required is an aquatic treadmill.

An example of this kind of investigation is found in the work of
Pugh and Edholm (1955), who measured the oxygen consumption of
Channel swimmers. A moderate breast stroke demanded 2·11 litres per
minute and a crawl of 58 strokes per minute 2·97.

MAN UNDER PRESSURE

Many of the changes occurring in man under water are due to the
increase of pressure in the respired gases. These conditions can be
simulated by exposing man to pressure alone in a chamber. The

chamber must be of sufficient strength to withstand the pressure difference between the maximum working pressure within and the atmospheric pressure outside. Such strength is usually achieved by making the chambers cylindrical.

A high-pressure air supply is needed, usually from a compressor and a battery of storage bottles, and this air must be filtered and free from impurities. Care must be taken to ensure its freedom from oil vapour and carbon monoxide, impurities which may easily be introduced from a motor-driven compressor especially if there is any possibility of exhaust gases entering the compressor's air inlet.

(This warning should also be given to any underwater swimmer who may use some form of internal combustion engine and pump to recharge the bottles of his breathing set. It is essential to remember that the concentration of any impurity such as carbon monoxide is multiplied by the number of atmospheres of pressure under which it is being breathed.)

In designing a pressure chamber it is desirable to have inlet valves with which the rate of increase in pressure can be controlled manually from outside, to enable very rapid or very slow compression to be applied. The comfort of the occupant is increased if the incoming air is distributed between a large number of jets rather than rushing in through a single orifice. Similarly it must be possible to reduce the pressure either rapidly, in some cases explosively, or in a slow bleed-off. Pressure gauges are essential and for convenience should be graduated in 'equivalent depth', i.e. in feet according to the pressure within. This avoids the confusion of a gauge reading pressures of 1 atmosphere less than the absolute pressure.

It is desirable also that the chamber should be fitted with an air-lock, an additional compartment large enough to hold a man, so that persons can be passed into or out of the large chamber without altering its pressure. A much smaller air-lock is also usually incorporated so that small items such as food or instruments may be passed in or out without wasting compressed air. Quick-opening doors are also an advantage. Warm clothing should be provided within as temperature falls considerably during decompression.

Users must be aware of the increased fire risk under pressure. The partial pressure of oxygen being increased encourages any combustion. A cigarette is gone in a few puffs and a match strikes with a great flame. Electrical fittings must be specially enclosed and no apparatus which could form a spark should be admitted as, for example, an electric motor. Where recording drums are used they should be clock-work driven. All woodwork should be rendered fireproof. Failure to observe these simple fire precautions has resulted in explosion and tragedy. Matches should never be taken inside and watches (unless specially made) and fountain pens should also be left outside.

Pressure chambers are also used in the training of divers and submariners, for surface decompression and for the treatment of decompression sickness. They vary in size from small portable ones, which will take one man lying down, to larger ones which will hold a dozen, seated or standing. Though any may be used in research some are constructed primarily for this purpose. In this country the largest collection of experimental chambers is to be found at the Royal Naval Physiological Laboratory at Alverstoke in Hampshire, where three are available for human experimental work and two are usually reserved for work with goats.

In addition this laboratory possesses a wide range of small portable chambers designed to study the effects of pressure on animals varying in size from rats and mice to cats and dogs. Most of the animal experimental work, however, is carried out with goats in the larger chambers as they produce results more compatible with those of man. (Figs. 9, 10 and 11.)

The largest of these chambers is 10 ft. long and 8 ft. in diameter. It is fitted with seats and can accommodate 12 men. It has a battery of accurately reading 'Bristol' pressure gauges and an equivalent depth may be reached at 100 ft. per minute. Evacuation can be accomplished slowly or at a similar rate. Its maximum equivalent depth is 300 ft. though a depth of 600 ft. might be reached in an emergency. It can also be adapted for use as an altitude chamber being fitted with an evacuating pump which will produce a pressure within equivalent to an altitude of 30,000 ft. It has an air-lock of $4\frac{1}{2}$ ft. by 4 ft.

The remaining three chambers are of similar size, 8–10 ft. long and 4–5 ft. diameter but without the large air-lock. Their maximum working equivalent depth is also 300 ft. Each will take two men. One of them is wired to a six-channel electro-encephalograph and recordings under pressure can be made very satisfactorily. A large three-compartment chamber capable of simulating a depth of 800 ft. has recently been installed.

All the chambers are fitted with observation ports and telephones are available for human experiments.

The pressure chamber is certainly the most valuable tool in underwater medical research. It is doubtful if any real progress could be made without it. Though referred to formally as 'The Chamber', so familiar is

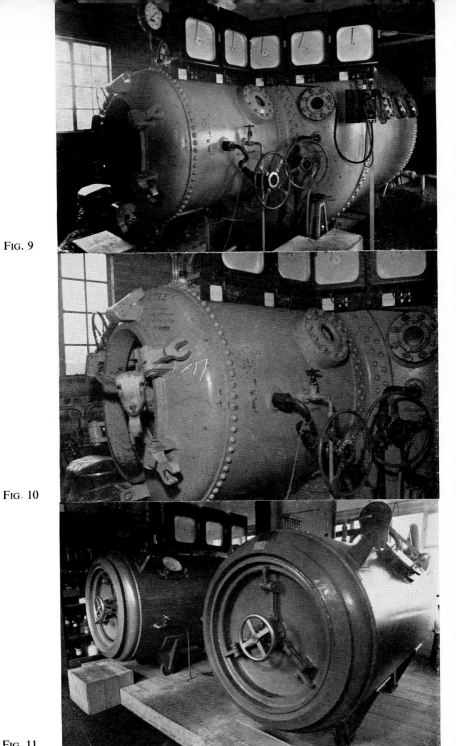

FIG. 9

FIG. 10

FIG. 11

Pressure chambers at R.N. Physiological Laboratory

it to all connected with the underwater environment, that it is known affectionately as 'The Pot'. On one occasion a telephone call for the author could not be accepted because, as the confused operator told the caller—'Dr Miles is in the Chamber Pot'!

Another and very valuable source of information of the effects on man of 'dry' pressure is the work done in such undertakings as the construction of tunnels beneath rivers and estuaries, and the laying of foundations for bridges. It is the practice in such undertakings to carry out the excavations under high air pressure either in tunnels or caissons, such pressure holding back the seepage water and keeping the workings dry. Under such conditions there are many opportunities to observe the effects of pressure on large numbers of workmen and much of the present knowledge of the causes, pathology, clinical picture and treatment of 'Caisson Disease' has evolved from this source. 'Caisson Disease' is a form of Decompression Sickness, an occupational hazard of all who work under pressure be it dry or wet. In most cases today the companies responsible for such projects welcome the advice and help of experts in the study of the effects of the working conditions on the men. A good example is the construction of the new Dartford Tunnel under the Thames, where a careful investigation is already yielding most valuable information as a result of close and effective co-operation between Industrial Medical Officers, Academic Physiologists, Radiologists and Naval Scientists (Golding, Griffiths, Hempleman, Paton and Walder, 1960).

A recent advance in medical treatment is the use of high-pressure oxygen together with X-ray therapy in the treatment of certain forms of cancer. This is achieved with small pressure chambers just large enough to take the patient lying down. In this technique relatively low pressures are used and the chambers are lightly built. Even perspex has been used. Though this is essentially a treatment facility, it is used under expert supervision and must be regarded as a potential source of further information on man's reaction to pressure and particularly to high-pressure oxygen.

Under high pressure the effects of some anaesthetics may be enhanced without the risk of anoxia and, for example, nitrous oxide, which, if used under pressure in a chamber, may approach the ideal anaesthetic. Heart operations have also been performed in a pressure chamber when the accumulation of oxygen in the tissues following pressurization, breathing oxygen, may be sufficient to maintain vital centres for the duration of the operation, thus dispensing with the need for a heart-lung machine.

MAN IN WATER UNDER PRESSURE

The next step in the approach to reality which can be achieved in the Laboratory is to observe man both under water and under pressure.

If depth of water is to be used to produce pressure, then a high water tower would be needed with observation ports at various depths. The Royal Navy has such a facility at the submarine base, H.M.S. *Dolphin* at Gosport, which was built for the training of submarine personnel in methods of escape. This can be, and is, used for experimental observations of men under pressure and under water but the subjects are not

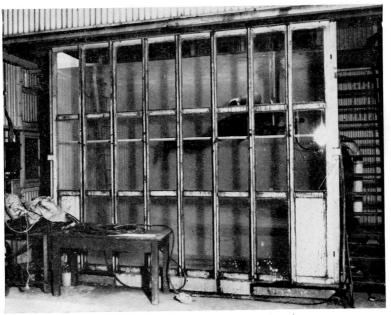

FIG. 12. A glass-sided experimental tank

conveniently accessible and visibility through observation ports is limited. It has, however, a diving bell which can be lowered through the water. This bell has a domed roof under which air is trapped and an observer can descend breathing this air and look through ports also in its roof. This bell was used to make the tracing of breathing pattern in Figure 6. Electrocardiograph tracings have also been obtained from subjects at the bottom of this tower. It is essential to make the electrodes watertight with dry contacts. The results are far from perfect but may have some value.

A more simple underwater observation tank has been constructed at the Admiralty Experimental Diving Unit in H.M.S. *Vernon* at Portsmouth. This is 15 ft. deep with one side constructed entirely of glass panels which gives unrestricted vision of the man underwater but here again instrumentation is limited by the water and the depth is not great (Fig. 12). Both the *Dolphin* and *Vernon* tanks, however, are widely used.

Underwater pressure can, however, be simply achieved without resort to depth. If a tank of water is taken into a pressure chamber and the pressure increased, then the water will be under the same pressure as that of the chamber. If the chamber pressure is raised to four atmospheres, that of the water is similarly raised and a man in that water would be subjected to exactly the same conditions as if he were immersed in water at a depth of 99 ft. Such an arrangement has the advantage that the subject can be kept near the surface of the water and is accessible for all manner of apparatus and instrumentation. Furthermore, observers can enter the chamber, remain dry, and be in close contact with the subject. An additional safety factor is that the man, if in trouble, can be immediately removed from the water.

To use a tank within a pressure chamber does, however, greatly restrict the volume of water that can be used, and thus limits considerably any activity within the water. The principle involved, however, can be applied more realistically and there is, in fact, beneath the 100 ft. column of water in the Navy's submarine escape tower a further compartment which can be flooded to a convenient depth, and air pressure applied above it to achieve equivalent depths up to 100 ft. This compartment is large enough to enable men to swim around in it and even carry out specific tasks. Facilities for instrumentation, however, are extremely limited.

Where, however, underwater research is the primary object, special 'wet' pressure chambers can be constructed for this purpose. Such a chamber is available at Messrs Siebe Gorman's diving research unit at Surbiton and has been extensively used in Naval Medical Research particularly for study of decompression schedules. The classical work of Donald on oxygen poisoning (referred to in a later chapter) was carried out in this chamber.

The Siebe Gorman 'Wet' Chamber consists of an upright cylinder containing water 7 ft. deep with an air space above and a seat for an observer. It is possible for two divers to work within it and be observed from above. A simulated depth of 200 ft. can be attained. This chamber has made, and is still making, a valuable contribution to underwater medicine. Unfortunately it is small and instrumentation is difficult.

The requirements for full research in underwater medicine demand

Fig. 13.
Deep diving
unit at R.N.
Physiological
Laboratory

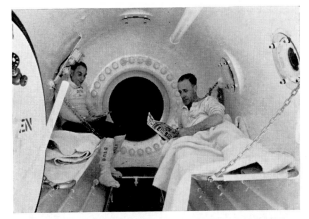

(a) Inside dry
section

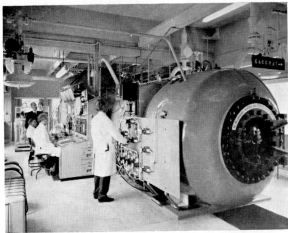

(b) Control
panels

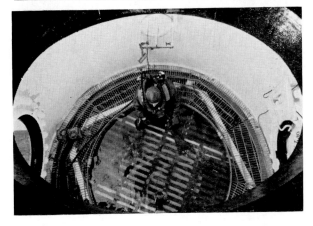

(c) Inside wet
section

the use of a combined wet and dry chamber with adequate facilities for observation and recording. In 1964 a new self-contained all purpose chamber was completed at the Royal Naval Physiological Laboratory. This consists of a vertical cylinder of 10 ft. diameter containing water to a depth of 8 ft. Above the water is a cat-walk for observers and instruments, and leading off horizontally from the top of the wet chamber is a dry chamber 11 ft. long and 6 ft. internal diameter. It is possible to use the wet and dry chambers together or separately, and each has its own air-lock. Special glands are fitted to take cables for instrumentation up to a total of 24 circuits. Simulated depths up to 1,000 ft. can be produced. All the necessary services and equipment with a small laboratory are provided in the building housing the chambers. Such a much needed facility provides an immense scope for further underwater research and a provisional experimental programme has already been visualized. (Fig. 13.)

SEA TRIALS

Finally, trials must be repeated in the natural environment, either in the sea or other natural waters. Though in the laboratory a close approximation to the environment may have been produced, there still remain subtle differences which only the real thing can provide. Differences in location and background temperature, currents and waves, and the boundlessness and enfolding expanse of the sea all play a part in the final setting.

The Royal Navy has modified one of its smaller ships, H.M.S. *Reclaim* (Figs. 14 and 15) as a diving research and training vessel. This ship has carried out many valuable sea trials and from her, in Norway in 1956, Lieutenant George Wookey achieved a world-record diving depth, in a flexible suit and helmet, of 600 ft. *Reclaim* is especially adapted for deep diving of the conventional form where the breathing mixture is supplied and control maintained from the surface. She has facilities for providing mixtures of helium and oxygen for very deep diving, and an observation chamber which can be lowered to a depth of 1,000 ft. or more. A large pressure chamber is provided which has three separate sections which can be used to accommodate divers at different stages of decompression. A further facility is a submersible decompression chamber (Fig. 16), which, by increasing the pressure of its air supply, can be lowered into the ocean to pick up a diver at the pressure equivalent to his depth and then be sealed to raise him to the surface without further reduction in pressure. From the submersible decompression chamber he can be directly transferred, remaining under pressure, to a larger fixed pressure

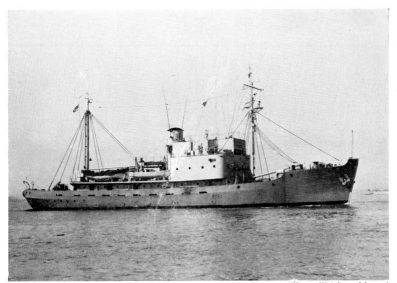

(*Photo: Wright and Logan*)

FIG. 14. H.M.S. *Reclaim*

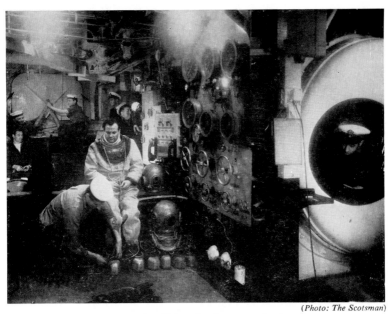

(*Photo: The Scotsman*)

FIG. 15. The diving flat in H.M.S. *Reclaim*

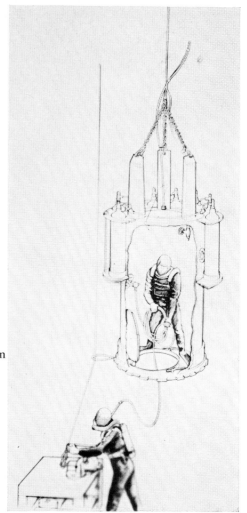

FIG. 16
Submersible decompression
chamber

chamber wherein he can be decompressed as necessary in comparative comfort. Facilities for maintenance of equipment are, of course, also provided and a small laboratory is available for simple gas analysis.

With the main interest swinging from the helmeted diver to the self-contained underwater swimmer, smaller craft with fewer crew and less maintenance costs are being used, and for this purpose the fundamental requirement is simply a pressure chamber.

However, such equipment is the *sine qua non* of professional underwater research. For the amateur with no more than his own underwater equipment there is much to be studied of his reactions and behaviour in the new environment. It is rare, too, for the underwater swimmer to be working alone in what is essentially, especially in the interests of safety and economy, a group practice. Underwater groups usually have professional advice available and with such help useful and interesting programmes of research and investigation can be planned to be run in conjunction with whatever is the main objective. As an extreme example may be cited an organization of underwater swimmers in Sydney, Australia, who, impressed by the need for further knowledge, have formed themselves into an 'Underwater Research Group'. Their object is to study the effects on man of activity underwater. Already they and similar organizations have made some very worthwhile contributions and have set an example which others may profitably follow.

Findings in research frequently result from determined and controlled observations, but on the other hand many quite startling and important discoveries are the results of pure chance. Perhaps the most valuable contribution every underwater swimmer or diver could make would be the careful compiling and maintenance of a personal 'log' book. In this should be recorded full details of every dive, location, weather conditions, depths, times, apparatus, breathing mixtures, personal impressions and any pertinent observations of companions. Such a log book grows in interest and value with every entry and may, one never knows, ultimately be the key to some profound advance in knowledge.

It is inevitable that in the practice of underwater swimming or diving accidents will sometimes happen. All too often the tragedy of the event masks the need to find out the real cause. Many are frequently dismissed as drowning or misadventure. There is no greater contribution to be made to underwater medicine than that every accident, however serious or however trivial, should have the fullest possible and expert investigation. Much may be learnt which would save repetition of the accident and often too, some information may be forthcoming which may place another piece in the jig-saw of understanding. This is particularly true of underwater accidents for here, unlike their counterparts on land or in the air, where final mutilation of tissues often masks the true cause, the body may be gently cradled in the water until recovered, when the underlying fault may be more easily found. No appeal for the fullest and most careful investigation, analysis and recording of the details of these accidents can be too strong.

The facilities for underwater research are thus seen to consist not only of the special technical laboratory facilities but to extend to every stretch of water which man explores. It begins with the toddler who puts his first exploring toe into the strange and frightening ocean and will not end until the bounds and abyss of the seas and the living things therein are fully explored and tamed by man. In this vast enterprise, man has far to go, but the trail is already being blazed.

RECENT ADVANCES

As was to be expected underwater research has in the past ten years gathered a great deal of momentum. The increased operational depth and time at sea of submarines and the need to retrieve missiles or air-craft accidentally lost at sea has greatly increased the naval need to develop search, diving and rescue techniques. The finding of stores of natural gas and oil under the sea-bed has given an additional com-mercial boost. Academic, cultural and recreational interests under water have grown to such an extent that many amateur underwater clubs have put their resources at the disposal of university depart-ments.

Useful studies of marine growth are progressing as for example the 'Operation Kelp' organized by Bellamy and Whittick (1968) of Durham University. The historians have also learnt much from the current search for the treasure in Sir Cloudesley Shovell's flagship sunk off the Isles of Scilly in 1707 (Gayton, 1967).

Underwater research however can be extremely expensive though much less so than that into space. Major enterprises need government or commercial support. These are being obtained in many parts of the world and include, as well as the growing British effort at Alverstoke, the American Navy's Deep Submergence Systems Project (Craven, 1967) concerned with deep ocean technology, Deep Submergence Vehicles (Feldman, 1967) and Sealab III (Bond, 1967). The French Navy too has facilities for deep diving research in Toulon at the 'Groupe d'Etudes et Recherches Sous-Marine' (Barthelemy, 1967).

Commercial enterprises include the Ocean Systems Inc. Tonawanda Research Laboratory in New York where simulated saturation diving at 650 ft. has been studied.

Two other projects which have stirred the imagination are Captain Cousteau's long range research programme and Ed Link's joint effort with the University of Pennsylvania 'Man in the Sea'.

Though large scale, imaginative and costly enterprises are producing advances in knowledge and rapid progress the efforts of smaller groups and indeed individual divers continue to contribute in no small way to the over all picture. In the final reckoning it will be the individual and personal relationship between the diver and his environment which will hold the secret of his ultimate mastery.

READING AND REFERENCES

Barthelemy, L. (1967). 'French Naval Activities in Diving Physiology'. Proc. 3rd. Symposium on Underwater Physiology. Williams and Wilkins Co., Baltimore.

Bellamy, D. J. and A. Whittick (1968). 'The Kelp Project'. *Triton 13*, 16.

Bond, G. F. (1967). 'Sealab. III'. *Astronautics and Aeronautics;* July, 1967. p. 80.

Cousteau, J. Y. (1964). 'At Home in the Sea'. *National Geographic 125*, 465.

Craven, J. P. (1967). 'An Assessment of the Future of Deep-Ocean Technology'. *Astronautics and Aeronautics;* July, 1967. p. 36.

Feldman, S. (1967). 'Developing a New Breed of Deep Submergence Vehicles' *Astronautics and Aeronautics;* July, 1967. p. 44.

Gayton, J. B. (1967). 'The £1 million Treasure of Sir Cloudesley Shovell'. *Triton 12*, 160.

Golding, E. Campbell, P. Griffiths, H. W. Hampleman, W. D. M. Paton and D. N. Walder (1960). 'Decompression Sickness during the Construction of the Dartford Tunnel'. *Brit. J. Indus. Med.* 17, 167.

Link, E. A. and R. Stenciet (1965). 'Outpost Under the Sea' and 'The Deepest Days'. *National Geographic 127*, 530.

Ocean Systems Inc. (1966). 'Saturation Diving to 650 ft.' Tonawanda Research Lab. *N.Y. Tech. Memo.* B.411.

Pugh, L. G. C., and O. G. Edholm (1955). 'The Physiology of Channel Swimmers', *Lancet, 269*, 761.

Underwater Research Group, N.S.W. (1959). 'Deep Diving after Hyperventilation'. *R. N. Diving Magazine*, Vol. 7, No. 1.

U.S. Navy (1957). 'General Description of the U.S. Naval Medical Research Laboratory'. Report issued by Submarine Base, New London, Conn., U.S.A. September, 1957.

PART II

The Hazards of the Environment

CHAPTER V

The Effects of Increased Pressure

IN THE chapter heading the definite article has been introduced before 'increased pressure' to emphasize that in the underwater environment, the pressure is always greater than that of the atmosphere and because man may be moving up or down within it, both rises and falls of pressure must be considered.

It is important, too, that a clear differentiation should be made between the direct physical effects of pressure changes and the secondary complications of abnormally high quantities of respiratory gases dissolving in the blood and tissues. The first of these, the physical effects, are included under the broad term 'BAROTRAUMA'. The more elusive secondary reactions, which are not collectively grouped, but carry such individually descriptive titles as 'Nitrogen Narcosis', 'Oxygen Poisoning' and 'Decompression Sickness', will receive special attention in subsequent chapters. The immediate interest is in the direct influences of changes in pressure on man in water and the damage this may do, namely the barotrauma.

It has already been stated that, provided the air in all the air-containing cavities of the body is maintained at the pressure of the surrounding tissues, i.e. at the pressure of the water at the depth at which the individual is placed, the direct effects of pressure on the individual are of no consequence. This is certainly true for the present depth range in which man has operated, and as far as is known is likely to be so for very much greater depths still.

It is when, for some reason or other, a situation arises where the pressure of air or gas in a cavity becomes different from that of the surrounding tissues, that trouble begins. Since man under water is generally dependent on artificial means, frequently under the control of his attendants, failure to maintain pressure equalization is usually due to inadequacy of the means, neglect on the part of the attendants or occasionally, a weakness in the man himself. Before these means are considered, however, it is as well to look at changes which can take place in a man who undertakes a dive beneath the surface sustained solely by the lungful of air he takes beforehand. This, the simplest of all dives, will be familiar to all who have attended aquatic sports and watched the experts gathering armfuls of plates from the bottom of the deep end of the swimming pool. A more practical application is that of the

73

pearl-diver whose technique is the most primitive form of commercial diving.

All the gas- or air-containing cavities must be considered, but as, without doubt, the most serious complications result from disturbances of pressure equilibrium in the respiratory system, these will be studied first and fully.

EFFECTS OF INCREASED PRESSURE IN A FREE DIVE

The free diver, for example the pearl-diver, is limited in his activity by the time for which the breath may be held. In order to obtain the maximum proportion of this period working on the bottom it is a common practice to enter the water holding a weight, such as a heavy rock, to accelerate descent. This is abandoned when the bottom is reached.

Though it is possible to prolong the breath-holding time by hyperventilation, this is a dangerous practice and should be strongly discouraged for reasons which will be given later.

Before entering the water, a full inspiration is taken and, as far as the effects of pressure are concerned during the dive, it will be assumed that the diver enters the water with the chest and lungs fully expanded, i.e. with 100% vital capacity.

In the average man this may be taken as 4·5 litres. To this must be added a residual volume of 1·5 litres, for it is essential to consider the effect of pressure on the total lung volume which in this case is 6 litres. As he descends through the water the pressure on the chest increases, and since the chest is able to contract, the pressure of the contained air may be likewise increased by a corresponding decrease in volume. When a depth of 33 ft. is reached, the pressure being doubled causes the contained air volume to be halved and similarly at 99 ft. it is reduced to one quarter.

The following table illustrates these changes for the average man, the small man and the large man:

		Average Man litres	Small Man litres	Big Man litres
SURFACE	Vital capacity	$4\frac{1}{2}$ } =6	3 } =4	6 } =8
	Residual air	$1\frac{1}{2}$	1	2
33 ft.	Lung contains	3	2	4
66 ft.	Lung contains	2	$1\frac{1}{3}$	$2\frac{2}{3}$
99 ft.	Lung contains	$1\frac{1}{2}$	1	2

The striking fact about these figures is that in each case at 99 ft. the total respiratory volume has been reduced to the residual volume. In practice this implies that the free diver who enters the water following full inspiration, by the time he reaches about 100 ft. will be in a state of full expiration without having lost any air as far as chest content is concerned. Conversely, when he surfaces from his depth the decreasing pressure will ensure that he does so, as he entered, in full inspiration; provided, of course, there is no voluntary or accidental expulsion of air whilst under water.

It is not known how much below residual volume a healthy chest may be compressed. It is certainly likely to be very little and for convenience it may be assumed that the two volumes are the same. When man reaches that depth, i.e. pressure, when the respiratory volume has reached the physical minimum, there can be no further diminution in volume and therefore, as far as the air is concerned, no further increase in pressure. The outcome of continued descent would be that the air in the lungs remains at constant volume and pressure whilst the pressure of the pulmonary circulation and tissue continues to rise, thus creating a pressure difference. At first fluid would pass from the alveolar capillaries, pulmonary oedema, to be followed by, if the difference continued, burst vessels and pulmonary haemorrhage. It would be possible in an extreme case for the ribs to crack and the chest wall cave in. It is obvious, therefore, that free diving to a depth much in excess of 100 ft. could be quite disastrous. Reference back to Figure 2 will make the understanding of this problem easier.

In such a deep free dive as this the pressure changes are gross. The respiratory system is, however, sensitive to quite small changes in pressure, and the significance of this is also important.

EFFECT OF SMALL PRESSURE CHANGES

Figure 6 showed how when a man was lowered into water the tidal volume range moved towards expiration. This effect occurred immediately on immersion and implied an increase in the inspiratory reserve volume and a decrease in expiratory reserve.

This may be appreciated by considering the example of a man upright in water with the head only breaking surface. (Fig. 17.) Apart from the small fluctuations due to resistance to respiratory air flow the pressure in the lungs remains the same as that of the atmosphere, say 760 mm.Hg. The pressure gradient in water is so very much steeper than in air that even with the depth of the upright chest the additional pressure will be effective. At the lower margin of the chest this would be about 30 cm. of water added to that of the atmosphere and at the upper level perhaps 10 cm. The net effect of this additional pressure on the chest is to disturb the underlying balance between chest elasticity and lung elasticity so decreasing chest volume. In fact from 300–400 ml. of air may be driven out by immersion of the chest. It will also be found that the vital capacity measured under these conditions is less than when measured with the whole body out of water. This external pressure gradient between mouth level and lower chest level is equally important when the body is totally immersed in the upright position and must be taken into account when

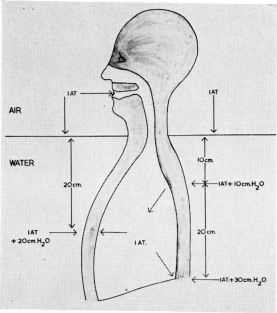

Fig. 17. Pressure gradient in the submerged chest

breathing apparatus is being designed. The pressure of the mixture and the position of any breathing bag must be carefully adjusted to give maximum comfort in breathing. The site of any relief valve on the breathing bag must be carefully chosen to ensure that changes in positions do not adversely affect its release pressure setting.

The simplest way of keeping a man totally immersed would seem to be the provision of a tube from his mouth to the surface. This method has, in recent years, become very popular as an aquatic recreation in the form of the 'Schnorkel' tube. It has, however, very strict limitations and may indeed be dangerous.

LIMITATIONS OF THE SCHNORKEL TUBE

If a long tube is taken and one end placed in a bucket of water, it is quite impossible, by forced inspiratory suction, to draw the water higher than about 45 inches. Similarly, if a tube extends below the surface of water, air cannot, by forceful expiration, be blown down the tube further than about 60 inches. These figures can only be achieved by starting with full expiration or full inspiration respectively. If the experiment is attempted with the lungs already containing half the vital capacity these distances would be reduced to 30 inches and 40 inches respectively.

These results represent the pressures obtained by forceful inspiration and expiration and are far and away above the pressures against which continuous breathing could be maintained. Silverman and his colleagues (1945) in an extensive series of experiments concluded that to maintain efficiency in active conditions which may be compared with swimming, the inspiratory resistance should not exceed 8·2 cm. water and the expiratory resistance 5·3 cm. water.

What these figures mean is simply that, when breathing through a 'Schnorkel' tube, if the centre of the chest is more than about 8 cm. below the surface, there will be some loss of efficiency which will increase if the chest gets deeper. By 'centre' of the chest, in this context, is meant the horizontal plane of equal pressure at the level of mean external pressure. In the upright position this plane may pass through the sternal notch and in the prone position through the anterior folds of the axillae.

In the upright position with the top of the head just below the surface the mean pressure plane would be at least 30 cm. below the surface and though war history books give instances of soldiers being concealed under water and breathing through reeds, respiration in such cases would be difficult and exhausting. It is the depth of the chest below the water which is important, rather than the length of the tube.

In practice the breathing tube is used with the swimmer in the horizontal position. It enables the positively buoyant person to lie face down in the water effortlessly floating with perhaps a few square inches of posterior scalp above water when, if goggles are worn, there is good visibility below the surface. Most tubes have a float valve so that when under water they will not be flooded and can be used effectively for shallow water spear-fishing and diving. They should not be used when in the upright position.

Length of tube, though less important if the chest is near the surface, does, however, add to the respiratory dead space and resistance. Unless the outfit is so constructed that the tube is used solely for inspiration, and few of them are, this must be seriously considered. Since the tube is used with the swimmer face down in the water it must be constructed to bend from the mouth and pass vertically beside the head. In order to prevent flooding a further 180° bend is needed to accommodate the float valve. These two bends must add considerably to the overall length of tube. The simplest way to overcome the disadvantage of a long tube is to use it solely for inspiration with valves either side of the mouth-piece ensuring that expired air escapes into the water or up a second tube.

The 'Schnorkel' tube gives the users a great deal of pleasure and is valuable as an introduction for potential skin-divers to their new medium. The tube should always be as short as practically possible and in no circumstances should it be used for breathing except with the body horizontal and floating awash or swimming on the surface.

PRESSURE DIFFERENCES WITH BREATHING APPARATUS

In standard or helmet diving, failure to maintain an air pressure equivalent to depth may result in the respiratory air pressure being higher or lower than the depth pressure. Both these situations produce unfortunate results well known to divers as follows:

1. *Air Pressure Greater than Depth Pressure.* This is not a very common occurrence but a situation may arise where in preparing to ascend a diver may tighten up the escape valve in the helmet to increase the volume of air in the suit giving greater buoyancy. He may then begin to ascend, and if his attendants were not alert and failed to reduce his air pressure or the diver did not re-open his outlet valve fully, the falling external pressure would result in still further inflation of the suit and acceleration upwards. The excess pressure within the suit would cause it to become quite rigid so that the diver would become spread-eagled within it and unable to help himself by releasing the helmet valve. He would rise with great speed and might damage himself against surface objects. If he reached the surface safely he would lie there inflated and helpless. Fortunately rupture of the suit would be prevented by escape of some excess air past the elastic cuffs of the sleeves. In such a state the diver is said to be 'blown up' and care must be taken in his recovery. (Fig. 18.) If an enthusiast slashed the suit he might sink before the slack of his life-line could be hauled in. The results of this would be disastrous. He should be secured and quickly deflated by opening the helmet valve and letting air out of the cuffs. It is a frightening experience for the diver and alarming to the attendants and may be complicated by

the development of acute decompression sickness or even a 'burst lung'.

2. *Air Pressure Lower than Depth Pressure.* Theoretically a sudden failure of the supply of compressed air to a diver working under water would result in the pressure in his helmet and respiratory system dropping to that of the atmosphere, whereupon the pressure difference so created would result in his being crushed by the surrounding water against his rigid breast plate and helmet. That this does not occur in

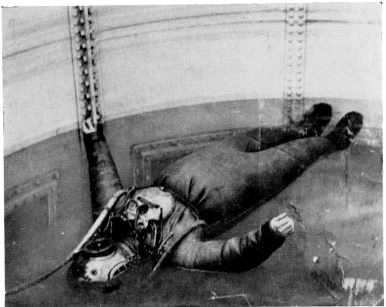

(By courtesy of Sir Robert Davis)

FIG. 18. A blown-up diver

practice is due to the fitting of a non-return valve at the entrance of the air supply pipe to the helmet. If the air supply fails, this valve traps the air already under pressure within the helmet and suit. This is of sufficient volume to meet respiratory needs provided he is surfaced without delay, or the air supply is quickly re-established.

There is, however, another circumstance in which the crushing effect may occur. If, for example, a diver, working from an underwater plat-form on the side of a ship or dock, accidentally steps off that platform he may, unless his attendants above are very alert, fall through the water before being checked by his life-line and air pipe. In such a fall it would be unlikely that those working the pump would be able to increase the air pressure to keep pace with requirement. Under these conditions the pressure in the helmet and respiratory system would remain equivalent to the depth of the working platform, unless the volume it occupied could be proportionately decreased, whilst that on the body would rapidly increase. The decrease in volume of the air plus the increasing external pressure would force the diver into his helmet and if the fall was great enough profound physical damage would occur, possibly fatal. The excess pressure in pulmonary tissue and circulation would result in pulmonary oedema and haemorrhage and similar effects may occur in other surfaces exposed to the air, particularly the conjunctiva where oedema and subconjunctival haemorrhage would be likely. This unfortunate accident is known amongst divers as a 'SQUEEZE', a very expressive term.

The damage caused by a squeeze is, of course, proportional to the distance through which the diver falls. In addition the outcome is profoundly affected by the depth at which the fall occurs. This may be illustrated by comparing two similar falls at different depths. A diver falling from 33 ft. to 66 ft. would be subjected to an increase in pressure from 2 atmospheres to 3 atmospheres. This would necessitate a decrease in the volume of air in the suit and respiratory system to $\frac{2}{3}$, i.e. a $33\frac{1}{3}\%$ reduction if the pressure equilibrium is to be maintained. Such a large change could not occur without gross crushing. If, however, the diver fell from 132 ft. to 165 ft., the same distance, the increase in pressure would be from 5 atmospheres to 6 atmospheres. This corresponds to a reduction in volume to $\frac{5}{6}$, which is only $16\frac{2}{3}\%$, i.e. half as much. It is highly probable that this reduction in volume could be accepted with little or no damage remembering of course that the volume at the start of each fall is the same. It follows therefore that, distance for distance, the nearer to the surface the fall occurs, the more dangerous is the squeeze.

PRESSURE DIFFERENCES IN 'SELF-CONTAINED' DIVING

The conditions just described are those of sudden increase or reduction in air pressure as they may occur in the standard diver. They have their counterparts in the self-contained diver though the picture and outcome is somewhat different. The same rules of distance and depth apply but the volume of air concerned is very much smaller. Suits, if worn, are close fitting and contain relatively little air, though contraction of this may cause bruising. The volumes to consider in these cases are those within the respiratory system and others which may be contained within the semi-rigid frame of goggles or a face mask.

Increase in Air Pressure (or whatever breathing mixture is used) is unlikely to present a problem for the self-contained diver whilst the set is in use. Only if it fails and must be abandoned does the danger occur as described below.

When a *Decrease in Pressure* occurs, as with an unconscious diver falling through water, the air in the respiratory system usually maintains

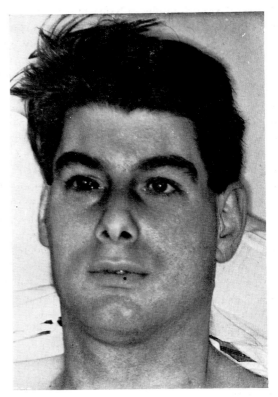

FIG. 19. An example of 'squeeze'

its pressure equilibrium by the action of the demand valve or the contraction of the air in the breathing bag. However, if the face-piece or goggles have a rigid frame to support the glass they cannot collapse on to the contours of the face. This results in the conjunctiva being exposed to a low pressure causing oedema and rupture of capillaries with subconjunctival haemorrhages and local bruising (Fig. 19).

6

BURST LUNG

This formidable sounding condition may be the result of gross distension of the lung following relative increase of intra-pulmonary pressure. On land this could only be achieved by active positive pressure inflation of the lungs. In water, however, if ascent is undertaken with the lungs full of air and release of this air is resisted then, as the surrounding pressures fall, the air, if it cannot expand, will remain at a pressure which as the ascent continues becomes increasingly higher than that of the tissues. This excess of air pressure over tissue pressure may steadily expand the lungs and chest until the former rupture allowing air to escape into the interstitial tissues, the pleural cavity or be drawn into the circulation. The results of this accident, burst lung, are technically described as PULMONARY BAROTRAUMA.

The common situation in which this may arise is when a man ascends through water holding his breath. This is particularly dangerous if at the commencement of the ascent the lung is full. In practice there are two situations in which the risk of Pulmonary Barotrauma may be present. The first is during training for submarine escape (or indeed in escaping from a sunken submarine should this rare event actually occur) where the trainees leave a pressurized air-lock after taking a full inspiration. They are, of course, taught to breathe out steadily and continuously whilst rising through the water, but very occasionally this is not done and for some reason or other the breath may be held. The second situation is one which may overtake the self-contained diver. Should he find for some reason or other that his breathing set is faulty, he may wish to abandon it and return to the surface without it. Details of these techniques and further reference to Burst Lung will be made in the chapter on 'Free Ascent'. (See Chapter XX.)

Essentially then the predisposing factors to 'burst lung' are breath holding with decrease in environmental pressure. It is while nearing the surface that the hazard increases for here the relative pressure volume changes are greatest.

The condition was first reported by Adams and Pollak (1932) who described a fatal accident during Submarine Escape Training in America. Since then many other observers have recorded similar incidents, fortunately by no means all fatal, both in submarine escape training and diving (Peirano, Alvis and Duffner, 1955). Lambert (1958) in an account of the former in this country, pointed out that 34,000 ascents had been made with only 12 cases of Pulmonary Barotrauma. This may seem a very small proportion, but so potentially dangerous is the condition that every effort must be made to eliminate it completely.

MECHANICS AND PATHOLOGY OF BURST LUNG

When air is trapped by breath holding or laryngeal spasm, the sequence of events, as the individual ascends through the water, is first that as the surrounding pressure falls the contained air will expand the lungs and chest to their fullest capacity. This expansion is brought about by pressure from within, which unlike normal inspiration will tend to displace blood from the pulmonary vascular bed and may expand the lungs to a greater extent than is reached in maximum inspiration. Lung tissue is stretched and breaks in the continuity of the alveolar membrane occur. Air may then leak into the pleural cavity or infiltrate the connective tissues of the mediastinum and superficial tissues of the neck to produce an interstitial emphysema. When the subject reaches the surface of the water he is able to resume normal respiration usually commencing with a profound exhalation. This release of compressed air results in a fall to normal of the intra-pulmonary pressure. The pulmonary circulation is restored and if, as frequently happens, some of the tears in lung tissue have involved pulmonary blood vessels, air, often in surprisingly large quantities, may be drawn into the pulmonary circulation. This passing to the left side of the heart will be distributed therefrom in the peripheral circulation. Such air may pass through the circulation in the form of bubbles—AIR EMBOLI (Figs. 20 and 21)— which may become lodged in smaller arterioles producing infarcts. The dangerous sites for these air emboli to lodge are the cerebral and coronary circulations, the former producing a wide variety of signs and symptoms of acute cerebral impairment, the latter heart failure (Miles and Wright, 1963).

There is little doubt that the lung damage is caused not by the direct effect of increased pressure but by over-distension and stretching. This is supported by the work of H. C. Wright who, using tracheotomized rabbits, showed that when subjected to decompression with the trachea clamped a much greater survival rate occurred if the chest and abdomen were firmly bound. Even an abdominal binder alone offered some degree of protection. (Malhotra and Wright, 1960 a and b.)

In an attempt to find just where the lung damage was occurring Wright carried out further investigations on fresh unchilled cadavers. He found that the intra-tracheal pressures required to produce trauma were 80 mm.Hg in an unbound corpse, 93 mm.Hg with an abdominal binder and from 133–190 mm.Hg in those where both chest and abdomen were bound. In the unbound body rupture of the visceral pleura occurred where basal pleural adhesions were present and in the remainder pulmonary interstitial emphysema occurred. (Malhotra and Wright, 1960 c.)

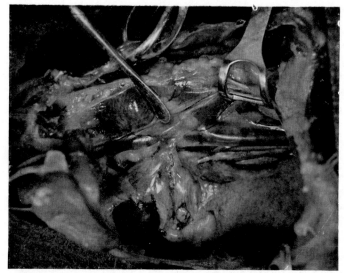

Fig. 20.

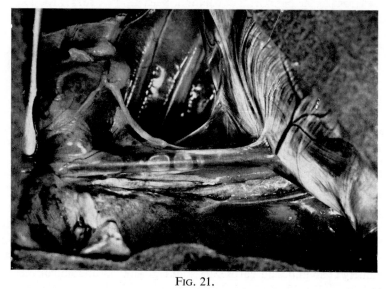

Fig. 21.

Examples of 'air embolism'

Further support for the belief that it is stretching rather than excess pressure which causes the lung damage comes from the well-established fact that very high intra-pulmonary pressures, such as those which occur in violent coughing, can be tolerated without harm. In such instances there is marked muscular resistance to over-expansion. In addition the weakness of the Hering-Breuer reflex in man may be a further factor in permitting over-expansion without muscular resistance.

So far only those cases where the obstruction to the free escape of air is at the larynx have been considered. Theoretically it is possible that an obstruction in one of the smaller branches of the bronchial tree may trap air beyond the obstruction so that a small volume only of lung may be involved. Such an isolated volume of trapped air would be most likely to rupture since if the remaining lung was venting freely the expansion of the trapped volume would be virtually unimpeded. One such case where obstruction was found due to calcified gland having eroded into and blocked a bronchus is mentioned in Lambert's paper (1958). Evidence, however, on the true mechanics of many of the cases is very sparse and there is an urgent need for more information, especially with regard to local intra-pulmonary obstruction which potential danger no amount of training in free ascent technique will remove. Similarly, structural weaknesses in the lung such as emphysematous bullae may well be a predisposing factor.

THE CLINICAL PICTURE

The three syndromes which pulmonary barotrauma may present are PNEUMOTHORAX, INTERSTITIAL EMPHYSEMA and AIR EMBOLISM. Usually only one of the three is present but mixed syndromes may occur. Malhotra and Wright (1960 b) in their animal experiments found greater quantities of air in the circulation when interstitial emphysema was present than with pneumothorax.

Of the three presentations Air Embolism is far and away the most important demanding immediate action if life is to be saved. No time can therefore be wasted in elaborate examination and treatment usually commences before the diagnosis is confirmed.

The clinical picture of air embolism depends upon the final resting place of the offending bubble and this must largely be one of pure chance. The most serious sign is that of loss of consciousness immediately on reaching the surface or soon after. Convulsions have occurred, spastic or flaccid paralysis and visual changes are quite common while less dramatic symptoms such as vertigo and limb tingling may be the only signs. The rule must be that after free ascent any abnormality, however trivial, without an immediate and simple explanation must be attributed to an air embolism. The treatment routine must be introduced immediately and maintained until a diagnosis is established.

Pneumothorax and Interstitial Emphysema may cause the sufferer, when he leaves the water, to complain of pain in the chest or abdomen. A cough is also commonly present very often accompanied by a nose bleed or small haemoptysis. Again no time is available for a complete diagnosis for here again is a man who has just completed a free ascent and shows some abnormality. It may look like a pneumothorax or interstitial emphysema but to produce this there is a burst lung and air may be in the circulation also. Treatment for this possibility must be started at once. There will be ample time and opportunity to establish the diagnosis while treatment is going on.

In thirty cases of pulmonary barotrauma the presenting signs or symptoms were:

Unconsciousness	—	16
Pain in the chest	—	13
Weakness and paralysis	—	13
Disorientation	—	9
Cough	—	6
Visual impairment	—	4
Convulsions	—	3
Breathlessness	—	2
Cyanosis	—	2

TREATMENT

Wherever possible the facilities for treatment should be immediately to hand. Under no circumstances should men undergo practical free ascent training either for submarine escape or for surfacing after abandoning a breathing set unless these facilities are available.

Fortunately, though any form of embolism is a dangerous event, the air embolism is the most easily resolved. Being air it will respond to pressure and immediate compression of the patient will cause the embolism to shrink until it may slip past its point of obstruction and even through the capillary network or, if it remains an embolism, be so small as to produce a negligible infarct. Furthermore the increase in pressure will cause much of it to dissolve in the blood. Adequate treatment therefore needs a pressure chamber situated near the point where the men surface. In practice it has been found that a chamber within a few minutes of the water is unsatisfactory. The patient must be under pressure within seconds. Once inside the chamber pressure is rapidly applied until the patient's symptoms disappear or he reaches a pressure of 6 atmospheres absolute. As soon as possible a doctor is also 'locked' into the chamber and should be able to make a diagnosis upon which will depend subsequent treatment.

For an air embolism prolonged and slow decompression may be needed in order that the bubble shall not form again. Schedules for these accidents have been established and are published as 'Therapeutic Decompression' Tables. A severe case may take as long as 38 hours to decompress safely. Having dealt with the emergency of burst lung by immediate recompression and having diagnosed an air embolism subsequent procedure follows the same lines as the treatment of a severe case of Decompression Sickness and reference to Chapter XI should be made for details of the various methods. On completion of the decompression it is wise to admit the patient to hospital for full medical examination and observation. An electro-encephalograph taken immediately on admission may give an indication of a focal intra-cranial lesion.

When a pneumothorax or interstitial emphysema is found subsequent treatment may be different. The interstitial emphysema is usually retrosternal and may by virtue of this position become an embarrassment. When decompression is commenced the gas trapped in the pleural cavity or connective tissue may expand once more to produce pain, respiratory distress and cardiac embarrassment. Absorption of air from these sites is slow and other means for its removal must be adopted. A slow 'bleed off' of pressure may be more satisfactory than reduction by stages but most effective when practical is to remove the air directly from the patient. In the case of a pneumothorax a cannula may be introduced into the pleural cavity from where the expanding air can freely escape. The lung of course is likely to remain collapsed and subsequent hospital treatment is necessary. Oxygen should be available for use if there is cyanosis but this is unlikely where air pressure is increased.

With the retro-sternal emphysema removal of the air is more difficult. With patience and prolonged decompression success may be achieved without surgical interference. However if the reduction of pressure involves expansion of air in the retro-sternal area with pressure on and embarrassment of the mediastinal contents it may be necessary to free the trapped air. Extreme care is needed to avoid damage to vital structures and a slightly curved very blunt cannula should be used.

In the treatment of an uncomplicated pneumothorax or interstitial emphysema the immediate compression is unnecessary but unfortunately there is never time to ascertain that this is so and full emergency treatment must be given in all cases.

Quite a few will turn out to be false alarms or hysteria. When this happens and the possibility of embolism has been ruled out a relatively rapid decompression routine may be used depending on the equivalent depth reached and the time involved. It could in fact be treated as a simple dive and decompressed accordingly.

There is some justification for saying that no two cases of 'burst lung' are alike. Consequently it is not easy to give firm advice to those responsible for their care. Much is to be gained however from practical experience when it will become possible to give a good assessment of damage and in some cases take short cuts in decompression treatment. For the inexperienced however a strict adherence to the instructions in the Therapeutic Decompression Tables is essential. The physician examining the patient in the chamber is working under difficulties. As well as the general noise and cramped position there is the added complication that under pressure the sounds of percussion and auscultation are considerably altered and only gross abnormalities can be detected by these means.

The above methods can only be used for accidents which happen during organized training, when the full facilities are present. Where, in the sea or inland water, a diver surfaces having abandoned a faulty set, and showing evidence of a burst lung, his treatment is a very difficult problem. If circumstances permit he could be put into a diving suit or given a breathing apparatus and with a companion be lowered down into the water again for recompression. Failing this pneumothorax and Interstitial Emphysema may be treated along conventional lines, e.g. rest, evacuation of air and oxygen if necessary. The danger of an air embolism must be considered and if immediate recompression is not available treatment must be aimed at keeping the air bubble away from such vital areas as the cerebral and coronary circulations. Air in fluid will of course rise and the bubbles in the blood-stream are no exception. Thus the body should be positioned so that any bubbles will rise away from the danger areas. The position of choice is between the prone and left lateral and with the body sloping so that the head is kept low. In this position the chances of the bubble missing the cerebral and coronary circulations are most favourable. This practice should also, as far as possible, be adopted when treatment is being carried out in a pressure chamber.

The patient should also be kept at rest and sedatives may help. Having started postural treatment in the absence of a pressure chamber the decision has then to be made whether or not the patient should be transferred to the nearest chamber. If there is reason to suspect that there is air in the circulation then without doubt the patient should be taken to a chamber if this can be accomplished without undue distress. Having got the patient there his condition can be reviewed, usually in consultation with experts, and even if he is not compressed it is comforting to know that the facility is on hand if things take a turn for the worse. If air transport is used low flying or a fully pressurized cabin is necessary to avoid any further bubble expansion or formation.

For large organizations where many divers are employed the possibility of having mobile pressure chambers should be studied. Indeed some already exist. It would of course be greatly preferable if in a 'burst lung' accident the chamber could be brought to the man. This may one day be possible if underwater activity grows and the ultimate service may well be one where a collapsible fabric chamber is quickly transported by helicopter.

As has been said, even with free ascent from an abandoned breathing apparatus, 'burst lung' is a very rare accident. This rarity, even though the condition is extremely dangerous, makes the introduction of any general emergency treatment service at the present day uneconomical and quite out of the question. All that can be recommended is for users of underwater breathing apparatus to become familiar with the technique of free ascent and for them and their colleagues to know what recompression facilities are available in their locality.

PREVENTION OF BURST LUNG

In brief, for this will be fully considered in Chapter XX, the best safeguard is to have had proper training so that panic may be avoided and the ascent made with the mouth and larynx completely relaxed and open allowing the expanding air to escape unhindered in a prolonged expiration to avoid lung distension.

A further safeguard is to eliminate from underwater activity all those who have clinical or radiological evidence of lung pathology, e.g. cysts, adhesions or emphysema.

PRESSURE CHANGES AND THE EARS

As well as the respiratory system other spaces must be considered and meriting second place is the middle ear. The air in the middle ear is normally separated by the tympanic membrane or ear drum from the air in the external auditory meatus and by the closed Eustachian tube from that in the naso-pharynx. The Eustachian tube is only lightly closed and usually opens during the act of swallowing. Its function is to allow air in or out of the middle ear to maintain an equal pressure on each side of the drum as may be necessitated by changes in barometric pressure. In the healthy individual the opening of the tube during swallowing is quite sufficient to maintain the necessary adjustment to small changes without conscious awareness. In a number of persons,

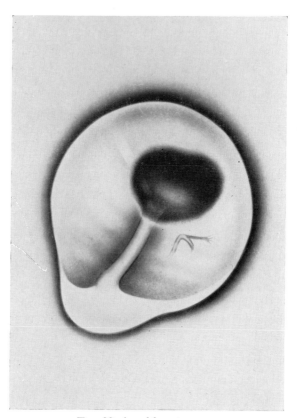

FIG. 22. Aural barotrauma

however, the Eustachian tube does not open freely and when external pressure rises it will not admit air from the naso-pharynx to provide an appropriate rise in pressure in the middle ear. If the pressure rise continues an inward bulging of the drum occurs with stretching, pain, haemorrhage and ultimately perforation (Fig. 22). There must be few people who have not at some time sensed discomfort in the ears during a steep descent from a high mountain or the landing of an aeroplane.

In diving the steeper pressure gradients make the problem much more acute.

In most cases the difficulty in equalizing the pressure results from a catarrh of the Eustachian tube which may be temporary, as during a common cold, or more or less permanent as with a chronic respiratory catarrh. When passing through an environment of increasing atmospheric pressure the repeated adjustments of middle ear pressure are noticed as a change in tone of general background noise and an improvement in hearing and comfort. If the Eustachian tube fails to 'clear' readily discomfort and pain may occur. The clearing of the tube can, however, be assisted by various active manœuvres. Of these swallowing is the simplest and it is to increase natural swallowing that boiled sweets are often issued to air liner passengers prior to landing. If this fails more violent action may be needed such as holding the nose and swallowing, rotatory movements of the jaw with the mouth wide open, or, with nose and mouth closed, increasing the intra-naso-pharyngeal pressure. This is usually successful but has always the danger of forcing infected material up the Eustachian tube towards the middle ear.

Underwater descent of a few feet will cause acute discomfort in an ear which is not 'clearing'. Inability to clear the ears makes all forms of diving intolerable and continued descent results in the inward bulging of the drum, tearing of capillaries with stretching and acute pain which would only be relieved by perforation. In ears of men who have made repeated attempts to dive but failed to clear the ears it is not unusual to see evidence of this in an inflamed drum behind which is haemorrhage into the middle ear. The acute pain is usually sufficient to prevent the diver going deep enough to produce perforation but this has happened in emergency pressurizations as in the case of an attendant accompanying a burst lung casualty during emergency treatment. The procedure would not be stopped for a painful ear but the speed of compression would very quickly translate the pain of the bulging drum into the comparative relief of a perforation. On the other hand the unconscious victim in such a case might well escape ear damage for it is generally found that the ears of an unconscious person clear readily under pressure.

Examples given have been those where the external pressure is increasing above that in the middle ear. When the opposite is happening, i.e. when the external pressure is falling below that of the middle ear as when a diver ascends, there is usually no difficulty in the expanding air of the middle ear escaping into the naso-pharynx to maintain pressure balance. The Eustachian tube stoppage when it does occur is usually one against entering air.

It is a wise precaution that anyone proposing a dip under water should first make sure that both Eustachian tubes will clear freely with pressure changes. Beginners quite often have considerable trouble in doing this but with time and experience the process can be relegated to the subconscious when the pressures either side the drum will be equalized at frequent intervals, almost continuously. This ensures the drum freedom from damage and is much more satisfactory than periodic forceful blow-throughs. In the winter when colds and catarrhal conditions are prevalent there is much more time spent 'off diving due to ears' than at other times of the year. But some help may be obtained from intranasal decongestant drops or sprays.

REVERSED EARS

If an underwater swimmer dives with a tight fitting rubber hood or cap, air may be trapped in the external auditory meatus. As water pressure rises the hood is pressed firm against the ear until the contained air volume can shrink no further. Meanwhile as environmental pressure increases so will that of the tissues and the air in the respiratory tract. If the Eustachian tube opens this pressure will be passed to the middle ear. The resulting situation will be one in which the air pressure in the

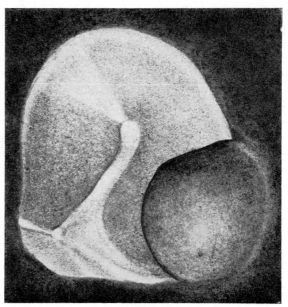

FIG. 23. 'Reversed ear'

outer ear is becoming increasingly lower than that of the surrounding tissues and middle ear. It is in fact equivalent to attaching a suction pump to the outer ear. There will of course be outward bulging of the drum but Jarrett (1961) has shown that the common presenting sign is oedematous swelling of the lining of the meatus with blebs and large haemorrhagic blisters. Pain is not a prominent feature. (Fig. 23.)

In the rare event of this external plugging occurring with a Eustachian tube which failed to open in spite of increased pharyngeal pressure there would be a low pressure in both middle and external ear relative to surrounding tissues. The drum would not move but in addition to the suction effects in the meatus a similar action would be occurring in the middle ear with oedema and haemorrhage.

This condition of 'Reversed Ears' should not occur in practice if care is taken always to ensure that there is no barrier to pressure equalization between the external ear and the surrounding water or if an overall hood is worn with connection between the ear and the naso-pharynx.

ALTERNOBARIC VERTIGO

This rather formidable condition was first described by Lundgren (1965) as a diving hazard following a questionnaire sent to 550 Swedish divers. Twenty-six per cent of them had, at one time or another, experienced vertigo or dizziness. Coles and Knight (1961) questioned 61 Naval Divers of whom 14 had dizziness underwater. They believed that some link might exist between this and difficulty in clearing the ears. Of this group thirty were questioned but only three experienced any dizziness when clearing their ears on land.

Further interest was aroused by a press report (Evening Post, Jersey, 20th October, 1964) of a civilian underwater swimmer who pleaded 'not guilty' to charges of dangerous driving on the grounds that his co-ordination had been impaired by his diving. An expert witness stated that it would be very difficult to discount diving as a contributory factor to this accident. As a result the man was acquitted but the Magistrate indicated that 'the same defence could not hold good in future and where a person was not fit to drive due to something he had inflicted upon himself he was not generally absolved from liability but as this was the first case of its kind in a British Court the accused could not have been expected to know the risk he was taking in driving a car immediately after underwater swimming'. It would thus appear that the common charge for those in trouble with their cars and the police might even be 'he was under the influence of drink, drugs or diving'.

This was followed up by an inquiry amongst British and Rhodesian divers organized by the magazine 'Triton' (January, 1965). In the majority of cases there seemed to be some slight association between the attacks of dizziness and difficulty in clearing the ears, or the presence of an upper respiratory tract infection. It also appeared more common in the more adventurous diver and some of the individual reports were quite frightening, one man being so dizzy during his ascent that he actually found himself returning to the bottom head first.

The wave of interest in dizziness has in recent years subsided. This may be due to better training and a realization that the condition exists and may be dangerous. It cannot however be lightly dismissed. It is worthy of further serious investigation.

PRESSURE AND THE SINUSES

The air-filled sinuses of the cranium are normally connected by channels to the naso-pharynx. This enables a pressure equilibrium to be established and maintained between them and the rest of the respiratory system. When one of these channels becomes blocked as in an attack of sinusitis air cannot pass in or out. If the sufferer attempts to dive, or undergo pressure increase in any way, the pressure of the surrounding tissues will exceed the pressure within the sinus, its lining will swell and haemorrhage may occur. This event is usually sufficiently painful to cause the individual to abandon the dive forthwith. Polyps too may give trouble. In a diver going down a nasal polyp may be pressed against the entrance to the maxillary antrum blocking it and giving pain. Coming up a polyp in the antrum may do the same from the other side.

The rule must be that any person suffering from sinusitis or polyps must not dive or go under pressure.

PRESSURE AND BAD TEETH

Round the roots of various teeth may be found small pockets of gas resulting from fermentation. These being isolated would during compression shrink and the space they occupied possibly fill with blood and tissue fluid. On surfacing the bubble would expand again and with its erstwhile space occupied with fluid a local increase in pressure would be set up. The result—pressure on the nerve and—ouch! The moral—don't dive with decaying teeth!

INTESTINAL GASES

Generally speaking the volume of the gaseous content of the visceras is decreased by the pressure of the dive and returns to the same volume on decompression or surfacing.

However, there are many occasions when fermentation will continue while the diver is working to produce additional gas. This, when he surfaces, will produce abdominal distension, discomfort and embarrassing flatulence. Meals taken under pressure in a chamber have produced so much distension on decompression as to cause syncope.

The inexperienced or anxious diver may, whilst descending or working under water, swallow air, sometimes in copious amounts. On surfacing this swallowed air expands producing extreme discomfort and inconvenience.

Once this possibility is appreciated it is less likely to be really troublesome. Intelligent restriction of diet before entering the water is a good insurance against subsequent inflation and good training and the achievement of confidence and poise under water will lessen the risk of air swallowing.

PRESSURE AND CLOTHING

Though clothing will be discussed with equipment there is one pressure effect which is important. In ensuring that the underwater swimmer is kept warm whilst operating, insulating garments are usually provided. These generally depend on pockets of trapped air for insulation as is the case with foam-rubber. The effect of depth and pressure is to reduce the volume of the cells and increase the density thus greatly diminishing the insulating property. A suit which would keep a swimmer warm on the surface might well be useless at depth. This simple fact must be considered when underwater suits are being designed or chosen. The shrinking of air pockets in an undergarment may result in a deep impression of the garment on the skin.

THE PARALLEL IN AVIATION MEDICINE

It is intended to do no more than remind the reader that in Aviation Medicine a parallel pressure problem exists, the difference being that the directions are reversed, decrease in pressure first then increase on return to ground level. Respiratory and ear problems are present and the aviator who leaves the ground after large quantities of champagne will know the meaning of abdominal distension when the environmental pressure is reduced.

In many ways common ground must be studied, as for example with decompression sickness, a hazard of both fields.

In apparatus design, in pressure breathing and oxygen problems there is even closer co-operation but when a plane crashes in the sea the techniques for saving the pilot call upon the resources of both aviation and underwater medicine.

EFFECT ON TISSUES OF VERY HIGH PRESSURES

Earlier in this chapter, and also in Chapter II, the impression has been given that provided the gas pressures in the body cavities can be equalized with the pressure of the immediate environment the body tissues themselves are unaffected by increase in hydrostatic pressure. This has been universally accepted in diving practice, certainly with regard to the depth in which man is likely to operate in the forseeable future.

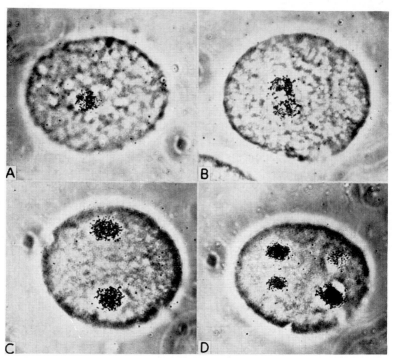

Fig. 24. Autoradiographs of *Arbacia* eggs which were immersed in ^{3}H thymidine (a precursor of DNA) for 60 min., starting at metaphase.

A and B, eggs were given 5,000 lbs/ in ^{2}pressure (20°c) at the beginning of the ^{3}H-thymidine incubation, two autoradiographic patterns are shown. In A, the grains are situated in one mass; in B, the chromosomes separated, and the grains separated into two groups. C and D, Control eggs were also treated with ^{3}H thymidine for 60 min. but were kept at *atmospheric pressure*. In C, both nuclei are labelled, and in D, a more advanced cell, all four nuclei exhibited incorporation. These photomicrographs illustrate that cells can synthesize DNA under pressures of 5,000 lbs/in^2.

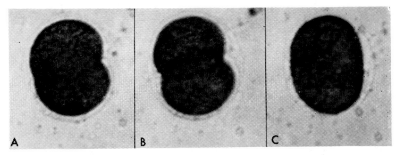

Fig. 25. Effects of pressure on a dividing marine egg (*Arbacia*). The cell was photographed through the windows of a pressure chamber with the use of a specially designed microscope. In A, at atmospheric pressure the egg is just starting to divide. B, is a photomicrograph of the cell at 6,000 lbs/in² of hydrostatic pressure for a duration of 1·75 minutes. The same egg is shown in C after 9 minutes of compression. Note that the furrow has completely aborted.

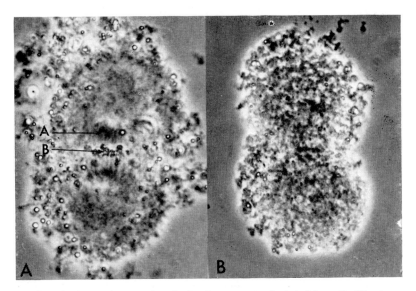

Fig. 26. Photomicrographs of mitotic apparatus isolated from fertilized sea urchin eggs (*Arbacia*).
(A) Control mitotic apparatus shows linearly oriented mitotic spindles (A) and chromosomes aligned along the metaphase plate (B).
(B) A representable mitotic apparatus which was isolated from a fertilized egg at metaphase which was subjected to 10,000 p.s.i. for a duration of one minute. This photomicrograph shows loss of linear and radial organization in the spindle and aster region.

At a recent underwater conference in Kiel however, Professor Zimmerman, a Zoologist at the University of Toronto, reported changes that had appeared in preparations of living cells subjected for short periods to very high degrees of hydrostatic pressure. Small stainless steel chambers were used in which a thermostatically controlled temperature 20°C. was maintained during exposure to pressures ranging from 2,000 to 10,000 p.s.i. The pressure could be built up in under 2 seconds and released instantaneously. Relatively short exposures were used.

In his earlier experiments Zimmerman (1963) studied the effect of very high pressure on the synthesis of D.N.A. in living sea urchin eggs and found by autoradiographic studies that in fact the synthesis is interrupted at certain stages as was incorporation of 3H-thymidine into D.N.A. from a solution containing it. Exposure varied from 15–60 minutes to be effective according to the stage of fertilization of the eggs. A casual reference to a 'biological clock' at molecular level being slowed by the pressure is a fascinating claim.

In later papers with other workers (Zimmerman and Marsland 1964 and Zimmerman and Silberman, 1965 and 1967) similar results were obtained with the marine eggs. Very high pressure was shown to produce a drastic disorganization in the dividing cells though recovery seems possible (Figures 24, 25 and 26).

These exciting experiments may seem far away from the practical problems of diving medicine and highly academic. Nevertheless if hydrostatic pressures of 2,000 to 10,000 p.s.i. can affect the internal chemical process or reproductive activities in living cells the possible significance of this as far as man is concerned must not be overlooked.

These pressures do however represent colossal depths of 4,500 ft. to 22,000 ft. They do nevertheless exist and moreover the exposures involved have only been minutes. Man is already approaching the 1,000 ft. region and may in time be exposed for hours. At the moment he would appear safe from these effects. They must not be forgotten as they may become significant and perhaps even lend scientific support to the 'old wives tales' that too much diving may adversely affect a man's virility or that divers wives tend to produce an excess of girl children. Thank you Professor Zimmerman for drawing the attention of underwater physiologists to this biological effect of their environment. Its potential influence on human tissues will be watched.

READING AND REFERENCES

Adams, B. H. and I. B. Pollak (1932). 'Traumatic Air Embolism in Submarine Escape Training'. *U.S. Navy Med. Bull.* 30, 165.

Coles, R. R. A. and J. J. Knight (1961). 'Aural and Audiometric Survey of Qualified Divers and Submarine Escape Training Tank Instructors'. M.R.C. Report R.N.P. 61–1011.

Jarrett, A. S. (1961). 'Ear Injuries in Divers'. *J.R.N. Med. Service.* 47, No. 1.

Lambert, R. W. J. (1958). 'Submarine Escape'. *Proc. Roy. Soc. Med. 51,* 824.

Lundgren, C. (1965). 'Alternobaric Vertigo—a Diving Hazard'. *Brit. Med. J. 2,* 511.

Malhotra, M. S., and H. C. Wright (1960a). 'Air Embolism during Decompression Underwater and its Prevention'. *J. Physiol.* 151, 32P.

—(1960b). 'Air Embolism during Decompression and its Prevention'. *M.R.C. (R.N.P.R.C.) Report U.P.S.* 188.

—(1960c). 'The Effect of a Raised Intrapulmonary on the Lungs of Fresh Unchilled Bound and Unbound Cadavers'. *M.R.C. (R.N.P.R.C.) Report U.P.S.* 189.

Miles, S. and H. C. Wright (1963). 'Pulmonary Barotrauma' Modern Medicine, May, 1963, p. 359.

Peirano, J. H., H. J. Alvis and G. J. Duffner (1955). 'Submarine Escape Training Experience'. *M.R.L. Report* 264, U.S. Navy Dept.

Silverman, L. G., Lee, A. R. Yancy, L. Amory, L. G. Barney and R. C. Lee (1945). 'Fundamental Factors in the Design of Protective Respiratory Equipment'. *O.S.R.D. Report No.* 5339, U.S.A.

Zimmerman, A. M. (1963). 'Incorporation of 3H–Thymidine in the Eggs of Arbacia Punctulata'. *Expt. Cell Research 31,* 39.

Zimmerman, A. M. and D. Marsland (1964). 'Cell Divisions—Effects of Pressure on the Mitotic Mechanisms of Marine Eggs'. *Expt. Cell Research 35,* 293.

Zimmerman, A. M. and L. Silberman (1965). 'Cell Division—The Effects of Hydrostatic Pressure on the Cleavage Schedule in Arbacia Punctulata. *Expt. Cell Research 38,* 454.

—(1967). 'Studies on Incorporation of 3H–Thymidine in Arbacia Eggs under Hydrostatic Pressure'. *Expt. Cell Research 46,* 469.

CHAPTER VI

The Problem of Density

THERE are many ways in which the effect of increasing air density on the comfort and efficiency of a man working under water may be demonstrated but perhaps the most expressive description comes from an experienced diver who, following a period of fairly heavy work on a wreck, was asked what the breathing was like.

'You don't breathe,' he said, 'you have to suck air in and then you have to blow it out again.'

Many of the phenomena of increased density can be observed in a pressure chamber as increasing depth is simulated. One of the first of these is the character of the voice which is greatly altered. Whistling, too, becomes impossible. To what extent these voice changes are due to increased density is not yet clear for no measurable relation between voice change and density has been established and it is known that the pressure of a gas does not influence the rate at which sound passes through it. Voice production involves far more than air passing over the vocal cords and changes in density may well alter resonance and articulation.

A more positive indication of the increasing density is found, if whilst under pressure a sheet of paper is wafted fanwise. The increased resistance to the paper's movement can actually be felt. It would take a very warped mind to imagine falling rose petals in a pressure chamber but could such a situation be pictured at a depth of say 100 ft. or more, without a doubt those petals would fall to the ground more slowly and more gently than ever before. Even hardened divers playing a quick game of solo whilst doing a 'pot dip' find the cards which they eagerly fling on the table seem to land with an air of nonchalance.

Sitting in the chamber under high pressure, playing a quiet game of cards, trying to whistle or wafting sheets of paper may not bring home the true significance of increased density. The individual who really does know what it is all about is the common house fly who might have the misfortune to be caught up in the experiment. The behaviour of the fly is quite instructive and level flight seems impossible. A quick buzz of the wings on the thick air and up he goes, again and again the same, bobbing along like 'spring heel jack' unable to adapt to the new environment and maintain level flight.

The limiting effects of increased density can be well shown by changes which take place in the Maximum Breathing Capacity. Cotes (1954) measured this in groups of men at simulated altitudes of 10,000, 17,000 and 27,000 feet and showed increases above sea-level value of 12%, 24% and 36% respectively. As this effect had been attributed to a decrease in density it seemed appropriate to repeat the experiment with increasing density. A simple low resistance apparatus designed by C. B. McKerrow (1953) was used to measure the maximum breathing capacity of men in a pressure chamber at pressures of 2, 3 and 4 atmospheres. In this series the sea-level maximum breathing capacities were decreased

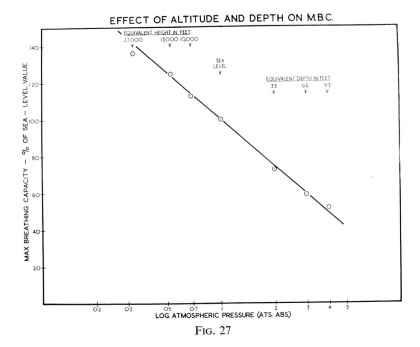

FIG. 27

by 28%, 40% and 49% respectively, which in fact means that the maximum breathing capacity of a man in compressed air at an equivalent depth of 99 ft. is halved.

If the results of these two quite independent trials are taken together and the maximum breathing capacities at altitude and depth plotted against absolute atmospheric pressure they follow the same curve (Fig. 27).

In this figure a logarithmic scale was used for the atmospheric pressure to represent the fact that changes in density for equivalent depth are greater near the surface and decrease with depth. Extension of this line however would suggest that at 12 atmospheres (363 ft.) the M.B.C.

would be zero. Although undoubtedly a depth can be reached where the air is so dense that the work done by the muscles of respiration demands more oxygen than the air they move can supply this is known to be much deeper. The logarithmic scale is therefore not really satisfactory.

In a further series of experiments, measurements of the maximum breathing capacity were carried out at equivalent depths of 33, 66, 99, 150 and 200 ft. A curve showing the mean relationship between M.B.C. and depth is shown in Figure 28.

It is not easy to apply a simple formula to such a complicated system of forces, masses and movement as occurs in the respiratory system

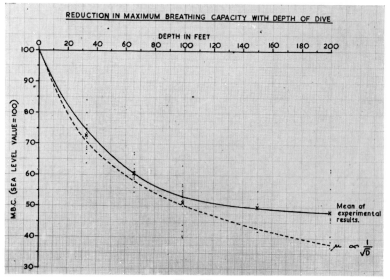

FIG. 28

during a breathing cycle. It may however be assumed that during the M.B.C. measurements the flow of air is entirely turbulent and density therefore the important factor.

A well-known formula is

$$P = \tfrac{1}{2}mv^2$$

where P is the force, required to move mass 'm' with velocity 'v'. If P is the work done in breathing and represents a maximum effort throughout it may be taken as constant whence—

$$v \propto \frac{1}{\sqrt{m}}$$

The volume of air moved, other things being equal is dependent on the velocity and the mass in unit volume is directly proportional to density thus.

$$MBC \propto \frac{1}{\sqrt{D}} \text{ where } D = \text{density.}$$

If such a relationship is plotted on the same graph (Fig. 28) a quite similar curve is obtained.

That the experimental curve shows a lesser reduction in M.B.C. is difficult to explain especially in view of the fact that the resistance of the recording apparatus, though negligible at the surface, was found to be 5 cm. H_2O at 100 ft. for a flow rate of 100 litres per minute. With the decreased ventilatory volume however the inspiratory and expiratory excursions would be much less under which conditions the respiratory muscles and chest elasticity would be relatively more efficient.

Whether or not such a simple mathematical application is justified for so complicated a system, it is however most convenient in practice. The assumption that respiratory volume, for the same muscular effort, varies with the inverse of the square root of the density is a useful guide in assessing the effect on respiratory efficiency of, not only depth alone, but depth in conjunction with various forms of breathing apparatus and mixtures of gases other than air.

DENSITY AND DEEP DIVING

An example of the use of such a curve is shown in Figure 29. This shows that air, if breathed at 600 ft., would produce a very considerable reduction in breathing capacity of 75% even with no breathing apparatus, i.e. the maximum breathing capacity for air at this depth would be 30 litres per minute which could be sustained for but a few seconds only. The maximum working volume would be much nearer half this amount allowing very little active work. Breathing then would be a serious embarrassment. A diver who actually achieved this depth used a mixture of 8% oxygen in helium which only reduced the breathing capacity by 60% which is equivalent to breathing air at about 150 ft., which is within the diver's comfort range for moderate exercise.

Helium, being about $\frac{1}{7}$ the density of nitrogen, can be used to great advantage as an alternative diluent of oxygen in deep diving. With it density is no problem in the depths so far reached but if ever man considers diving to 1,000 ft. or even deeper, the question of the increased density will need reconsideration. At 1,000 ft. the pressure would be about 31 atmospheres and here of course the oxygen content could be still further reduced. Even a percentage of 0·75 oxygen would give a more than adequate partial pressure of 177 mm.Hg. Such a mixture of

0·75% oxygen in helium would have a density of approximately $\frac{1}{7}$ that of air which even at this depth could be breathed with ease. However a very much lighter mixture could be obtained if the oxygen was diluted with hydrogen. A mixture of 0·75% oxygen in hydrogen would have a density of approximately $\frac{1}{14}$ that of air. This mixture at 1,000 ft. would be breathed as easily as air at about 40 ft. and might well be the mixture of choice if such depths were ever contemplated.

It has been said that in producing the artificial atmosphere for the man under water every effort must be made to ensure that all the variables present are kept within their normal surface limits. This is of

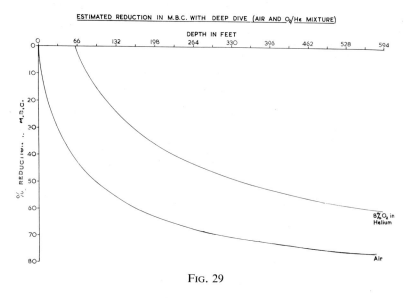

FIG. 29

course not always possible to achieve but at least the ranges should be limited to those in which the body will function without loss of efficiency and without prejudice to safety and health.

Density is one factor which must be regarded in such a light. As density increases with depth, when air is breathed, so does efficiency lessen and if this is unavoidable the work rate must be reduced. At atmospheric pressure in a healthy individual muscular effort is limited by cardiac output. No physical activity can be great enough to need a respiratory minute volume anything like the maximum breathing capacity. Work rates of 1660 Kg. metres per minute on a bicycle ergometer needing 3500 ml/min. oxygen have been described by Silverman and his co-workers (1951) which would presumably require a minute volume of at least 70 litres. To attempt such work under pressure would result in great distress. At an equivalent depth of 100 ft. this ventilatory requirement would be almost equivalent to the maximum breathing capacity. A situation would therefore arise where a task which was within the capacity of the individual's muscles and cardiac output could not be performed because of an inability to achieve adequate ventilation. Breathing capacity now becomes the limiting factor to muscular effort, a situation foreign to the healthy individual. Under such circumstances an accustomed task may be accompanied by unaccustomed respiratory embarrassment. The inexperienced diver may find this respiratory distress alarming and his anxiety may lead to hyperventilation when he has given up his work, with its attendant disturbances and sometimes dangerous results.

It is absolutely essential to accept, when breathing air or mixtures of increased density, the restriction which is placed on physical effort. To work flat out in the face of respiratory discomfort is foolish and may be dangerous. Knowing the restriction exists will remove the risk of finding the breathing difficulty alarming. Experience will enable the diver to set a work rate well within the limits of his respiratory comfort zone.

DENSITY AND SHALLOW DIVING

It has been seen that as far as the deep diver is concerned considerable depth can be reached without density being a serious problem but it must be remembered that the diver with a rigid helmet is supplied with air or mixture at the correct pressure surrounding his head and there is no resistance problem other than that of his own respiratory system. With self-contained diving where he may have to breathe through a mouth-piece, tubes, valves, or even a carbon dioxide absorbing canister, these will produce additional resistance.

As depth adds to personal resistance so it will increase any additional resistance of the breathing apparatus. It therefore becomes essential to construct apparatus to have the minimum resistance. This may be largely achieved by using wide smooth bored tubing, carefully designed low-resistance valves and optimal shape, volume and granule size in absorbing canisters. The end result must however be a compromise for consideration must also be given to robustness, bulk and absorbing efficiency. If an open face mask is used which is continually supplied with a free flowing gas mixture external resistance can be almost completely removed but such a system would be most wasteful and unacceptable from an economic and endurance point of view. A valve which has no resistance has not yet been designed but in some closed circuit sets

4*

valves may be dispensed with provided a carbon dioxide absorbing canister is used but this of course has its own resistance.

To measure resistance at atmospheric pressure is comparatively easy. Personal resistance will vary from one individual to another but a convenient working figure is one of 4 cm. water, per litre flow per second. One of the earlier underwater air breathing sets had a resistance at the surface also of 4 cm. H_2O/1./sec. giving an overall resistance when in use at atmospheric pressure of 8 cm. H_2O/1./sec.

To estimate the working resistance of man with apparatus at depth a simple formula may be used. Whereas the volume of air moved was

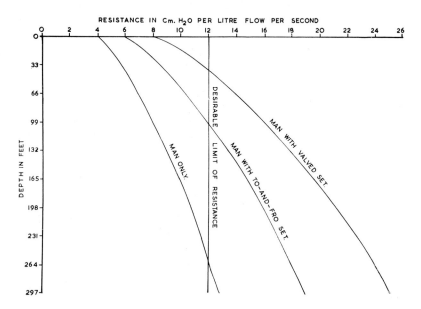

FIG. 30. Resistance to breathing at depth

proportional to the inverse of the square root of the density, the resistance, other things being equal may be taken as proportional to the square root of the density.

$$R \propto \sqrt{D}$$

It must be remembered that this is a practical guide and not an accurate mathematical formula. The application is well seen in Figure 30, which compares resistance in cm. H_2O per litre flow per second with depth in feet. The surface density is taken as unity in which case it will be 2 at 33 ft., 3 at 66 ft., and so on.

The left-hand curve represents the resistance for man's respiratory system alone, and that on the right the combined resistance of man and the breathing set with valves which has the same resistance as man at the surface. Between them is the curve for a closed circuit to and fro breathing set with a canister and no valves. It will be observed that all the resistances increase with depth.

It is necessary for convenience to establish some acceptable limit for total resistance. The ideal would be one below which activity could be carried on without any loss of efficiency. No two physiologists will agree just what this limit should be and it will of course vary to some extent from one person to another.

Silverman and his colleagues (1951) have extensively studied the resistances of breathing apparatus at atmospheric pressure and Mead (1955) has investigated the problem under increased pressure. From the results of these and other workers it would seem reasonable to accept a figure of 12 cm. H_2O per litre flow per second as being the desirable limit. This limit will of course not change with depth and is therefore shown as a vertical line on the graph (Fig. 30). The practical importance of the limit is that where the total resistance exceeds it there is the risk of increasing carbon dioxide retention, discomfort in breathing, loss of efficiency and ultimate exhaustion. The limit however is a guide and does not imply that breathing apparatus should not be used if the resistance is beyond the line. In experienced men who are trained to work under these conditions it is quite certain that the limit of tolerance is very much greater.

The principle will be found useful when the design of breathing apparatus is under consideration and may serve as a guide to circumstances where full working efficiency should not be expected. The ideal is to keep the combined resistance to the left of the line. The deeper one goes the less is available for the resistance of the set until at 264 ft. the human resistance reaches the line. With careful design of the breathing apparatus and in extreme cases by using respiratory gases of lower density the problem of resistance need not prejudice efficient underwater activity.

The problem of density is one which is often overlooked. It is well worth while considering, for there are many occasions under water when it may be responsible for discomfort and distress which if the circumstances are appreciated could be avoided.

In spite of all the disadvantages there is a slight bonus which increasing resistance may give to the underwater swimmer. When the breathing flow rate pattern is considered (Fig. 5) it is found to change in shape with increasing resistance. The 'sine' curve is flattened which means that the maximum flow rate is decreased but the same volume is maintained by the higher flow rates of the curve being prolonged. This means that the maximum flow rate demanded is less and absorption of carbon dioxide through a canister will be more efficient.

INSPIRATORY AND EXPIRATORY RESISTANCE

So far no distinction has been made between inspiratory and expiratory resistance. Silverman (1951) however has shown that for very heavy work without loss of efficiency the added inspiratory resistance should not exceed 7·5 cm. $H_2O/1./sec.$ and the added expiratory resistance 2·9 cm. $H_2O/1./sec.$ He goes on to state that expiratory resistance should never exceed inspiratory resistance and apparatus should be designed where necessary to draw air through a canister with inspiration. Where man is upright under water the local pressure gradient between mouth and lower chest does assist the elastic forces of expiration and so helps to lessen the gap between acceptable inspiratory and expiratory resistance.

In practice it is often difficult to keep expiratory resistance below that of inspiration though the former being an elastic recoil and the latter muscular effort this is a logical procedure. The best to be hoped for is usually that they should be equal. Where breathing sets have been constructed with a carbon dioxide canister on the inspiratory side of a closed circuit this has been found unsatisfactory and in general it is best for both inspired and expired air to pass through the absorbent.

It may seem contrary to recommend a lower expiratory resistance when it is well known that one can blow harder than one can suck but the aim is to meet the requirements of natural breathing and to disturb as little as possible the balance between active inspiration and passive expiration.

This observation gives once more the opportunity to stress the underlying aim in adapting man to a new environment. For efficient activity the stresses of the environment must be brought within those limits in which man is developed to operate. To some extent man's limits may be widened by experience and training but the approach must be unhurried and controlled.

READING AND REFERENCES

Cotes, J. E. (1954). 'Ventilatory Capacity at Altitude.' *Proc. Roy. Soc. B.* *143*, 32.

McKerrow, C. B. (1953). 'Assessment of Respiratory Function.' *Proc. Roy. Soc. Med. 46*, 532.

Mead, J. (1955). 'Resistance to Breathing at Increased Ambient Pressures.' *Proc. Underwater Physiol. Symposium.* National Academy of Science—National Research Council, U.S.A. Publication No. 377.

Miles, S. (1957). 'The Effect of Changes in Barometric Pressure on Maximum Breathing Capacity.' *J. Physiol. 137*, 85P.

— (1958). 'The Effect of Increase in Barometric Pressure on Maximum Breathing Capacity.' *M.R.C. (RNPRC) Report U.P.S.* 174.

Silverman, L., G. Lee, T. Plothin, L. H. Sawyer and A. R. Yangy (1951). 'Air Flow Measurements on Human Subjects with and without Respiratory Resistance at Several work rates.' *Arch. Ind. Hyg. & Occ. Med. 3*, 461.

CHAPTER VII

Nitrogen Narcosis

'DESPITE their chemically unreactive nature, the noble gases at certain pressures display all the typical properties of anaesthetic agents.' This most important and possibly surprising statement was made by Dr Frank Carpenter in a paper on Inert Gas Narcosis at a symposium on Underwater Physiology held in Washington in 1955.

Of these gases nitrogen is the one most intimately and continuously associated with man comprising 79% of the air he breathes. Had it not been for the experience of divers, who between the two world wars exceeded depths of 200 ft. with compressed air, nitrogen might still be accepted as wholly inert and unworthy of attention. As it was, the alterations in mood and responsiveness which such divers (Damant, 1930) described led Behnke to suspect that nitrogen under pressure might be responsible (Behnke, Thomson and Motley, 1935).

Since this relatively recent incrimination nitrogen has been shown, fairly conclusively, to be responsible for a condition of progressive narcosis in persons exposed to it under increased pressures. Nitrogen Narcosis has become a recognized syndrome, a specific disorder peculiar to those who are subjected to high air pressures, and a hazard to deep divers.

It is rare to find any report on nitrogen narcosis which does not refer to it with the apt and descriptive words of Cousteau (1954), '*L'ivresse des grands profondeurs*' usually translated as the 'rapture of the deeps'. Nothing could be more true, or more French. Unromantic British divers simply call it 'Narks'. There are those, however, who object to the name 'narcosis' claiming with some justification that this implies sedation (Unsworth, 1960) whereas in fact the nitrogen effect first shows a degree of excitation. An alternative of 'Nitrogen Intoxication' is suggested, but as the general and important effect is one of progressive narcosis it is preferable to retain the well-known and accepted title. Euphoria is not an uncommon prelude to narcosis.

The condition of nitrogen narcosis was first encountered in the standard helmeted diver and was regarded as little more than a nuisance, sometimes a pleasant one, where if the diver's behaviour became alarming he could be brought up towards the surface by his attendants. With the free swimming self-contained diver a much more serious view must be taken for should he be affected he might well lose his sense of reality and act in such a manner as to prejudice his safety.

SIGNS AND SYMPTOMS OF NITROGEN NARCOSIS

Like so many conditions where the effects are largely subjective it is most difficult to give a concise account of the symptomatology and cases vary very much one from another. Experience too plays an important part and it might help to imagine as examples two extreme cases, a class of novices being exposed to pressure in a chamber for the first time, and an experienced diver doing a deep dive.

The class would probably first have had a medical examination, with ear drum inspections and all watches, pens and matches taken away. They could not really know what to expect and when the heavy door is clamped behind them many would be very very anxious. Grinning faces peering at them through the ports would not help and the air comes in with a startling roar. Most likely before the equivalent depth of 12 ft. is reached some would be complaining of ear pain for which compression must be stopped until sticky Eustachian tubes are cleared. There may be those who cannot do so in which case the pressure must be released to let them out of the chamber. However once the ears are sorted out pressure can be increased steadily—usually for beginners a rate of descent of about 20 ft. per minute might be used giving them time to settle down. As they approach the 100 ft. mark one of them may start to speak or try to whistle at the suggestion of the instructor, who of course is with them. The inability to whistle and the strange distortions of the voice (slurring, high pitched and sometimes quite ridiculous) are the signal for laughter, garrulousness follows and the group resembles a happy gathering of revellers. Gone is any real interest in the physics of the pressure chamber and as the depth approaches the 200 ft. mark, a few may be incoherent and all are a little hysterical. This is deep enough for a start and on return to the surface all may be a little sheepish and rather tired.

Quite different is the effect on the experienced diver going to the limit to carry out some urgent task. He would descend to 250 ft. keeping a firm grip on himself knowing what to expect and at 300 ft. may find tasks such as shackling wires difficult as his hands are clumsy. He would have difficulty in remembering quite simple and familiar routines. The job would take longer and probably not be quite so well done and he may resent helpful advice from the team up top. However with his experience and sufficient motivation his will power would fight back the narcosis and somehow the work would be done though he may finally surface and remember very little about it. Such a diver might keep going even at 350 ft. until he passed into unconsciousness.

These extreme examples may well be used to set the limits of tolerance in depth when breathing air to 150 to 200 ft. for novices and 300 ft. for veterans. Between them are all stages of reaction and adaptation and some attempt may be made to tabulate the sequence of events for the average man as follows.

100–150 ft. Light headed, increasing self-confidence, loss of fine discrimination and some euphoria. (The voice changes which appear at this stage are not due to the narcosis.)

150–200 ft. Joviality and garrulousness. Perhaps some dizziness.

200–250 ft. Laughter may easily be uncontrolled and approach hysteria. Power of concentration is lessened and mistakes made in simple practical and mental tasks. May be peripheral numbness and tingling. Less attention paid to personal safety. Delayed response to signals and stimuli.

300 ft. Depression, and loss of clear thinking. Impaired neuro-muscular co-ordination.

350 ft. May be approaching unconsciousness but in addition there is the added danger of oxygen poisoning and little reliable information is available.

ON RETURN TO SURFACE—Where there has been a considerable degree of narcosis, amnesia lasting for several hours may follow. Extreme sleepiness is very common.

PREDISPOSING FACTORS

Anxiety is, in the inexperienced, likely to advance the onset of symptoms especially if alone. When a group is exposed anxiety may be somewhat alleviated by numbers but this is more than out-weighed by the infectiousness of the earlier symptoms of excitement. Alcohol if taken prior to pressurization greatly enhances the nitrogen effect the two being almost additive.

Fatigue will render a man more prone to nitrogen narcosis as will any circumstance causing retention of carbon dioxide such as very rapid compression.

AMELIORATING FACTORS

Experience, strong will and frequent deep diving all help to increase tolerance to nitrogen narcosis and there is some evidence that some anti-hallucinatory drugs might be effective. There is some suggestion that a man who can take alcohol and remain clear headed has therefore some similar resistance to the narcosis. True some divers are quite hard drinkers but this stems from the desire to balance the loneliness of their underwater world with the companionship of the saloon bar, not for the purpose of acclimatizing themselves to deep dives.

TREATMENT OF NITROGEN NARCOSIS

This is no real problem for when the pressure is released the excess nitrogen leaves the tissues and recovery is complete, except in severe cases for some temporary amnesia, and in all cases tiredness, due to pressure.

No specific treatment other than normal surfacing or reduction of pressure need be prescribed. In the rare cases where profound depression or unconsciousness has occurred observation in hospital for a further 24 hours is a wise precaution.

PREVENTION

Limiting the depth of compressed air diving to 150 ft. for the inexperienced and 250 ft. for the expert is a wise precaution.

Where these limits need to be exceeded the nitrogen must be replaced wholly or in part by a less narcotic gas. For this, helium which is about $\frac{1}{8}$ as narcotic as nitrogen has been extensively used for deeper diving, including one to 600 ft. As far as the narcotic effect is concerned a depth of 1,500 ft. could possibly be reached with helium. Figure 31 shows the advantage gained by using a mixture of equal parts air and helium.

Recent work by Bennett (1963) suggests that certain drugs, antipyretics, hypnotics and sedatives, may lessen the narcotic effects of nitrogen and Buhlmann (1961) stated it could be prevented by assisted ventilation.

RESEARCH INTO THE PROBLEM OF NITROGEN NARCOSIS

The picture so far given has been one of a condition which is largely manifest by changes in behaviour. Nothing positive or measurable has been suggested. Many workers have however attempted to find alternative and more definite means of measuring the narcotic effect in the hope that the mechanisms involved may be discovered.

One of the earliest attempts was that of Schilling and Willgrube (1937) who gave a battery of simple arithmetical tests and measured reaction times in a group of men exposed to a series of pressures up to an equivalent depth of 300 ft. They found that as depth increased there was a steady worsening in ability to get correct answers and an increase in time taken. Much worse results were obtained in inexperienced men as compared with experienced ones. The changes in reaction times were very much less marked, the mean increase at 300 ft. being only $7\frac{1}{2}\%$. These workers also stated that the effect was due to nitrogen at increased pressure, a conclusion which was supported by many others (Case and Haldane, 1941; Zetterstron, 1948; Burjstedt and Severin, 1948; and Rashbass, 1955).

8

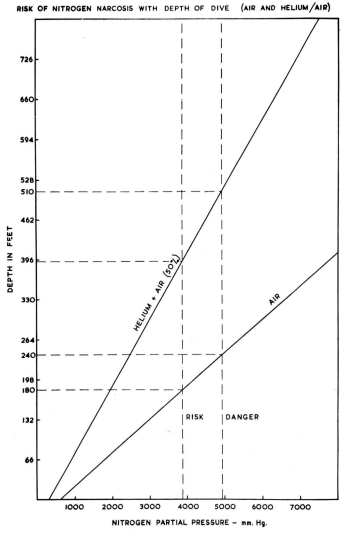

RISK OF NITROGEN NARCOSIS WITH DEPTH OF DIVE   (AIR AND HELIUM/AIR)

DEPTH IN FEET

NITROGEN PARTIAL PRESSURE – mm. Hg.

FIG. 31

Bean (1950), however, took a different view and claimed that the effect was due to a retention of carbon dioxide in the tissues which is especially marked if the compression is applied rapidly. This he claims causes (i) an increase in CO_2 partial pressure in the alveoli as a result of compressing the gases, (ii) the inflow of air into the chest to hinder the escape of CO_2, and (iii) difficulty of diffusion of the CO_2 due to increased density. In support of this theory he found the alveolar CO_2 concentration of rapidly compressed dogs to be raised from 5% to 10%.

Though the effects described by Bean do occur and it is agreed that CO_2 retention increases the narcotic effect it would seem wrong to exonerate nitrogen from blame entirely. Rashbass (1955) carried out a convincing series of experiments in which a group of 26 subjects were each rapidly compressed to an equivalent depth of 250 ft. Previously they had been given a sheet of simple multiplication sums (two figures by a single number) and a record was kept of the number of correct answers achieved in two minutes. This test was repeated immediately on reaching the chosen pressure. After this half the subjects hyperventilated for a further five minutes in an attempt to get rid of any accumulated carbon dioxide and the remainder did not. At the conclusion of this five-minute period the arithmetical test was repeated.

All the men showed a reduction in score immediately after reaching 250 ft. to 70% of the surface score. Five minutes later both groups, the hyperventilators and the normal breathers had almost identical scores of 75% of the original. Alveolar carbon dioxide measurements showed a surprisingly small increase under pressure, the only significant change being a drop of $1\frac{1}{2}$% after hyperventilation. From this experiment it was concluded that carbon dioxide had very little to do with any deterioration in performance other than possibly worsening the effect during the period immediately following compression. It is furthermore the general experience amongst divers that a very rapid compression gives a severer degree of euphoria than a slow one. This lasts only for a short while when it reverts to the degree achieved by slower compression.

THE EFFECT OF NITROGEN ON THE CENTRAL NERVOUS SYSTEM

The nature of the condition suggests that as far as nitrogen narcosis is concerned the most profitable system to investigate is the central nervous system.

To this end Bennett and Glass (1957 a and b) working with one of the pressure chambers at the Royal Naval Physiological Laboratory have investigated the effect of increased atmospheric pressure on the response of the electro-encephalograph (E.E.G.) to mental problems. This work is a major contribution to underwater medicine and may well be the key to the complicated problem of nitrogen narcosis.

These two workers used as a basis for their experiments the well-recognized effect that mental activity has on the 'alpha' rhythm of the electro-encephalograph as described by Golla, Hutton and

Grey-Walter (1943). The alpha rhythm in the E.E.G. is the basis of the normal tracing, with a frequency of 8–12 cycles per second and a strength of 10–50 micro-volts This rhythm is best seen when the subject is relaxed with the eyes shut. If the subject is then given a mental problem say a moderately difficult multiplication, the alpha rhythm will in a large number of persons disappear. This effect is known as 'alpha blocking.' If this test is done on large numbers of persons it can be shown that the population is divided up into three groups which are—

    (i) 'M' TYPE OR MINUS where the alpha rhythm is very small and is not blocked by opening the eyes or doing problems (29% of population).

    (ii) 'P' TYPE OR PERSISTENT where the alpha rhythm is of normal size

THREE PHYSIOLOGICAL TYPES OF E.E.G RECORD

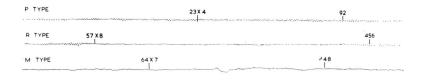

R & P TYPES ARE ASSOCIATED WITH IRREGULAR & M TYPES WITH REGULAR
RESPIRATION   M TYPES ALSO TEND TO THINK VISUALLY.
CLASSIFICATIONS OF THIS KIND MAY BE OF USE IN THE SELECTION OF
MEN FOR DIVING & OTHER UNDERWATER WORK.

(BENNETT AND GLASS 1957)

FIG. 32

and frequency and again is not blocked by eye opening or mental problems (19%); and

    (iii) 'R' TYPE OR RESPONSIVE in which a normal alpha rhythm is blocked when the eyes are opened or there is mental exertion (52%).

Examples of these three types are given in Figure 32.

Bennett and Glass showed that the E.E.G. of man exposed to raised atmospheric pressure was abnormal when a subject of type 'R' was used. If he was exposed to a high enough pressure for a long enough time the alpha blocking effect was abolished, i.e. the alpha rhythm continued unchanged throughout the effort of solving the mental arithmetic. Unfortunately this could of course only be applied to the 'R' types which therefore denied the investigators of 50% of their available subjects. Nevertheless, at last here was something that could be measured. Equivalent depths and time of exposure were accurately controllable, the alpha

EFFECT OF 4 ATS PRESSURE ON ALPHA BLOCKING (BENNETT AND GLASS 1957.)

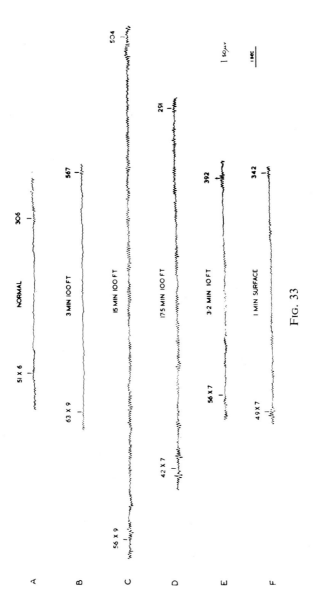

FIG. 33

blocking could be seen visually and the time of its onset recorded. This was a yardstick free from the vagaries of subjective reporting.

A typical example of the abolition of alpha blocking is shown in Figure 33. Great patience is needed in this sort of work if accurate results are to be obtained and care must be taken to ensure that subjects arrive for a trial run, alert, co-operative and free from the effects of previous nicotine, alcohol or pressure. The effort that has been put into this project has been extremely rewarding and it is possible to plot for any individual a time depth relationship for the abolition of alpha blocking. One example only need be quoted, a man who was on seven separate occasions exposed to equivalent depths of 50, 75, 100, 125, 150,

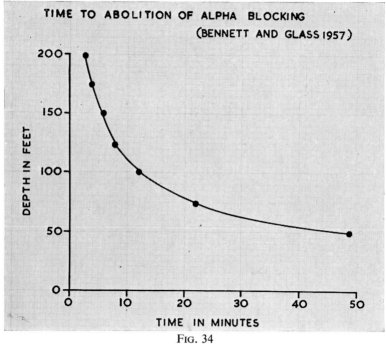

FIG. 34

175 and 200 ft. At each depth the time taken for the abolition of alpha blocking was measured and the results were found along a curve from 50 mins. at 50 ft. through 12 mins. at 100 ft. to 4 mins. at 200 ft. (Fig. 34).

It is advisable at this stage to stop and consider the implications of these very important findings.

Firstly the wide variation in times which were found in different individuals for abolishing of alpha blocking under identical conditions, e.g. at equivalent depth of 150 ft. one subject took 18 minutes and another only 4. This suggests a different degree of sensitivity or different rate of absorption into the central nervous system. Two factors are thus involved. In the nervous centres responsible for the alpha rhythm phenomena it may be assumed that a certain local build-up of nitrogen is needed to abolish the blocking, i.e. there is a nitrogen threshold. In addition the rate at which that threshold is reached will depend on the head of pressure which the nitrogen is exerting and the rate at which it can diffuse into the tissue.

In an individual of the 'R' type where there is alpha blocking at the surface there must be a critical depth, or pressure increase, where provided time is allowed for nitrogen saturation the alpha blocking is abolished. This saturation may take many hours especially if the tissue involved is avascular. This is of course the nitrogen concentration threshold which is independent of time and diffusion characteristics. At depths or pressures greater than this critical value the threshold concentration will be achieved in a shorter time because the external pressure head is greater. Where this pressure difference is large the threshold concentration is rapidly reached giving a shorter time to alpha blocking abolition. For small pressure increases it may take many hours to establish a threshold. Thereafter at increasing depths or pressures the shortening of the time for abolition would give an indication of the rate of diffusion of nitrogen through the tissue.

It must not be forgotten that the base line from which these experiments start is not zero nitrogen pressure but atmospheric nitrogen pressure ($\frac{4}{5}$ atmospheres absolute).

At this pressure 50% of the population show no alpha blocking to mental effort (the 'P' and 'M' types). Does this mean that the alpha rhythm blocking has been abolished because the nitrogen threshold is exceeded by a pressure of $\frac{4}{5}$ atmospheres? Does this mean that if nitrogen could be entirely eliminated all human electro-encephalographs would show the reactions of the 'Responsive' type? This is an interesting thought which could be tested in an altitude chamber at about 35,000 ft. where oxygen could be breathed at a partial pressure equivalent to sea-level and in time all the body nitrogen eliminated. It is however unlikely that such a change would be present for the difference between the 'M', 'R' and 'P' types of E.E.G. reaction is believed to be due to the balance in thought processes between visual and auditory perception. Also later work by Bennett (1960) using a different technique has shown similar nitrogen effects with the 'M' and 'P' types.

These changes in E.E.G. are repeatable in the individual but vary quite considerably from one person to another. There is often a parallel between the sensations felt by, and impairment in mental activity of the subject and the time taken for the abolition of alpha blocking. When pressure is released the blocking of alpha rhythm is restored and a similar result can be achieved if whilst still under pressure the air is replaced by an oxy-helium mixture.

The work of Bennett and Glass strongly supports the view that nitrogen narcosis is indeed due primarily to the nitrogen effect. They consider the diffusion delay too great to indicate action on the vascular grey matter and suggest that synapses are particularly sensitive to raised pressures of inert gas, e.g. the reticular activating system and cortical apical dendrities.

Bennett (1958 and 1960), not satisfied with the wastage of subjects caused by the suitability of 'R' types only for his tests, investigated the use of 'flicker fusion frequency' as an alternative. He fitted his chamber with a small flickering neon light the rate of flicker of which could be increased until a subject within indicated that it had become a steady light. After a short time under pressure it was found that the frequency at which the flicker became constant changed to a new level. The time taken for the establishment of the new threshold was found to vary with the pressure so that pressure multiplied by the square root of the time was a constant. This ratio was the same as that occurring in the abolition of alpha blocking. Indeed, in the same individual at a given depth, the time to the onset of the maintained alteration in the fusion frequency of the flicker was (if he were an 'R' type) the same as the time to the abolition of alpha rhythm blocking. Table 1 is an example of the close correlation. Bennett also used an argon oxygen mixture in his trials. Argon is known to be about twice as narcotic as nitrogen and it was found to produce the flicker fusion change and the E.E.G. response in just half the time taken in air at the same depth.

There seems to be little doubt that nitrogen is responsible for the narcotic effect when air is breathed under pressure and with evidence available it is possible to speculate as to the mode of action.

A very long time ago the Meyer-Overton theory was introduced (Meyer, 1899) and it is still applied today. This law states that any inert substance will act as a depressant in the central nervous system provided the amount of it dissolved in the lipid part of the cell reaches or exceeds a certain threshold. The solubility of the substance and the ratio by which it is distributed in solution between fat and water (the partition coefficient) are important factors determining the final effect. The gas breathed under pressure must first dissolve in the blood and then be

TABLE 1.

A comparison between time of onset of abolition of Alpha Blocking (E.E.G.) and Depression of Flicker Fusion Frequency (F.F.F.)

SUBJECT	DEPTH (Ft.)	F.F.F.	E.E.G.
A	50	38	37
A	100	19	18
A	150	9	9
A	175	12	12
B	100	19	19
B	150	15	15
C	100	12	10
C	125	8	8
D	150	21	21
E	150	8	6
F	150	8	6
F	125	11	9

rapidly transported to the central nervous system where, according to its partition coefficient, it is distributed between aqueous and fatty tissues.

It is instructive to compare the solubility and oil/water partition co-efficient of some of the anaesthetic and so-called inert gases. They have been put in the generally accepted order of narcotic efficiency:

GAS	(A) SOLUBILITY ml. gms. per ml. water at 37%	(B) PARTITION COEFFICIENT $Ratio\left\{\dfrac{gas\ in\ oil}{gas\ in\ water}\right.$	(A)×(B)
CYCLOPROPANE	0·204	35	7·14
XENON	0·097	20	1·91
NITROUS OXIDE	0·549	3·2	1·76
KRYPTON	0·051	9·6	0·49
ARGON	0·029	5·3	0·15
NITROGEN	0·013	5·2	0·068
HYDROGEN	0·016	3·1	0·048
HELIUM	0·0085	1·7	0·014

It will be seen that cyclopropane has a fairly high solubility and a very high partition coefficient making it an efficient narcotic and anaesthetic.

Nitrous oxide though almost twice as soluble has a much smaller co-efficient. It is difficult with this gas to obtain a good anaesthetic effect without risk of anoxia but if used under pressure it is most effective.

In producing the narcosis the effect must depend on the local concentration of the substance in the lipid factor of the responsible nervous tissue. To get there it must travel via body fluid its concentration in which is dependent on the partial pressure it exerts in the lung alveoli. When the concentration of argon for example in the lungs is represented by 1·0, the proportion in the blood will be 0·029 which will give a proportion of 0·154 in the lipid tissue. For nitrogen the figures would be 1·0, 0·013 and 0·068, which shows that for the same external pressure there is 2·25 times as much argon in the lipid tissue as there is nitrogen which supports very closely the subjective finding that argon is twice as narcotic as nitrogen.

A useful guide to the comparative narcotic effect of these substances is obtained by taking the product of the solubility and the oil/water partition coefficient. This is included in the table on p. 121.

It will be seen that helium is placed at the bottom of the table. Some workers however claim that helium is more narcotic than hydrogen. This seems most unlikely as helium is both less soluble and has a lower oil/water partition coefficient than hydrogen. Claims that this is so should be re-examined for it is indeed most difficult to see how the narcotic effect of hydrogen could be realistically examined in view of the explosive nature it exhibits in the presence of even small quantities of oxygen. If indeed, in spite of this difficulty, it is shown to be less narcotic than helium this may well be due to the possibility that its behaviour, once it is absorbed into the blood stream, is more active than the inert helium. It may well enter into chemical combination with constituents of the blood and less of it reach the lipid focus. Any hydrogen ions would be immediately absorbed. It is an element which occupies a unique place in the atomic table and is relatively active in many ways.

A very important clue to the activity of inert gases has been given by Ebert, Hornsey and Howard (1958), who studied the effect of inert gases on radio sensitivity. They showed, by measuring the effects of X-ray on the growth of bean roots, that increasingly high concentrations of the inert gases decreased the sensitivity until an anoxic level was reached. It was suggested that their action was to displace oxygen from sites within the cell, the oxygen being responsible for the radio-sensitivity. Cyclopropane and nitrous oxide were not used but the other gases were placed in order of activity which was the same as that for narcotic effect in the table on p. 121 with Xenon first and Helium last.

Taking into consideration all the work that has been done on inert gas narcosis and radio-sensitivity it would seem that the effect is ultimately due to an histotoxic anoxia. Much more work is needed and as interest grows no doubt the answer will be found.

ADAPTATION TO NITROGEN

With practice and experience divers most certainly improve their resistance to nitrogen narcosis. The adaptation is by no means permanent and to maintain it dives to 300 ft. once a week are recommended. This can be done in a pressure chamber and only a few minutes at depth is needed.

It is interesting to consider how man in his process of evolution from an aquatic animal achieved his adaptation to the atmospheric nitrogen. It can be assumed that the body fluids of a fish are in the equilibrium with the sea water as far as dissolved substances are concerned. If this is so, a transfer to a land existence would present no problem and no change in tissue nitrogen would be expected. There could, however, be no adaptation to pressure changes for in the sea depth does not substantially alter the concentration of dissolved gases. They have no increased partial pressure so that fishes (except of course the aquatic mammals) would not be subject to the risk of nitrogen narcosis.

Man would therefore be conditioned to quite a small range of tissue nitrogen saturation. There is ample evidence to show what happens if this tension is increased. What effect will removal of nitrogen from the tissues have?

Arguing on purely theoretical grounds from what has been said of the intimate action of narcosis, removal of nitrogen from the intracellular sites of adsorption might allow its replacement by oxygen molecules with some increase in alertness and perhaps of radio-sensitivity of the cell. Increased central nervous activity might be expected. An even more simple general deduction might be that, if excess nitrogen produces narcosis its removal should give the reverse effect. Bennett in his experiments has shown that even relatively small increases in nitrogen partial pressure will show evidence of change in response. It would be unusual if this was a one-way effect.

In practice it is not difficult to remove tissue nitrogen. The simplest way is by breathing pure oxygen. When this is done about 75% of the body nitrogen is removed within an hour. Thereafter elimination becomes progressively slower and it may take twelve hours to reach complete elimination. Complete, that is, as far as present recording techniques show, but it is possible that absolute denitrogenation may take several days. Removal of nitrogen by this method is unsatisfactory if nitrogen loss is being studied because the effects of breathing pure oxygen are themselves quite marked.

A more satisfactory procedure is to place a subject in an altitude chamber at a pressure of 160 mm.Hg, i.e. about 37,000 ft. At this pressure he could breathe 100% oxygen which would be presented at the same partial pressure as ground level and therefore have no complications. Preliminary trials under these conditions have been carried out on a small number of subjects but the results are conflicting.

Just as Bennett and his colleagues were able to find some method of measuring the effects of excess nitrogen so one day someone may develop a technique to measure the changes produced by nitrogen elimination.

Subjectively there is some flimsy evidence to suggest that a lowering of tissue nitrogen levels may enhance nervous activity. At altitude the nitrogen partial pressure is lowered and according to the height, the total body content will be reduced. At 10,000 ft. almost $\frac{1}{3}$ would be lost. The elation of altitude is well known. Philosophers retreat into lofty hide-aways to indulge in profound mental activity and visitors to high mountain regions are conscious of an increased clarity of mind. Could it not be that the enfolding expanse of nitrogen, which dilutes the oxygen we breathe and tempers its vitality, does in some subtle way shield the delicate mechanisms within the nerve cell nuclei against the consuming of undiluted oxygen? In such a role the 'nitrogen blanket' would play a vital part in the regulation of man's nervous activity, putting the brake on dynamic reaction, soothing, softening and mellowing. Might not the fat man be rather placid because of a high intracellular load of nitrogen containing lipids whilst his lean and fiery brother is ever restless and excitable for lack of the dampening nitrogen?

Yes, of course there are many other quite reasonable explanations which can be offered for these rather indefinite reactions but it is relaxing at the end of a chapter on the complicated story of nitrogen narcosis to dream and speculate a little. The 'nitrogen blanket' may well be non-existent and the last few sentences just idle thoughts. But thoughts they are!

Unfortunately it has not been possible to support this theory experimentally. Hall and Kelly (1962) exposed men to 100 % oxygen for 5 days at a simulated altitude of 34,000 feet without significant effect. Individual difference in the nitrogen narcosis threshold nevertheless have not been adequately explained.

THE NARCOTIC EFFECT OF HELIUM

The growing use of helium to replace nitrogen in the breathing mixture for very deep diving has naturally given rise to some speculation as to whether the gas has any narcotic properties.

Bennett (1966) in his monograph 'The Aetiology of Compressed Air Intoxication and Inert Gas Narcosis', makes frequent reference to the weak narcotic effect of helium which he calculates should become apparent when used at depths in excess of 450 feet. Marked decriments in performance were found in 20 minute exposures with men breathing 5% oxygen in helium at a simulated depth of 800 ft.

Under these conditions tremor, nausea and occasional vomiting have been described (Bennett, 1967). It is not clear however whether these effects are due solely to helium narcosis. At such depths the oxygen partial pressure may be higher than the ideal leading to hypoventilation with some carbon dioxide retention. This would point to the need for strict attention to the partial pressure of oxygen in the mixture.

Undoubtedly though helium is making deeper diving possible it introduces new specific problems which need careful study. Narcosis may be one of them but, as so often happens in human situations, it is rarely a single factor which leads to difficulties. It is often the summation of many. At these depths even with helium, increased density is also becoming a problem.

Helium is thus not the perfect gas to replace nitrogen in very deep diving. It may be the best we have unless the very great risks of explosion with hydrogen oxygen mixtures can be satisfactorily controlled. It certainly seems that the improved facilities today available may well be limited in their use by physiological restrictions imposed by the properties of the respiratory gases available.

READING AND REFERENCES

Behnke, A. R., R. M. Thomson and E. P. Motley (1935). 'Psychological Effects from Breathing air at Four Atmospheres Pressure.' *Am. J. Physiol. 112,* 554.

Bennett, P. B. and A. Glass (1957 a). 'The Electroencephalograph and Narcosis under High Partial Pressure of Nitrogen and Isonarcotic Concentrations of Nitrous Oxide.' *M.R.C. (RNPRC) Report U.P.S.* 170.

— (1957 b). 'High Partial Pressures of Nitrogen and Abolition of Blocking of the Occipital Alpha Rhythm.' *J. Physiol. 138,* 18P.

Bennett, P. B. (1958). 'Flicker Fusion Frequency and Nitrogen Narcosis. A Comparison with E.E.G. changes and the Narcotic Effect of Argon Mixtures.' *M.R.C. (RNPRC) Report U.P.S.* 176.

— (1960). 'Inert Gas Narcosis.' *Ergonomics. 3,* 273.

— (1963). 'Neuropharmacoligic and Neurophysiologic Changes in Inert Gas Narcosis.' Second Symposium on Underwater Physiology. National Academy of Science. National Research Council (U.S.A.) Publication 1181.

Bennett, P. B. (1966). 'The Aetiology of Compressed Air Intoxication and Inert Gas Narcosis'. Pergamon Press, London.

Bennett, P. B. (1967). 'Performance Impairment in Deep Diving Due to Nitrogen, Helium, Neon and Oxygen'. Proceedings of 3rd. Symposium of Underwater Physiology (Editor, Lambertson). Williams and Wilkins Co., Baltimore, U.S.A.

Bennett, P. B. and A. V. Cross (1960). 'Alterations in the Fusion Frequency of Flicker Correlated with Electroencephalograph changes at Increased Partial Pressures of Nitrogen.' *J. Physiol. 151,* 28P.

Buhlmann, A. A. (1961). 'The Respiratory Physiology of Deep Sea Diving.' *Schweiz. med. Wschr. 19,* 774.

Burjstedt, H. and G. Severin (1948). 'The Prevention of Decompression Sickness and Nitrogen Narcosis by the use of Hydrogen as a Nitrogen Substitute.' *Milit. Surgery. 103,* 107.

Carpenter, F. G. (1955). 'Inert Gas Narcosis.' Underwater Physiology Symposium, National Academy of Sciences. National Research Council (U.S.A.) Publication 377.

Case, E. M. and J. B. S. Haldane (1941). 'Human Physiology under High Pressure.' *J. Hygiene. 41,* 225.

Cousteau, J. Y. (1954). *The Silent World.* Hamish Hamilton Ltd., London.

Damant, G. C. C. (1930). 'Physiological Effects of Work in Compressed Air.' *Nature. 126* (2), 606.

Ebert, M., Shirley Hornsey and Alma Howard (1958). 'Effects on Radiosensitivity of Inert Gases.' *Nature. 181,* 613.

Golla, F., E. L. Hutton and W. Grey-Walter (1943). 'The Objective Study of Mental Imagery.' *J. of Mental Science. 89,* 216.

Hall, A. L. and H. B. Kelly (1962). 'Exposure of Human Subjects to 100% Oxygen at Simulated 34,000 ft. Altitude for 5 days'. Report No. NMC–TM–62–7, U.S. Navy Missile Center, Point Mugu, Ca.

Meyer, H. H. (1899). 'Zur Theorie der Alkoholnarkose.' *Arch. exp. Path. u. Pharmakol. 42,* 109.

Rashbass, C. (1955). 'The Unimportance of Carbon Dioxide as a cause of Nitrogen Narcosis.' *M.R.C. (RNPRC) Report U.P.S.* 153.

Schilling, C. W. and W. W. Willgrube (1937). 'Quantitative Study of Mental Reactions as Influenced by Increased Air Pressure.' *U.S. Nav. Med. Bull. 35*, 373.

Unsworth, I. P. (1960). 'Nitrogen Narcosis. Some aspects.' *St Mary's Hospital Gazette. 66*, 272.

Zetterstrom, A. (1948). 'Deep Sea Diving with Synthetic Gas Mixtures.' *Milit. Surgery. 103*, 104.

CHAPTER VIII

Oxygen

HAVING isolated oxygen Joseph Priestley (1774) wasted no time in breathing it and reported his experience with the following memorable words—

'The feeling to my lungs was not sensibly different from that of common air but I fancied that my breast felt peculiarly light and easy for some time afterwards. Who can say but that in time this pure air may become a fashionable particle in luxury? Hitherto only two mice and myself have had the privilege of breathing it.'

Priestley's observation has frequently been confirmed but his suggestion for the future use of oxygen has not been realized. Many mice and quite a few men have suffered from breathing pure oxygen and some indeed have died.

In underwater practice where pressures are increased and where there is a dependence on artificial means for air supply there are many occasions when, if things go wrong, disastrous results may occur from excess oxygen on the one hand or from too little on the other. Both must therefore be considered.

THE EFFECTS OF INCREASED OXYGEN TENSION. HYPEROXIA AND OXYGEN POISONING

The importance of partial pressure in the study of underwater respiratory gas problems has been emphasized in Chapter II. The partial pressure of oxygen at sea-level is 160 mm.Hg and this may be increased in two ways. Either (i) the mixture breathed may be enriched with oxygen until only oxygen is present, giving a maximum partial pressure of 760 mm.Hg or (ii) the pressure of the air or oxygen mixture breathed may be directly increased by which means there is theoretically no upper partial pressure limit. The most effective increase can of course be achieved for less environmental pressure if 100% oxygen is used as the table on following page shows.

With air the partial pressure of oxygen reaches 760 mm.Hg (that of 100% oxygen on the surface) at a depth of 124 ft.

Whichever way the increase in partial pressure is accomplished the effect of the oxygen on body function will be the same. What is more difficult to establish is at what pressure adverse effects may be expected. There is some evidence that small increases may be beneficial. Bannister and Cunningham (1954) found that muscular exercise could be considerably improved by breathing 60% oxygen but with 100% oxygen the improvement was very much less. There is a vast amount of literature on the effects of excess oxygen on animals, much of it contradictory, but, as far as man is concerned, it is reasonable to assume that in the healthy individual breathing concentrations up to 60% (partial pressure 456 mm.Hg) can be continued indefinitely without harm.

Of the work which has been done on oxygen toxicity that of Bean and of Donald is quite outstanding. Bean (1945) studied all the available reports, balanced up the evidence both in man and animals and presented a full account of the problem. Donald (1947), as a result of a large series of human experiments, was able to give a clear picture of the clinical aspects of oxygen poisoning, the predisposing factors and the variability of reaction. Limits of tolerance were also established which are today still accepted in diving practice. Much of what follows is based on these two reports.

As with other toxic gases not only must the partial pressure be considered, but also the time for which man is exposed. Where there is a threshold for reaction, time must elapse before this is reached and the higher the pressure the shorter will be this time.

In practice it is found that two distinct conditions occur. A relatively low oxygen concentration (say 500 mm.Hg to 1000 mm.Hg) continued for many hours will produce a chronic poisoning the presentation of which is very different from that resulting from a brief exposure to very high tensions of 1500 mm.Hg and above. These two forms, chronic and acute, can well be studied separately.

CHRONIC OXYGEN POISONING

Lorrain Smith (1899) observed that animals exposed to high oxygen pressure developed degenerative lung changes which he regarded as a

Atmospheric Pressure	Equivalent Depth in Water	Partial Pressure of Oxygen mm.Hg	
Atmospheres	Feet	Breathing Air	Breathing 100% Oxygen
1	SURFACE	160	760
2	33	320	1520
3	66	480	2280
4	99	640	3040
5	132	800	3800
6	165	960	4560

protective reaction to the irritant effect of the oxygen. His name is frequently associated with this form of oxygen poisoning. In animals quite gross changes and death may occur. Few organs escape but the lungs suffer most showing inflammatory reactions, congestion, oedema and bronchitis. Cardiac enlargement may also be present. Such reactions can occur with 100% oxygen in as little as six to eight hours.

Man however seems to be more resistant requiring many days to produce severe distress. Though it is not possible to expose man experimentally, cases have been reported of patients dying from pneumonia where the lungs of those who had been given continuous oxygen showed more inflammatory reaction than those who had not.

Certain general effects observed in man include a slowing of the pulse, lowered pulse pressure, and evidence of vaso-constriction in the central nervous system and retinal vessels.

Common and early symptoms may be fatigue, a feeling of soreness in the chest especially on deep inspiration. Occasionally a dry cough may develop.

Exposure of newborn infants to pure oxygen for long periods in incubators has resulted in cases of retrolenticular fibroplasia. If a 40% to 60% mixture is used the benefit of oxygen can be obtained without risk.

Remembering that in deep diving it is only necessary to descend to 124 ft. breathing air to produce an oxygen partial pressure of 760 mm.Hg, it becomes possible to expose the diver to a chronic oxygen poisoning risk. In practice few deep dives are of sufficient duration to present a serious hazard, but there are occasions when, following decompression sickness, it is necessary to keep a diver under pressure in a chamber for 24 hours or more. Such treatment may well be complicated by pulmonary irritation with dry cough and respiratory discomfort.

A much more common danger in diving is that of—

ACUTE OXYGEN POISONING

Credit for the first reliable description of acute oxygen poisoning must go to Paul Bert (1878) who observed convulsive seizures in animals exposed to high oxygen pressure. He found marked variations between different animals finding birds more sensitive than dogs and also that the higher the pressure the shorter was the time required to produce convulsions.

Many interesting animal investigations followed. Mice, rats, guinea pigs, monkeys, cats, frogs, pigeons and an alligator were all used and generally speaking the warm-blooded animals convulsed. The higher up the animal scale they were the sooner they did so. The cold-blooded animals were immune to the pressures used. Before convulsions, some of which occurred under pressure and some immediately on release, there was occasionally restlessness, dyspnoea or muscular twitchings. In some as pressure increased a convulsion occurred followed by recovery then a final and continuous further convulsion. Recovery, in cases where pressure was released immediately on the appearance of the convulsion, was complete.

The first report of man suffering an oxygen convulsion was made by Thomson (1935) who described how two divers in 1933 breathed pure oxygen at a pressure of 4 atmospheres (p.p. 3040 mm.Hg). The first experienced severe twitching of the face after 16 minutes but recovered on breathing air. The second developed a tremor of the lips after 13 minutes but on turning over to air developed a general convulsion and lost consciousness.

Some years later Haldane (1941) breathing oxygen at 7 atmospheres (p.p. 5320 mm.Hg) for 5 minutes experienced a sudden and violent convulsion with little warning.

It is however to Donald (1947), who in 1942 commenced a large series of trials involving over 2,000 exposures, that credit must be given for our present knowledge of the clinical problem of acute oxygen poisoning and the introduction of reliable safety precautions for divers and others exposed to high pressures.

The work was carried out in a dry pressure chamber and in order to establish a tolerance level 36 men were exposed to a pressure of 3·7 atmospheres. An oxygen breathing apparatus was used giving in fact about 95% oxygen or a partial pressure of 2670 mm.Hg. Five of these men convulsed but the time taken varied from 19 to 35 minutes. The remainder were removed when severe symptoms were observed which included lip twitching, nausea, vomiting, vertigo and syncope. The time for onset of symptoms varied from 6 to 96 minutes.

The first difficulty encountered was the profound variation in individual tolerance.

Similar experiments were conducted using a wet pressure chamber with the subject completely submerged, under pressure and breathing oxygen at simulated depths from 25 ft. to 100 ft. Observations were made with the man at rest and exercising by repeatedly raising a heavy bag of weights with a rope and pulley, the weights being in air.

As a result of these painstaking observations a number of very important facts emerged.

(i) Variation in tolerance was not only extreme between individuals but the sensitivity of any one man may vary greatly from day to day. For example one diver at rest at an equivalent depth of 70 ft. (p.p. oxygen 2470 mm.Hg) showed an onset of toxic symptoms in 7 minutes on one day and 148 on another. His average time was 55 minutes and there seemed to be an increase in tolerance with the repeated dives.

SURVIVAL OF GROUPS OF INDIVIDUALS
BREATHING OXYGEN AT 90 FEET (3·73 ATS. ABS.)
IN THE DRY AND THE WET
(DONALD 1946)

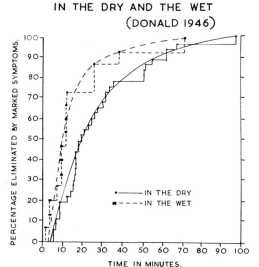

PERCENTAGE OF SUBJECTS ELIMINATED BY TOXIC SYMPTOMS AT 90 FEET (3·73 ATS: ABS·) BREATHING OXYGEN IN COMPRESSED AIR AND UNDER WATER (65°F) IN DIVING SUIT NO WORK PERFORMED DURING DIVES.

FIG. 35

(ii) The onset of symptoms occurred consistently sooner when experiments were done with men in water than with men in a dry chamber (Fig. 35).

(iii) The time of exposure before onset of symptoms became much less as the oxygen pressure was increased (Fig. 36).

(iv) When work was carried out the tolerance to the high pressure oxygen was greatly reduced (Fig. 37).

The wide variations of individual reactions made it very difficult to establish a safety limit but taking all the factors into account it seemed wise to state that all diving on pure oxygen below 25 ft. of sea water is a hazardous gamble.

SURVIVAL OF DIVERS ON PURE OXYGEN AT VARIOUS DEPTHS UNDER WATER

(DONALD 1946)

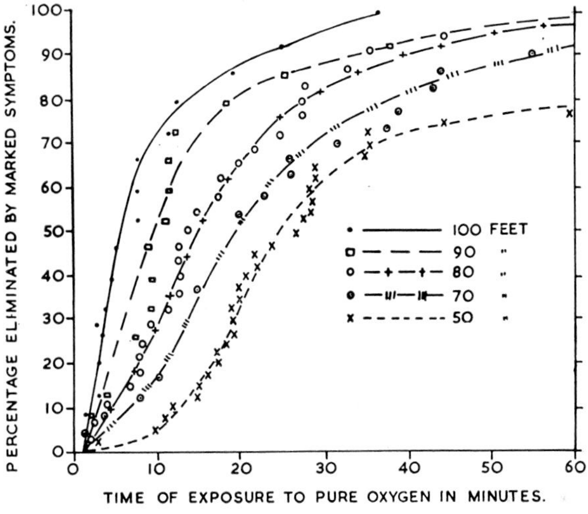

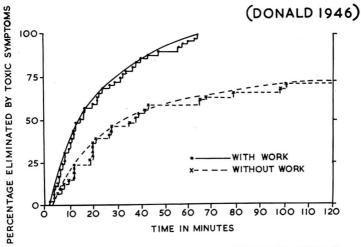

SHOWING THE PERCENTAGE OF DIVERS, ON OXYGEN, UNDER WATER
SURVIVING AT VARIOUS TIMES UP TO 1 HOUR AT 50 FEET, 70 FEET,
80 FEET, 90 FEET, AND 100 FEET OF SEA WATER
TEMPERATURE THROUGHOUT 65°F. NO WORK PERFORMED.
ACTUAL END POINTS PLOTTED.

FIG. 36

EFFECT OF WORK ON OXYGEN POISONING IN THE WET AT 50 FEET OF SEA WATER
(2·52 ATS : ABS.)

(DONALD 1946)

SHOWING PERCENTAGE ELIMINATED BY TOXIC SYMPTOMS AT 50 FEET IN
THE WET (2·52 ATS : ABS) DURING A PERIOD OF 2 HOURS WITH
& WITHOUT WORK. GROUP OF 46 DIVERS WORKING AND
41 NOT WORKING. TEMPERATURE THROUGHOUT 65°F

FIG. 37

Based on Donald's findings it is now current practice to limit oxygen diving when work or swimming is being done to a depth of 25 ft. though where there is no exertion a depth of 33 ft. may be allowed. The time factor is so variable that it is better not to introduce it. For deeper diving the oxygen must be diluted and the limit adjusted to cover the apparent oxygen depth, e.g. if a 40% oxygen mixture is used the working limit would be 113 ft. or if a 33% oxygen limit is used, 132 ft. (In mixture breathing diving practice allowance is made for oxygen consumption diluting the mixture in the breathing bag of the apparatus and for a 40% O_2/60% N_2 mixture the safe depth is actually 140 ft. This will be explained when breathing apparatus is being considered in Chapter XVIII.)

SYMPTOMS OF ACUTE OXYGEN POISONING

So uncertain and variable are the symptoms of acute oxygen poisoning that it would be dangerous to rely on them for warning of an approaching convulsion. In Donald's series it was the practice to remove men as soon as definite symptoms occurred. In spite of this precaution 6·8% convulsed without warning in the groups working under water. Where symptoms do occur these are in order of incidence, lip twitching, dizziness, nausea, choking sensation, dyspnoea and tremor— lip twitching occurring in about half the cases. Similar symptoms occur in water when no work is done except that there is less complaint of nausea and vertigo.

The convulsion itself lasts for about two minutes and is not repeated if air is breathed and in every way resembles a major epileptic fit even including the after effects of confusion and amnesia. In some cases a return to air produces a temporary worsening of symptoms.

TREATMENT AND PREVENTION

There is no treatment needed other than a return to air when symptoms disappear in a few minutes. Where possible this should take place before pressure is reduced to lessen exacerbation of the condition. Where the victim is a self-contained diver in open water there is grave danger that the convulsion may cause him to lose his mouth-piece and drown.

The restrictions which experience has placed on oxygen diving, which otherwise would be most economical, have stimulated research into methods of compromise. Taylor (1957) is attempting to find a drug which can be given to increase resistance to oxygen poisoning. Though some success is claimed the results are not at present available. Whatever drug is found to be effective some convincing reassurance will be needed that, if a convulsion can be postponed, there is no continuing under-lying toxic effect. A second proposed compromise, still under investi-gation, stems from the fact that, at depths not greatly in excess of the critical depth, a short time may be anticipated before symptoms occur and on release of pressure there is a quick return to normal. If this is so, it should be possible by repetitive dives, say 10 minutes below 30 ft. alternating with 10 minutes rest on the surface breathing air, to produce quite a worthwhile total underwater working time.

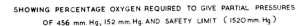

SHOWING PERCENTAGE OXYGEN REQUIRED TO GIVE PARTIAL PRESSURES OF 456 mm. Hg., 152 mm. Hg. AND SAFETY LIMIT (1520 mm. Hg.)

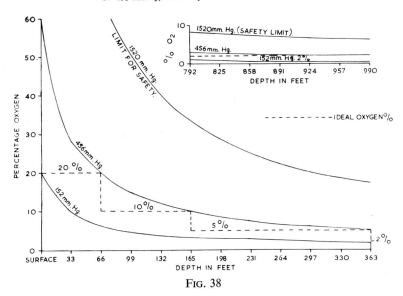

FIG. 38

Perhaps, however, the most satisfactory answer to the question of oxygen poisoning is to abandon pure oxygen for diving altogether or at least restrict it to the special uses for which it is most appropriate.

It has been stated over and over again that in the underwater environ-ment every effort should be made to present man with conditions as near to those of his land existence as possible. Therefore the aim, the ideal, which should be sought is to give the diver a mixture which is adjusted so that whatever his depth the partial pressure of the oxygen he breathes is between 152 and 456 mm.Hg (i.e. 20%–60% on the surface). Figure 38 shows the percentage oxygen range required to keep the partial pressures between 152 and 456 at different depths. In addition the absolute acceptable pressure for oxygen safety of 2 atmospheres absolute has been included.

A descent to 1,000 ft. keeping within the ideal limits would require a 20% mixture (or air) down to 66 ft., 10% from 66 ft. to 165 ft., 5% from 165 ft. to 363 ft., then 2% for the remainder. If it was only required to keep within the safety limit air could be used down to 200 ft. and 5% O_2 for the rest. In an actual dive down to 600 ft. air was used as far as 40 ft. and 8% oxygen thereafter. There is thus a reasonably wide safety margin for oxygen for deep diving provided accurate control of supply mixture is achieved. The big problem is finding a satisfactory diluent. Helium, though expensive, could be used to dilute air, a mixture of 1 part air with 6 parts helium giving a 3% oxygen equivalent. Such a mixture could be used from 200 ft. to 1,000 ft. with adequate oxygen and no nitrogen problems.

The prevention of oxygen poisoning thus is dependent on the ability of the equipment to keep the oxygen partial pressures within the safe limits which have been quite well established. It is a pity that high-pressure oxygen has this adverse effect for without it a self-contained underwater closed circuit oxygen breathing set without its depth limit would be a most economical and simple piece of apparatus.

THE MECHANICS OF OXYGEN POISONING

Two distinct mechanisms seem to be involved. A high excess partial pressure of oxygen, even in a short time, may produce high enough concentrations in the tissues to produce the acute effects, especially in the central nervous system. This is the acute oxygen poisoning, the 'Paul Bert' Effect which is reversible, i.e. there is no permanent damage. If on the other hand a smaller excess pressure is maintained for a considerable time there is an irritant effect on the lungs with local tissue damage. This is the chronic oxygen poisoning, the Lorraine Smith Effect which is not immediately reversible.

The difference between these two effects depends on the time-pressure relation. The central nervous system is very sensitive to excess oxygen but a certain threshold must be reached. Other tissues, the lung in particular, react to a continued though much lower increase in pressure. What happens within the tissues is the real puzzle.

At normal atmospheric pressure blood carrying oxygen from the lungs does so mainly by virtue of the haemoglobin. 100 ml. of blood will carry 19 ml. of combined oxygen and 0·3 ml. of dissolved oxygen. If the oxygen partial pressure is increased the oxygen carried by the haemoglobin will not exceed 20 ml.% which is saturation but that in solution will increase. If pure oxygen is breathed the amount of oxygen going into simple solution will increase to 2·03 ml.% which at 2 atmospheres would become 4·3 ml.%. As far as the tissues are concerned they will use the dissolved oxygen before calling upon that combined with the haemoglobin. As a result, according to the activity of the tissue, the combined oxygen may not be needed or if it is, much less will be required. This means there will be very little reduced haemoglobin available to assist with the removal of carbon dioxide and it will tend to accumulate. This has naturally led to the suggestion that carbon dioxide plays an important part in oxygen poisoning.

Taylor (1949 a and b) found a steady increase in tissue carbon dioxide in cats under high oxygen pressure, the oxygen tension first rising and then falling until convulsions or death occurred. He also found that adding CO_2 to the inspired air shortened the time to onset of convulsion and hyperventilation lengthened it. Lambertson and his colleagues (1953 a) on the other hand were unable to confirm this in men, dogs, rabbits and cats.

However, it is generally agreed that though carbon dioxide may lower the tolerance to high-pressure oxygen, it is not thought to be the main cause.

Lambertson's group (1953 b) also, on strong experimental evidence, considered that the rise in tissue CO_2 as a result of diminished haemoglobin reduction would, in fact, stimulate the respiratory centre and account for an increase in minute volume which they found. Indeed they showed (1953 c) that when pure oxygen was breathed at $3\frac{1}{2}$ atmospheres the actual carbon dioxide elimination was increased. It is also possible that the sensitivity of the respiratory centre may be improved and respond to stimuli from the local irritating effect of the oxygen in the lungs. Such increased ventilation would not occur in the earlier stages. A decrease in cerebral blood flow of 25% as a result of vaso-constriction is also described (1953 d). The effect of 100% oxygen on the cerebral circulation has also been studied by the use of radioactive Krypton (B. M. Lewis and others, 1956). A drop of 50% was recorded.

The important changes in man subjected to high oxygen pressure which occur before the onset of symptoms may be listed as:

   (i)   Slowing of heart rate.

  (ii)   Increase in ventilation. (Following a very short period of depression)

 (iii)   Diminished reduction of oxyhaemoglobin with impairment of CO_2 carriage.

 (iv)   Increased sensitivity of respiratory centre.

  (v)   Cerebral vaso-constriction.

(vi)   Reflex stimulation of the respiratory centre from pulmonary irritation.

These would in general seem to be an attempt on the part of the body to protect itself from the poisonous effects of too much oxygen.

The convulsion itself has been studied and in every way it resembles an epileptic fit even to the similarity of the electro-encephalograph pattern. It is a generalized convulsion involving the whole of the central nervous system.

Attempts have been made to investigate the biochemical changes involved and to this end Dickens (1946) exposed fresh slices of rat brain to high-pressure oxygen and suggested that an inhibition of pyruvic oxidase may be involved. This oxidase contains the sulph-hydryl group —SH which is inactivated by oxidation. Also shown to be inhibited by excess oxygen are Glyceraldehyde-3 phosphate dehydrogenase (containing reduced glutathione) and the acetylization of Choline (Haugaard, 1955).

Another clue to the puzzle of oxygen poisoning is found in the work of Gerschman and others (1954) who showed a similarity in action between high-pressure oxygen and X-irradiation. Both have a common mechanism in the formation in the tissues of oxidizing free radicals. This finding is of practical importance. The actions of X-rays and high-pressure oxygen are similar and will summate. This is made use of in the treatment of certain forms of cancer in which the diseased area is irradiated with the patient in a pressure chamber breathing oxygen under high pressure. (Other workers have shown that substances which will protect against the effects of X-irradiation will delay the onset of symptoms of oxygen poisoning. Such substances include Glutathione and Cysteine (Chapman, 1950; and Patt, 1949).)

Mention must be made of work by Stein and Perst (1956) who used a simple frog 'nerve-muscle' preparation in a sealed chamber. Compared with controls in oxygen at 1 atmosphere the effect of 12 atmospheres was a complete block of conduction in 4–5 hours. Adding 5% CO_2 speeded up the effect. In the early stages the block was partially reversible. The most interesting comment of these two investigators is that X-irradiation also produces a conduction block in the preparation.

Finally there is evidence that the pituitary-adrenal axis and sympathetic nervous system may be involved. In animals both hypophysectomy and sympathetic blocking agents will give some protection against oxygen lung damage and increase survival chances. High-pressure oxygen has produced hypertrophy of the adrenal cortex in experimental animals (Bean, 1955).

It is impossible from all these valuable snippets of information to be sure just what is happening in oxygen poisoning but it is encouraging that so many promising lines of investigation are being followed. Considering all available knowledge it would seem likely that the underlying mechanism is an inhibition of intracellular metabolism producing in fact a histo-toxic anoxia.

Acute oxygen poisoning, although its mechanism is of real academic interest, has in recent years been less of a problem to deep divers who are accepting the principle that the oxygen content of any breathing gas should be maintained at a partial pressure equivalent to its surface value in air, or at least within very narrow limits of this.

The increasing use of oxygen in therapeutic and resuscitative practice on the other hand has made physicians very conscious of the risk of its prolonged use even at atmospheric pressure.

Morgan (1968) has shown that the response of the lungs to excess oxygen is an increase in both pulmonary vascular resistance and the alveolar-arterial gradient with decreased compliance, atelectasis and pulmonary oedema.

Undoubtedly hypoxaemia must be treated with additional oxygen but it should be used with care. A 70% oxygen mixture breathed for a few days may be dangerous.

THE OXYGEN PARADOX

This is an interesting phenomenon described by Grandpierre and Franck (1952). When pure oxygen is administered to a person suffering from hypoxia there may be an immediate worsening of his condition with slowing of pulse, depressed respiration and a drop in blood pressure. If the patient is near to unconsciousness the impact of the pure oxygen might cause him to lose consciousness. These symptoms, and even the unconsciousness are purely temporary and the beneficial effect of the oxygen in the treatment of the hypoxia is very soon established.

This effect is possibly due to a sudden cerebral vaso-constriction with bradycardia temporarily reducing a critically low level of cerebral oxidation or to the temporary depression of respiration described by Lambertson (1963).

THE EFFECTS OF DECREASED OXYGEN TENSION—OXYGEN LACK —ANOXIA

Of much more practical importance in underwater medicine is lack of oxygen. Oxygen poisoning should be a rare event if simple precautions are taken but there are very many situations in which an inadequate supply may endanger an underwater swimmer's life.

At the outset it is necessary to clear up a question of terminology. Strictly speaking 'Anoxia' should be reserved for a complete lack of oxygen supply and 'hypoxia' used for all other occasions where there is a reduction only. However, it has become customary to call all conditions of reduced oxygen supply 'anoxia' and this practice—wrong though it is —will be maintained with sincere apologies to the pure physiologists.

The division of anoxia into acute and chronic forms is a purely artificial one which really depends on the rate of onset of the condition, the end result being the same in all cases—unconsciousness.

In acute anoxia (sometimes called instantaneous anoxia), such as might occur with an explosive fall in alveolar oxygen partial pressure, consciousness may be lost in a few seconds. This has been observed many times in physiological investigations on aviators. One of the best examples, with a series of ciné camera pictures is given in a paper by Luft and Naell (1956) who explosively dropped barometric pressure in a chamber from 760 to 70 mm.Hg. Unconsciousness occurred in 20 seconds of which 6 seconds was the time taken for the circulation to carry the effect from the lungs to the brain. A freezing of expression and posture precede the collapse which may be complete or heralded by a few quick convulsions. Recovery on restoration of normal oxygen supply is equally rapid but most significant is the amnesia for events immediately prior to the oxygen failure. This is important because a victim may recover from acute anoxia and be quite unaware of the cause, so much so that he might repeat the series of actions which brought about the anoxia.

The nearest approach to this condition under water occurs in the fortunately rare accident where the cylinders of the breathing apparatus have been mistakenly filled with nitrogen. A few breaths of this rapidly reduces the alveolar oxygen partial pressure and unconsciousness occurs within half a minute.

Unconsciousness results in all cases from a cerebral anoxia. This may be brought about by inadequate oxygen in the inspired air and poor oxygenation of the blood (anoxic anoxia), a failure of the circulation (stagnant anoxia) or a combination of both. Inadequate transport of oxygen (anaemic anoxia) would not be expected in the healthy individuals who go under water and the failure of intracellular oxygen metabolism (histotoxic anoxia) has already been mentioned in connection with nitrogen narcosis and oxygen poisoning.

SIGNS AND SYMPTOMS OF ANOXIA

Unconsciousness which is the important outcome of anoxia may actually be the first indication and it is almost impossible to train men to anticipate loss of consciousness from anoxia. Very often where the oxygen tension is slowly declining there is an abnormal sense of well-being and over-confidence. Even if a task is being done and increasing numbers of mistakes are made this is not recognized. In a recent series of experiments experienced divers breathed in and out of a large spirometer through a carbon dioxide absorbing canister so exhausting the oxygen supply. They were instructed to let go the mouth-piece and breathe the ambient air if they felt they were not getting enough oxygen. Not one in fact did so, they either quietly became unconscious or were told to let go by an observer. The percentage oxygen being breathed to produce unconsciousness was between 6% and 10%.

Provided there is no parallel accumulation of carbon dioxide, increase in ventilation need not accompany the anoxia. True it is well established that the chemo-receptors in the carotid body and aortic arch are sensitive to a lowered oxygen tension in the blood and in such circumstances will stimulate the respiratory centre. However a lowered oxygen tension will be present in the blood reaching the centre and the direct anoxic effect will render it less receptive to incoming stimuli. In the large number of subjects used in the above experiments the outcome of the struggle between the peripheral stimulation and central depression could be clearly seen. In 50% there was an actual diminution in ventilation in the few minutes preceding unconsciousness. In others there was increase in depth but not of rate, in some this was the other way round. Only a very few showed increase in rate and depth. Of particular interest were those which showed irregularity where periods of stimulation alternated with periods of depression.

From what is known about man's behaviour prior to loss of consciousness from anoxia one of the most important maxims in underwater medicine can be stated.

'Unconsciousness may be the only indication that an oxygen supply is failing or inadequate.'

Teaching the diver what to do in cases of anoxia is of very doubtful value. Teaching what to do to prevent anoxia is of paramount importance.

Of the many anoxic conditions which may affect man in water the simplest is syncope.

SYNCOPE IN WATER

If a person on land has a simple faint nobody worries very much. As often as not falling to the ground restores the circulation and he recovers.

In water the problem is much more serious. If loss of consciousness occurs the victim will drown unless immediately rescued. Furthermore in water the negation of gravity in the tissues is such that change in posture does not redistribute the blood. There is no rush of blood to the head when one is upside-down in water.

This fact gives rise to a second maxim—

'Loss of consciousness in water is a major emergency requiring immediate action.'

OXYGEN SYNCOPE—SHALLOW WATER BLACK-OUT

A number of cases have been reported where men swimming with closed circuit oxygen breathing sets have lost consciousness for no apparent reason. For lack of any specific finding the condition came to be known as Shallow Water Black-out.

There are however certain features which may be important: these are:

(i)   The condition occurs generally in the oxygen breathing set. It has rarely been reported using the open circuit air set.

(ii) It is very much more common in inexperienced men under training.

(iii) Its onset has no relation to the time in the water or the depth which is reached. It has occurred with men on the surface within a few minutes of entering the water as well as under water and after longer intervals.

Largely for lack of any alternative the condition was generally attributed to carbon dioxide poisoning. This is not very realistic for so many cases have occurred before any substantial build-up of CO_2 could develop and excess of CO_2 has not been found in the breathing bags when opportunities to examine their contents have been available. Nor did an improvement in canister design lessen the incidence.

More recently an investigation has been completed to investigate Shallow Water Black-out and the first question asked was—'Why should it be so exclusively associated with oxygen breathing?'

It is well known that syncope can be produced by a combination of hyperventilation, a sudden assumption of the upright posture and compression of the chest against a closed glottis. In this manœuvre cerebral anoxia is the result of a summation of effects. Hyperventilation lowers blood carbon dioxide which causes cerebral vaso-constriction. A sudden assumption of an upright posture causes blood to pool in the lower extremities at the expense of the cerebral circulation. An increase in intra-pulmonary pressure reduces filling of the left side of the heart and thus diminishes cardiac output.

In the laboratory a test was devised by which these syncope promoting factors could be controlled. The subject was placed horizontally on a 'tilt-table' and rested for 5 minutes. One minute of maximum hyperventilation followed on the completion of which the table was rapidly swung into the upright position and the subject instructed to blow forcibly into a rubber tube connected to a mercury manometer. The object was to maintain the mercury column at a height not less than 4 cm. for as long as possible. The test was so controlled that when breathing air syncope was approached but rarely complete.

In order to familiarize men with the routine this was in all cases first completed with the men hyperventilating from a mixture of 6% carbon dioxide in air. The presence of the CO_2 neutralized the CO_2 eliminating effect of hyperventilation and in no cases were any symptoms seen. Subsequently during the hyperventilation period subjects breathed from Douglas Bags filled with air and oxygen. In half air was first and in the remainder oxygen, separate tests being done with each.

In 130 men tested there were 18 cases where consciousness was lost of which 12 occurred when oxygen was breathed but not when breathing air. Six men lost consciousness when breathing oxygen and also when breathing air but there was no man who lost consciousness when breathing air who did not also do so with oxygen.

In addition 14 men showed evidence of approaching syncope of which 12 were breathing oxygen; one showed this effect when breathing both mixtures and one with air only.

There was no indication that testing with one or other mixture first made any difference and all had been familiarized previously with the CO_2 mixture.

This series of tests strongly suggested that in a number of persons breathing oxygen lowered the syncope threshold. This effect therefore could well be a factor in the cause of shallow water black-out.

The other important observation was that the condition most commonly occurred with inexperienced men during training. However good training methods may be, an element of anxiety must always be present in a man attempting to master a new technique in a strange and adverse environment. With anxiety there is hyperventilation. Furthermore experiments in the laboratory had also shown that beginners experienced marked hyperventilation when wearing a mouth-piece and nose clip. Hyperventilation thus may well be a further factor.

About the same time as this work was in progress physiologists of the Royal Canadian Air Force described a series of cases of Episodic Unconsciousness in pilots during flight (Powell, 1956). Here it was shown that unconsciousness had occurred as a result of the summation of two or more syncope promoting factors which alone would be unlikely to produce unconsciousness. These included hyperventilation due to anxiety (personal emotional problems or psychological stresses), the after effects of alcohol, hunger, pain and the incubating of a febrile illness.

Investigation of a large series of episodes with men in water showed that in addition to breathing oxygen such factors as Powell described were also present. The anxiety of the beginner and the unfamiliar use of a mouth-piece and nose clip was very common. Quite a few had entered the water late in the forenoon having had no more than a cup of tea for breakfast and an early supper the night before. Hangover, illness and personal problems also played their part. In one or two cases unconsciousness followed an action peculiar to diving, that of clearing the ears. Where this had been difficult forceful attempts had produced sudden increases of intra-pulmonary pressure sufficient with an already lowered threshold to cause syncope.

It is now firmly believed that this form of unconsciousness occurring in underwater swimmers using oxygen results from a summation of syncope promoting factors of which oxygen is the common one and the term 'Oxygen Syncope' is suggested.

Since the appreciation of these factors and the steps which have been taken to avoid or eliminate them the condition is now a relatively rare one. Complete replacement of oxygen apparatus by air or mixture breathing should remove it altogether.

LATENT ANOXIA

This condition is peculiar to the underwater swimmer who does not use breathing apparatus other than perhaps a Schnorkel tube. It has been observed in competitive aquatic sports and in spear-fishing. In the latter it is responsible for many fatalities.

A test of skill and endurance occasionally demanded in competitive water games is one of swimming under water as far as possible. On such occasions it is the practice for the swimmer to hyperventilate before entering the water to lower alveolar carbon dioxide pressure and prolong breath holding. There have been instances where a competitor completing an underwater swim of about 50 yards in a little over one minute has surfaced and lost consciousness and but for immediate rescue would have drowned.

This sort of trial should be strongly discouraged as a study of the circumstances will reveal. A hard swim of 50 yards would require a consumption of at least $2\frac{1}{2}$ litres of oxygen which is more than the lungs contain at the start of the swim. Even accepting an oxygen debt the alveolar oxygen tension will be very low.

A fall in oxygen partial pressure is much less of a stimulant to respiration than a build-up of CO_2 and if the latter is delayed by previous hyperventilation a dangerously low oxygen level may be reached before breath holding breaks. In the stress of such a swim the will to win may even delay the breaking stimulus so that the swimmer surfaces with his lung oxygen content critical. Before surfacing the swimming stops and in water this means a greater muscular relaxation than might occur after a run on land. With this sudden loss of muscle tone there may be a peripheral pooling of blood giving a diminished cardiac filling with slight reduction in cardiac output which, to an already hypoxic brain, may be just sufficient to cause unconsciousness. If this happens in water there is no postural aid to recovery. With brief sinking below the surface the anoxic situation is completed. Only quick rescue may give a chance of survival.

In the incident described it is assumed that the swimmer is not very far below the surface but depth may complicate the picture even further. Many cases have been recorded where a swimmer, usually after surface hyperventilation, goes under water to perform a difficult task or to chase a fish. On the way up after finishing the task consciousness is lost. At depth there is a more than adequate increase in partial pressure of oxygen due to the compression of the air in the chest. The alveolar carbon dioxide however follows a similar pattern to that on the surface being in equilibrium with that in the blood. It does not rise as would be expected due to increasing pressure for any excess is carried away by the blood flowing through the lung. The underwater effort may be extreme and, as in the chasing of a fish, the emotional urge may resist the desire to surface for breath. However, when the swimmer can continue no longer he turns to surface. At depth the oxygen pressure may still be adequate even with pooling of blood following cessation of activity. Unfortunately as the ascent continues the oxygen partial pressure must fall as the lung expands again and a pressure adequate to maintain consciousness at depth may rapidly become insufficient and produce unconsciousness before the surface is reached. This in water may well be the prelude to drowning.

10

Many cases of this 'latent' anoxia have occurred and it has become a recognized hazard of the spear-fishermen. Cabarrou (1960) has described the high incidence of what he calls 'masked anoxia' in spear-fishermen operating in the Mediterranean.

There is really no need for these tragic happenings. The underwater chase must be tempered with caution and respect must be paid to the role of carbon dioxide as the controller of respiration. The practice of hyperventilating to prolong breath holding for an underwater exploit cannot be too strongly condemned. It is even possible that a build-up of carbon dioxide under water could cause inhalation of water before the surface is reached.

Some authorities attempt to put a depth limit on this form of diving usually about 60 ft. Representatives of the Soviet Union diving organizations speaking at an international conference in Cannes in 1960 attributed their freedom from this sort of accident as being due to strict control. A depth limit of 20 metres (66 ft.) is applied and an experienced doctor is present. Only experts go deeper and then only if recompression facilities are available (Rallon 1960).

DILUTION ANOXIA

This further hazard is one which may beset the underwater swimmer who uses a closed circuit oxygen (or mixture) breathing set. Basically the principle of such a set is for the user to have a breathing bag of about seven litres capacity leading through a carbon dioxide absorbing canister to the breathing mouth-piece. In use the bag is filled up with oxygen and breathing from it through the canister removes carbon dioxide and as the oxygen is exhausted the bag is topped up from a small supply cylinder which is part of the set. Nothing apparently could be more simple but the following misuses have occurred resulting in anoxic death.

An adventurous diver with little knowledge obtains one such set, fills the bag with oxygen, puts on a nose clip, places the mouth-piece in position and enters the water. Gently swimming to the bottom he may become quietly engrossed watching fishes or studying other marine life. Quite soon without being aware of it he passes gently into unconsciousness on the sea-bed and peacefully dies.

The sequence of events commences with the fatal error. When he placed the mouth-piece in position and commenced to breathe from the set his lungs would contain air. If he started somewhere near full inspiration his own lungs might contain a total volume of 5 litres of air with 7 litres oxygen in the bag, i.e. 8 litres oxygen and 4 litres of nitrogen in all. As he continued quietly cruising under water he would gradually use up oxygen. There would be no warning carbon dioxide build-up as this is all absorbed in the canister. Ultimately the oxygen would be diminished until there was insufficient to support consciousness. No respiratory embarrassment would occur because the volume of nitrogen present would more than meet the needs of the tidal volume.

Such an example should be taken as a warning of the extreme danger of ignorance under water. There is no control over the sale or manufacture of breathing apparatus and indeed any enterprising handyman could make this simple set for himself. For the uninitiated it could be a death trap; for the experienced the acme of economy and safety.

Such a risk can of course be avoided if before using the set the diver takes three or four deep breaths of oxygen from the bag and breathes out into the open air so replacing the lung contents with oxygen and removing any nitrogen present. It is important to remember too, that should for any reason the mouth-piece be removed, as for example in talking to another diver on the surface, the lung washout procedure must be repeated before resuming breathing from the set.

There is in addition a further way in which this dilution anoxia may be brought about even when the correct action for removing lung nitrogen is taken. If the diver is breathing pure oxygen and has washed out all the nitrogen from the lungs the nitrogen partial pressure in the alveoli will have dropped to zero. In such circumstances dissolved nitrogen will escape from the tissue to the lungs. As much as 400 ml. may escape in half an hour and this of course will dilute the oxygen in the closed circuit. If the diver is engrossed in some quiet observation on the bottom (provided it is not too deep) it is very easy for his tidal volume to be less than this amount and possible for an anoxic level of oxygen diluted with this body nitrogen to develop before the breathing bag becomes empty enough to draw the user's attention to the need for topping up. This may not be a common happening but it has occurred. It is less likely with greater depth as increasing pressure slows the rate at which nitrogen leaves the blood.

The risk of onset of dilution anoxia can be avoided by a slight modification of the breathing apparatus. In the simple arrangement the user just fills up the bag as necessary from the supply cylinder. It is, however, a common practice and a wise precaution to introduce a reducing valve which gives a steady flow from the cylinder to the bag with a by-pass valve for topping up when necessary. A convenient figure for the flow rate of the reducer is $\frac{3}{4}$ litre per minute. Such a fitting ensures an adequate oxygen supply to avoid a risk of dilution anoxia although for hard work it may be necessary to keep topping up the bag.

This safeguard is not always popular with experienced divers nor can it be used if there is a need, in special circumstances, for a set which does not give off bubbles. At times when less than the by-pass flow is being used the excess will escape through the blow-off valve which is fitted to the breathing bag. This valve also allows expanding air to escape during ascent. The experienced diver may wish to make full use of his breathing bag as a buoyancy control filling it when he wishes to rise and keeping it fairly empty if he wishes to remain on the bottom. This he can do by manual control of the relief valve. Notwithstanding these objections it is considered that the fitting of the reducer with a by-pass for personal bag inflation is a desirable safeguard and for beginners essential.

OXYGEN REQUIREMENT UNDER WATER

Movement under water is a very inefficient use of muscular effort and it must be admitted that man was not designed for this activity. Even when fins are used on the feet the achievement is not remarkable. Efforts to achieve speed greatly increase the oxygen content and the underwater swimmer, to get the best out of his resources, should be content with gentle cruising using his legs with fitted foot fins as his means of propulsion. Little effort is required just to keep moving but the lack of streamlining, especially when a bulky breathing apparatus is worn, restricts speed. Extra effort is required in underwater breathing and respiratory muscles may well have to work twice as hard for the same ventilation as on the surface (Chapter VI).

A number of measurements have been made of oxygen consumption in both surface and underwater swimming under various conditions and all are in good general agreement.

Pugh and Edholm (1955) have published figures for the oxygen consumption of Channel swimmers. They found a slow crawl required 2·17 litres per minute, a rapid crawl 2·96 litres per minute and for a moderate breast stroke 2·10 litres per minute.

Donald and Davidson (1954) completed a large series of oxygen uptake measurements with divers in different rig carrying out various work rates or swimming. Those in boots walking through thick mud used as much as 2·35 litres per minute but their highest demands were exceeded by swimming divers. Swimming with fins at $1\frac{1}{2}$ miles per hour the highest recorded oxygen consumption was 4·15 litres per minute with a mean of 3·16 litres per minute. At a speed of approximately 1 m.p.h. the mean consumption was only 2·02 litres per minute.

Lanphier (1954) found that underwater swimmers moving at 0·9 m.p.h. required 1–3 litres of oxygen per minute. Above this speed there was also a diminution in efficiency. Similar results were obtained by Goff, Frassetto and Specht (1956) where speeds of 0·7 to 0·9 m.p.h. showed an oxygen expenditure of 1·3 to 1·9 litres per minute.

From these uniform recordings by reliable and experienced workers there is no doubt whatever that underwater swimming is a most uneconomical activity as far as oxygen consumption is concerned. Moreover as has been mentioned in an earlier chapter the speeds which can be achieved are frequently exceeded by tides and currents.

Wherever possible the man in water should conserve energy and be content with speeds not in excess of 1 m.p.h. Rapid action is wasteful of energy owing to displacement of water. Movements should be slow and purposeful and emergencies should be faced with deliberation and calm. Rushed movements of near panic will be exhausting in the extreme and lessen chances of survival.

Such relatively low rates of progress obviously limit very greatly the swimmer's range of activity. This restriction can be overcome by towing from surface boats or underwater power-driven units. Perhaps dolphins, which have pulled King Neptune's chariot, may be tamed and trained to pull sub-aquatic man. Even today in the bars of the underwater swimmers' clubs tales are told of adventurous rides on the backs of Manta Rays, of help from seals and even encouragement from sharks. But what a flop the sea-horse is!

READING AND REFERENCES

Bannister, R. G. and D. J. C. Cunningham (1954). 'The Effects on the Respiration and Performance during Exercise of Adding Oxygen to Inspired Air.' *J. Physiol. 125*, 118.

Bean, J. W. (1945). 'Effects of Oxygen at High Pressure.' *Physiol. Rev. 25*, 1.

— (1955). 'Hormonal Aspects of Oxygen Toxicity.' Underwater Physiol. Symposium. National Academy of Sciences—National Research Council (U.S.A.). Publication 377.

Bert, P. (1878). *La Pression Barometrique*. Masson, Paris.

Cabarrou, P. (1960). 'The Work of the Committee for the Prevention of Free Diving Accidents.' *Sous Marine*. No. 25. February/March 1960.

Chapman, W. H., C. R. Sipe, D. C. Eltzholty, E. P. Cronkite and F. W. Chambers (1950). 'Sulphydryl-containing agents and Effects of Ionizing Radiations.' *Radiology. 55*, 865.

Dickens, F. (1946). 'The Toxic Effects of Oxygen on Brain Metabolism.' *Biochem. J. 40*, 145.

Donald, K. W. (1947). 'Oxygen Poisoning in Man.' *Brit. Med. J. 1*, 172.

Donald, K. W. and W. M. Davidson (1954). 'Oxygen Uptake of Divers.' *J. Applied Physiol. 7*, 31.

Gerschman, Rebecca, D. L. Gilbert, S. W. Nye, P. Dwyer, and W. O. Fenn (1954). 'Oxygen Poisoning and X-irradiation. A Mechanism in Common.' *Science. 119*, 623.

Goff, L. G., R. Frassetto and H. Specht. (1956). 'Oxygen Requirements of Underwater Swimming.' *J. Appl. Physiol. 9*, 219.

Grandpierre, R. and C. Franck. (1952). 'The Paradoxical Action of Oxygen.' *J. Aviation Med. 23* (2), 181.

Haugaard, N. (1955). 'Effect of High Oxygen Tensions upon Enzymes.' Underwater Physiol. Symposium. National Academy of Sciences —National Research Council (U.S.A.) Publication 377.

Lambertson, C. J. (1963). 'Physiological Effects of Oxygen.' Second Symposium on Underwater Physiology. National Academy of Sciences—National Research Council (U.S.A.). Publication 1181.

Lambertson, C. J., M. W. Stroud, J. H. Ewing and C. Mack (1953 a). 'Oxygen Toxicity Effects of Oxygen Breathing at Increased Ambient Pressures upon pCO_2 of Subcutaneous Gas Depots in Men, Dogs, Rabbits and Cats.' *J. Applied Physiol. 6*, 358.

Lambertson, C. J., R. H. Kough, D. Y. Cooper, G. L. Emmel, H. H. Loeschcke and C. F. Schmidt. (1953 b). 'Comparison of Relationship of Respiratory Minute Volume to pCO_2 and pH of Arterial and Internal Jugular Blood in Normal Man during Hyperventilation Produced by Low Concentrations of CO_2 at 1 Atmosphere and by O_2 at 3·0 Atmospheres.' *J. Applied Physiol. 5*, 803.

Lambertson, C. J., M. W. Stroud, R. A. Gould, R. H. Kough, J. H. Ewing and C. F. Schmidt (1953 c). 'Oxygen Toxicity and Respiratory Responses of Normal Men to Inhalation of 6 and 100 per cent oxygen under 3·5 atmospheres pressure.' *J. Applied Physiol. 5*, 487.

Lambertson, C. J., R. H. Kough, D. Y. Cooper, G. L. Emmel, H. H. Loeschcke and C. F. Schmidt (1953 d). 'Oxygen Toxicity, Effects in Men of Oxygen Inhalation at 1 and 3·5 Atmospheres upon Blood Gas Transport, Cerebral Circulation and Cerebral Metabolism.' *J. Applied Physiol. 5*, 471.

Lanphier, E. H. (1954). 'Oxygen Consumption in Underwater Swimmers' Federation Proceedings (U.S.A.) *13*, 84.

Lewis, B. M., L. Sokoloff, R. W. Wechsler, W. B. Wentz and S. S. Ketz (1956). 'Determination of Cerebral Blood Flow using Radioactive Krypton.' U.S. Naval Air Development Centre, Bu. Med. and Surg. Report No. 8.

Luft, U. C. and W. K. Naell. (1956). 'Brief Instantaneous Anoxia in Man.' *J. Applied Physiol. 8*, 444.

Miles, S. (1957). 'Oxygen Syncope.' *M.R.C. (RNPRC) Report U.P.S.* 161.

— (1957). 'The Problem of Hyperventilation in Divers.' *M.R.C. (RNPRC) Report U.P.S. 165.*

— (1957). 'Unconsciousness in Underwater Swimmers.' *M.R.C. (RNPRC) Report U.P.S.* 172.

Morgan, A. P. (1968). 'The Pulmonary Toxicity of Oxygen' Anaesthesiology. *29*, 570.

Patt, H. M., E. B. Tyree, R. L. Straule and D. E. Smith (1949). 'Cysteine Protection against X-irradiation.' *Science. 110*, 213.

Perot, P. L. Jnr. and S. N. Stein (1956). 'Conduction Block in Peripheral Nerve Produced by Oxygen at High Pressure.' *Science. 123*, 802.

Powell, T. J. (1956). 'Episodic Unconsciousness in Pilots During Flight.' *J. Av. Med. 27*, 301.

Priestley, J. (1774). *Experiments and Observations on Different Kinds of Air*. J. Johnson, London.

Pugh, L. G. C. and O. G. Edholm. (1955). 'The Physiology of Channel Swimmers.' *Lancet 269*, 761.

Rallon, M. (1960). *'La plongée en Union Sovietique'* (From Report on Underwater Conference Cannes, 1960). *Sous Marine. 28*, 298.

Smith, J. L. (1899). 'The Pathological Effects due to Increase of Oxygen Tension in the Air Breathed.' *J. Physiol. 24*, 19.

Stein, S. N. and P. L. Perst (1956). 'Conduction Block in Peripheral Nerve Produced by Oxygen at High Pressure'. *Science 123*, 802.

Taylor, H. J. (1949 a). 'The Effect of Breathing Oxygen at High Pressure on Tissue Oxygen and Carbon Dioxide Tensions.' *J. Physiol. 108*, 264.

— (1949 b). 'Role of Carbon Dioxide in Oxygen Poisoning.' *J. Physiol. 109*, 272.

Thomson, W. A. R. (1935). 'The Physiology of Deep-Sea Diving.' *Brit. Med. J. 2*, 208.

CHAPTER IX

Carbon Dioxide and Other Gases

PLAYING so great a part in the physiology of respiration it is inevitable that Carbon Dioxide should receive considerable attention in underwater medicine. Unfortunately there has been a wide tendency to regard this versatile gas as the underlying cause of many of the accidents and illnesses encountered in diving. In turn it has been blamed for nitrogen narcosis, oxygen poisoning, shallow water black-out and as contributory even to decompression sickness. When in some mishap no obvious cause can be found it is not unusual to find the incident described as one of carbon dioxide poisoning.

Carbon dioxide is not used for any purpose in diving. If it is present in excess this is due to some failure in equipment, for the body under normal conditions is well able to get rid of this waste product of metabolism.

The conditions under which carbon dioxide poisoning may occur are those which involve exposure to comparatively high percentages. At atmospheric pressure air to which is added 3% of carbon dioxide can be breathed for several days without much more than slight slowing of reflexes and some loss of efficiency. A 6% mixture will produce a marked increase in ventilation in about 15 minutes and if continued will cause mental confusion and lack of co-ordination. Pulse rate and blood pressure are also increased and extreme exertion becomes impossible. Increasing the percentage to ten or more quickly results in toxic effects; a slowing of pulse rate and a drop in blood pressure, later followed by unconsciousness, paralysis of the respiratory and cardiac centres and death.

The onset of carbon dioxide poisoning may be recognized by the victim by the early increase in respiration which is more marked with exercise. Simple tasks may be grossly exhausting or impossible. A severe headache, steadily worsening is a constant accompaniment and vomiting may occasionally occur. A flush of vaso-dilation is usually seen.

Exposure to very high concentration, 20%–40%, will result in an immediate convulsion, extensor spasm and death if maintained. A few breaths of such mixtures have been used to produce therapeutic convulsions.

In diving and underwater swimming the effects of carbon dioxide poisoning are only likely to be severe in conditions where in a closed circuit breathing set the carbon dioxide absorbing canister is inefficient or exhausted. In the standard diver an inadequate air supply may allow the gas to accumulate within the helmet. Heavy work may even cause breathlessness causing the diver to rest a while until excess carbon dioxide has been washed out. In each of these conditions a trained diver should recognize the condition and take emergency action.

Though acute carbon dioxide poisoning should be a rarity it is the subtle changes in the body following rises in alveolar pressure that must be considered in relation to the other respiratory gases and their effects.

CHANGES IN PRESSURE AND CARBON DIOXIDE

The normal alveolar pressure of carbon dioxide remains pretty constant at 40 mm.Hg and consequently oxygenated blood leaves the lung with its carbon dioxide content in equilibrium with this pressure. Venous blood arrives with a CO_2 pressure of about 46 mm.Hg and rapidly loses the excess.

Carbon dioxide has the facility for very rapid exchange with the blood and is carried in three ways, each 100 ml. of arterial blood containing—

43 ml. combined as bicarbonate,

3 ml. combined with the haemoglobin as carbamino haemoglobin,

and 2·4 ml. in simple solution.

In venous blood these three values are increased to 46, 3·7 and 2·7 ml. so that as far as the carriage of this gas from tissues to lung is concerned, 75% is as bicarbonate, $17\frac{1}{2}\%$ by the reduced haemoglobin and $7\frac{1}{2}\%$ is solution. In circumstances where pure oxygen is breathed under pressure and owing to an abundance of dissolved oxygen the oxyhaemoglobin is not reduced, the tissues may lose $17\frac{1}{2}\%$ of the facility for removing their excess CO_2. The retention which occurs however will also be occurring in the cells of the respiratory centre where its stimulating effect will promote a compensatory hyperventilation.

When man is under pressure either in a chamber or diving so long as there is no carbon dioxide in the inspired air and ventilation is adequate the partial pressure of CO_2 in the lungs will be the same as on the surface, i.e. 40 mm.Hg, for this is determined by the venous tension which reflects the amount produced in the tissues. The mechanism which regulates the tension in arterial blood, the chemo-receptors, and the respiratory centre ensure this. To make this point quite clear the percentages and partial pressures of gases in the alveoli can be compared when dry air is being breathed at the surface (1 atmosphere) and at 99 ft. (4 atmospheres).

	Surface		99 Feet	
	p.p. mm.Hg	%	p.p. mm.Hg	%
OXYGEN	100	13·1	439	14·5
NITROGEN	573	75·4	2514	82·7
WATER VAPOUR	47	6·2	47	1·5
CARBON DIOXIDE	40	5·3	40	1·3
	760	100·0	3040	100·0

The important observation from this table is that the percentage of carbon dioxide in the alveolar air is decreased with depth, being at 100 ft. only $1·3\%$. This is significant in that $1·3\%$ CO_2 which could be breathed indefinitely at the surface would, if supplied to a diver at 100 ft., cause the same embarrassment as a $5·3\%$ mixture on the surface. This change is of practical importance when escape from a sunken submarine is being planned. The normal procedure involves flooding a compartment in a submarine to compress the air it contains to that of the surrounding water. If as commonly happens after prolonged submergence there is a high, though not dangerous CO_2 concentration in the atmosphere this may rapidly become dangerous during flooding up. A 3% CO_2 content at the surface which could just be tolerated would be rapidly fatal at a depth of 100 ft. or more. Submarines are fitted with breathing apparatus for use under these conditions to avoid exposure to the atmosphere within the vessel when compressed.

For the same reason special attention must be paid to all diving apparatus to ensure that the inspired air is in no way contaminated with carbon dioxide.

CARBON DIOXIDE AND THE FREE DIVE

The dive where no breathing apparatus is used is an interesting one in which to study the carbon dioxide changes. Such a dive is limited by the ability to hold the breath which is dependent primarily on the CO_2 partial pressure rising to a threshold of 60 mm.Hg in the alveoli. The alveolar pressure of carbon dioxide does not rise appreciably due to descent but is absorbed by the circulating blood to maintain the partial pressure about 40 mm., any rise due to metabolic CO_2 occurring much in the same way as a person holding his breath on the surface.

This rise in alveolar CO_2 in the surface breath holder is due to accumulation of the gas from metabolic processes which will of course similarly occur during the dive. It is easier to appreciate the pressure effect alone by supposing that during the dive no further carbon dioxide is being produced in the tissues. The diver starting from the surface with an alveolar CO_2 partial pressure of 40 mm.Hg would if no further carbon dioxide passed into the blood reach 100 ft. with a CO_2 pressure of 160 mm.Hg. This of course is impossible and more CO_2 will dissolve in the blood to establish a new equilibrium. If the alveolar volume was 4 litres at the surface reducing to 1 litre at 100 ft. then for a partial pressure of 160 mm.Hg 53 ml. CO_2 approximately would be needed. To bring this down to 40 mm.Hg 40 ml. CO_2 would have to enter the blood. This, assuming the blood volume to be 5 litres, would only increase the volume of CO_2 in the circulating blood by 0·8 ml. per 100 ml. of which 5% would be in solution and the rest combined. Thus the actual increase of alveolar CO_2 partial pressure due to the dive alone would not exceed 1 mm.Hg. This for all intents and purposes can be neglected. It is necessary of course to add the metabolic carbon dioxide which is continually being produced. The free dive therefore is little different from breath holding on the surface. During ascent, too, the fall in carbon dioxide tension due to drop of pressure and expansion will require very little from the arriving blood to maintain its normal level.

It should be remembered however that in such a dive as this the oxygen partial pressure will be increased at depth and excess oxygen allows a greater tolerance to rising carbon dioxide. This has the effect of giving a longer breath-holding time than on the surface. It can indeed be compared with the increased breath-holding time which pure oxygen will give at atmospheric pressure.

CARBON DIOXIDE AND THE CLOSED CIRCUIT APPARATUS

If an apparatus can be constructed to avoid the waste of oxygen in expired air its endurance is considerably increased. Many attempts have been made to achieve this with some measure of success. Whatever method is used, pure oxygen or mixture, some means must be provided for the removal of expired carbon dioxide from the circuit.

In designing the absorbing unit consideration must be given to many factors. It must be capable of removing all the carbon dioxide even when the respiratory flow is at its maximum (a rate which is very much in excess of the minute volume). The resistance of air flow must be the absolute minimum compatible with efficient absorption. Packing must be carefully carried out to ensure that there will be no shifting of granules during use, for a badly packed canister easily forms channels through which gas may pass without adequate contact with the chemical.

The substance used for this purpose is Soda-lime, well known as a carbon dioxide absorber in anaesthetic apparatus. Size of granule is important for the smaller the granule the greater the surface area and the greater the efficiency. However, very fine granules offer considerable resistance to air flow and so a compromise is needed. An acceptable size is in the range of 2–4 millimetres. The soda-lime should be stored in air-tight tins, and be thoroughly dry and free from dust when used.

The container should be of sufficient size to contain $1\frac{1}{2}$–2 lb. soda-lime. (Two pounds has a life for average work under water of about $1\frac{1}{2}$ hours but this varies greatly with activity.) The shape of the canister must be designed to give the maximum distribution of air flow. Where both inspired and expired air pass through the canister its diameter may be greater than its depth but with one-way flows the reverse is used.

Much study has been made of canister design, granule size and methods of packing which will be referred to when apparatus is described in detail.

CARBON DIOXIDE IN CONFINED SPACES

Great care must be taken to avoid accumulation of carbon dioxide in such confined spaces as diving bells, pressure chambers and submarines. It is usually possible by knowing the number of men in the space, the amount of work being done and the volume of the space to calculate both the CO_2 build-up rate and the oxygen requirement. In bells and chambers it is possible to maintain a steady air exchange or do periodic replacements without alteration of internal pressure. In the submarine artificial means are needed both for oxygen production and carbon dioxide removal.

ADAPTATION TO CARBON DIOXIDE

The response of man to relatively small increases in carbon dioxide is widely variable from one individual to another and even one individual may under certain circumstances show a marked change in response.

Under identical laboratory conditions the effect on ventilation pattern of breathing air containing 6% carbon dioxide for 15 minutes has been studied in a hundred divers. The differences were unexpectedly great in that 19 showed an increase in ventilation of less than 25% whereas 15 had an increase of more than 150%. Between these two the remainder were more or less equally distributed.

When experiments were repeated with 6% CO_2 in oxygen there was a general decrease in the ventilatory reaction, only 3 exceeding a 150% increase. (The 'median' dropped from a 75% increase to a 60% increase.)

This latter finding agrees with the results of many other workers, namely that in the presence of an increased oxygen partial pressure the respiratory centre is less sensitive to excess carbon dioxide.

Although it was not statistically significant there was some indication that the subjects whose initial ventilation showed a rapid shallow pattern were more sensitive to carbon dioxide than those whose breathing was slow and deep. Schaefer (1954) showed in a similar investigation that using 70 subjects it was possible for their response to $5\frac{1}{2}\%$ and $7\frac{1}{2}\%$ CO_2 to divide them into two groups (i) low ventilators with large tidal volume and slow respiratory rate and (ii) high ventilators with small tidal volumes and rapid respiratory rates.

Schaefer further showed that a group of experienced underwater swimmers had a greater tolerance to carbon dioxide than a similar group of laboratory workers not trained underwater swimmers.

A study of the breathing patterns of experienced divers shows that the best amongst them have a natural slow deep breathing rhythm. This indicates a general tolerance to carbon dioxide which may well come with practice. Under water the slow deep respiration is less exhausting and more compatible with chest movement and breathing denser air. Furthermore as any apparatus used will introduce additional dead space a slow deep rhythm will be more economical in that the dead space wastage for total volume breathed will be less.

In conclusion let it be said once more that provided carbon dioxide can be eliminated from the inspired air and efficiently absorbed in a closed circuit breathing apparatus it is of no primary importance as a hazard in underwater medicine.

That it may temporarily enhance the effects of nitrogen narcosis and hasten the onset of oxygen poisoning cannot be denied but with proper use of efficient apparatus these effects too may be largely avoided.

In the formation of bubbles which occur in decompression sickness it must play its part as one of the gases which come out of solution when too rapid decompression is applied.

HAZARDS FROM OTHER GASES

Text-books of Industrial Medicine contain long lists of gases which may be dangerous to man. Where values for toxic concentrations are given these are based on the experience of the factory where work periods are limited and ventilation is possible.

In underwater medicine two situations arise which introduce additional risk. In the submarine, especially the nuclear powered, men are totally enclosed with no connection with the atmosphere for days or

even weeks. Under such circumstances any toxic agent however slow its
rate of production will, unless steps are taken to remove it, build up to a
dangerous concentration. A simple example is the carbon monoxide
from smoking. Even a moderate tobacco consumption by the crew
would produce highly dangerous levels within weeks. In the submarine
therefore every known toxic compound must be considered and where
present eliminated. A watch must be continually kept for new and
unexpected poisons.

The second way in which toxic gases may become increasingly effective is by increase in pressure. The results of this with regard to nitrogen,
oxygen, carbon dioxide, and some anaesthetic and inert gases have
already been mentioned. Increasing total pressure by increasing the
partial pressure of the individual gas therefore proportionately multi-
plies the rate at which it dissolves in the blood and thus enhances its
toxic effect.

Where compressed air or a mixture of gases is used for diving it is
essential that a standard of purity be enforced stricter than would be
applied to air purification at atmospheric pressure.

This may present some difficulty in practice in the re-charging of
cylinders for underwater breathing sets. For the amateur this is often
an expensive and tiresome business for he must be conscientious and
insist on pure dry air. Compressors may have electric-, diesel- or petrol-
driven engines and in each case an inlet tube is necessary to admit the
air which is to be compressed. The siting of this inlet during use is most
important, the biggest danger, when internal combustion engines are
used, being that of drawing in the carbon monoxide containing exhaust fumes. Only small quantities of carbon monoxide are tolerable.
Air containing as little as 100 parts per million would produce percep-
tible effects in 4 hours. At 100 ft. this would be dangerous, at 300 ft.
it would cause death. (Ten p.p.m. should therefore be used as the upper
limit rather than the usual 100 p.p.m.)

CARBON MONOXIDE poisoning must therefore be included as one of the
occupational hazards of diving resulting from failure to ensure that the
air supplied, either from a pump or cylinders, is free from traces of this
gas.

The onset of this condition is heralded by increasing weakness, exhaustion with breathlessness, dizziness and fainting. The lips and
mucous membranes may appear bright red but elsewhere pallor is usual.

Oxygen is essential in treatment and where there is unconsciousness
artificial means for resuscitation may be needed. Adding 6% carbon
dioxide to the oxygen will assist the elimination of carbon monoxide by

increasing ventilation. Failure to respond to this treatment within an hour or so indicates some severe brain damage from anoxia.

Another risk that may occur with all forms of compressors is the introduction of oil vapour into the compressed air. Oil fumes give a very unpleasant taste to the mixture breathed and if used under pressure the concentration may be sufficient to irritate the delicate membranes of the lungs giving a troublesome cough or in extreme cases pneumonia.

It is not always easy to eliminate oil completely from the compressing machinery and therefore the compressed air before being supplied to the diver or put into storage cylinders should be passed through alumina filters or their equivalent.

Air which contains a little moisture is usually more pleasant to breathe but dry air is kinder to equipment. Storage bottles and delicate valves are less likely to corrode. The drying of the air can usually be accomplished at the same time as the filtration.

It is quite likely that as a result of an insistence on a supply of perfectly pure dry air one may be accused of being fussy and it may be pointed out that there are many situations in general daily life when quite noxious samples of air are breathed, heavy with tobacco smoke, exhaust fumes, dust and all the atmospheric pollution of modern cosmopolitan life. Be that as it may, the diver under pressure is very sensitive to minor changes in respiratory gases, the lungs may already be irritated by increased oxygen partial pressures and an abnormal exchange balance established. The least that can be done to mitigate the results of increased pressure is to ensure that the increase is not at the same time being applied to any additional commonplace harassing agent.

READING AND REFERENCES

Schaefer, K. E. (1954). 'Group Differences in Carbon Dioxide Response of Human Subjects.' *Fed. Proc. (U.S.A.)*. *13*, 128.

Miles, S. (1957). 'Respiratory Patterns of 300 Divers.' *M.R.C. (RNPRC) Report U.P.S.* 164.

CHAPTER X

Vision, Hearing and Special Senses

IN an environment so completely different from the natural one it is quite certain that few of man's systems will escape its influence. The respiratory system which is the bridge between the old and new has been given its deserved attention. Many of the surprises which lie ahead for the underwater adventurer are due to the inability of the sensory nervous system to interpret accurately different stimuli against a background of physical change. To show this the senses may be taken one by one.

VISION

Without the aid of artificial light vision is dependent on the clarity of the water and the penetration of daylight which is dependent on depth and time of day. At midday in clear water it is possible to see what one is doing as deep as 250 ft. A considerable absorption of light by water is thus taking place, so much so that the intensity of daylight is reduced to $\frac{1}{4}$ at 15 ft. and to $\frac{1}{8}$ at 50 ft. Descents in bathyscaphes have shown 1,500 ft. to be about the limit of penetration of sunlight.

Even at the best of times underwater visibility is very greatly limited (in the clearest water to 100 ft.) but quite often suspended matter, e.g. stirred up mud, may reduce it almost to zero.

Colours too are deceptive for the light is unevenly absorbed, so that objects on the bottom may have quite a different colour when removed from the water. Blue light penetrates further while red light is absorbed first as a result of which a dull looking pebble on the bottom might be bright red on removal from the water.

Comparative studies by Kinney, Luria and Weitzman (1967) show that the easiest colour to see in turbid waters is fluorescent orange followed by white, yellow, orange and red. In clear water fluorescent greens and white are best. Grey and black are most difficult to see and others with poor visibility are orange and red in clear water and blue and green in murky water. It is also more difficult to distinguish colours from one another e.g. black from red in clear water or blue from black in turbid water.

Artificial light can be and is in fact often used under water. The best colour is a mid-spectrum yellow which is a compromise between red which is largely absorbed and blue which is abundantly reflected from suspended particles. Even artificial light is not much help in muddy water but there is a simple device which can be used for inspection where necessary. The diver is supplied with a tapering tube, rather like a megaphone, 18 to 24 inches long with plain glass at either end. This is filled with clean water and with the eye against the narrow end objects near the larger end can be clearly seen. Clear water must be used rather than air which would make the instrument too buoyant and need extra strength to withstand pressure differences. (This very simple gadget was invented by a Dr Glass and is known by his diving friends as the 'Glass-Eye'.)

Underwater, not only is vision reduced by the diminished intensity of light but when water is in direct contact with the anterior surface of the cornea there is a considerable loss of refracting power so that a visual acuity of 6/6 is reduced to 6/60.

The eyes need some protection from the irritation and direct contact of water. This can be achieved with goggles, face mask or even contact lenses. Not only is the eye protected but if an air space is introduced in front of the cornea refraction is restored and visual acuity returns to normal.

The introduction of an air space in front of the eye does mean that

REFRACTION OF LIGHT WATER TO AIR

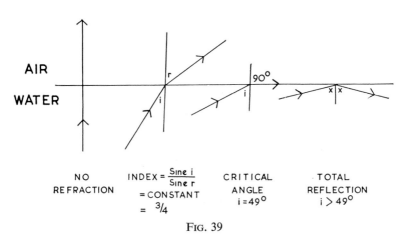

Fig. 39

light waves leaving an object in the water must before reaching the eye pass from water into air. The change in density at the interface causes all but perpendicular rays to be distorted. This change is known as refraction and is different for all media through which light may pass and dependent upon the REFRACTIVE INDEX of that medium. The refractive index is the ratio between the sine of the angle of incidence (sine i) and the sine of the angle of refraction (sine r). The index for the various media is obtained by passing light from a vacuum into the medium and for each the index is constant. (See Fig. 39.) The diamond owes its position as a precious stone to its high refractive index of 2·6 as compared with glass 1·5 and water 1·3. Air and gases in general have very low refractive indices (air is 1·0003).

Apart from the sparkle and the dancing colours of ruffled water, the refraction of light passing from water through air before reaching the eyes causes objects to be somewhat distorted and to appear nearer than they really are. The eyes follow back the light rays along the direction which they are taking as they enter the eyes. The angle of divergence of rays passing from water to air is increased by refraction so that they appear to be coming from a nearer point than their actual origin (Fig. 40). In fact they appear to be only about three-quarters of their actual distance away. Though at first the visual distortion presents a very strange and deceptive world the diver very soon learns to adjust his sense of distance and has little difficulty in carrying out his underwater duties.

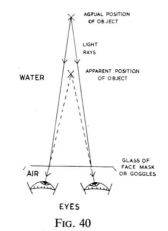

DISPLACEMENT OF IMAGE IN WATER

FIG. 40

GOGGLES AND MASKS

If the eyes are to be of any real use under water they must be protected by goggles or mask and aided by an intervening air space. Masks vary with apparatus and may be large to include the whole face (face masks), or small, covering only the area of the eyes and bridge of the nose (swim masks).

The windows of the goggles or masks must be flat, for a curved surface separating the water and air causes a fanning of refraction and gross distortion. In most cases they are single flat panes of glass or perspex in a rubber frame but in some there may be side pieces coming back at right angles to the front piece to give lateral vision.

VISUAL FIELDS IN WATER WITH GOGGLES

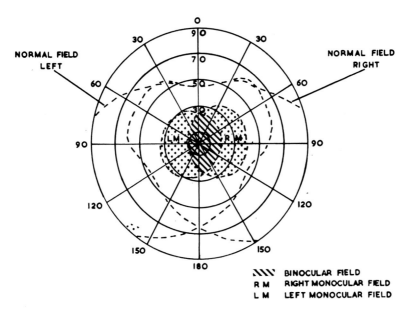

FIG. 41

In most forms of goggles and masks there is considerable restriction of the field of vision due to the frame as well as a diminution of field from refraction.

Barnard (1961) has modified a perimeter for use under water and has charted visual fields with goggles and swim masks in air and under water. Figure 41 shows the binocular and monocular fields of a subject wearing goggles under water. Compared with the normal fields the reduction is very marked. In Figure 42 the underwater visual fields have been plotted for the swim mask and although still greatly restricted the field is considerably larger than that with the goggles. It is interesting in

VISUAL FIELDS IN WATER. SWIM MASK

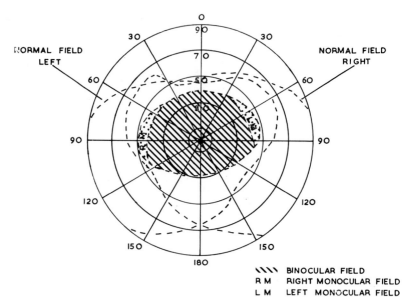

BINOCULAR FIELD
R M   RIGHT MONOCULAR FIELD
L M   LEFT MONOCULAR FIELD

FIG. 42

VISUAL FIELDS IN AIR AND WATER (GOGGLES)

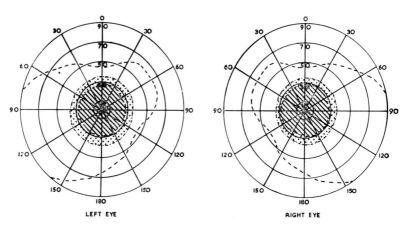

WATER
AIR

FIG. 43

this case to observe that owing to the lateral blinker effect there is a cross-over in monocular vision. Finally Barnard showed (Fig. 43) with goggles the extent the visual field is reduced under water. Luria (1968) also concludes that the loss of peripheral visual cues underwater is a significant cause of the drop in stereoscopic acuity.

Under water the swimmer, being horizontal, is particularly dependent on the upper zones of the visual fields and, compared with the normal, restriction is not great, particularly with the mask. The lower half of the field is much less important but in mask and goggle design there is need to improve the lateral vision. Wide vision face masks will to some extent help provided the distortion of a curved surface can be overcome.

Before leaving the problem of refraction it should be noted that no notice has been taken of any refraction occurring as light passes through the actual glass between the water and air. This change can be neglected as the refractive indices of water and glass are very close. Also many of the windows are made of perspex whose index is almost the same as water.

CONTACT LENSES

An obvious alternative to the goggles and masks would seem to be the contact lens. Even so the need still remains to present a flat surface to the water and to introduce a pocket of air between the water and the cornea. This means the construction of a special lens with an air pocket within, moulded to fit the eye yet having a flattened area in front of the pocket. Glass (1958) has experimented with such lenses and recommends that the fenestration, through which contact lenses normally allow the cornea to 'breathe', should include a tantalum gauze filter.

Whether or not there is a future for the contact lens under water is uncertain. Certainly it will give a good visual field but at present its manufacture is a costly process. Glass comments that 'whereas contact lenses could never replace goggles for general use they could be worn under water for several hours where circumstances make the use of goggles undesirable'.

HEARING

Sound in water travels at 4,700 ft. per second which is very much faster than its speed of 1,090 ft. per second in air. It also travels great distances, a fact which is made full use of in naval underwater listening devices and in echo sounding. A diver underneath a ship can hear very clearly the noises on board, the footsteps of men on metal plates, machinery, the clatter of dropped tools and even the mumble of voices. Underwater swimmers are able, if they are wearing face masks and can temporarily let go the mouth-piece, to talk to one another quite freely. Ships' engines and underwater explosions can be heard at great distances but there are also many natural underwater sounds, the breaking of waves, the shifting of shingle, whispering seaweed and even the faint crackling of crabs as they snap at food and scurry among the rocks. Fishes are said to communicate by sound but use frequencies above the range of the human ear.

In air man is able fairly accurately to locate the direction from which sound is coming. He does this by turning his head until both ears are equidistant from the source and the sound is synchronized in each. The increased speed of sound under water makes this virtually impossible. Attempts to counter this by using horn-like extensions in each ear have not been very successful.

Briefly then it may be said that sound in water has a greater range and speed but localization of the source is generally impossible.

In addition there is great scope for research into the effects and possible uses under water of supersonic and ultrasonic vibrations as aids to navigation, detection and communication.

COMMUNICATION

When air is breathed under pressure, changes in the voice, possibly in extreme cases exaggerated by nitrogen narcosis, make direct communication more difficult, especially over a telephone.

As deep diving and residence in pressurized compartments develops with the use of oxy-helium mixtures the distortion which this produces in the voice makes normal conversation extremely difficult. It causes an upward shift in the frequency spectrum. Although after a time there is some adaptation and improvement efforts are necessary to counter this inconvenience by artificial means.

Sergeant (1968) has shown that there are two possible ways in which a higher degree of intelligibility may be achieved. The first uses a high-fidelity microphone and recording system which is played back to the listener at half speed thus lowering the frequency. This has a disadvantage in the delay of message transfer. The second technique uses a commercial instrument, the 'Varivox' produced by the Kay Electric Company of New Jersey, which itself gives an 'on time' playback thus allowing instant communication. The quality however is not as good as that of the former method.

DEAFNESS IN DIVERS AND CAISSON WORKERS

The simplest, and a not uncommon form of deafness in divers results from a failure to obtain good equalization of pressure either side of the tympanic membrane, usually associated with some Eustachian catarrh or inexperience in 'clearing' the ears. Such deafness is incomplete and temporary, recovery being complete on pressure equalization. Repeated trauma may of course produce more permanent deafness but this is uncommon in experienced divers who quickly become conscious of the importance of efficient aural pressure equalization in their work.

Occasions have arisen too when, as a result of too rapid decompression, nitrogen bubbles have formed in the fluids of the inner ear. This again is usually a temporary condition.

Many reports have been made suggesting that deafness may be a risk in Caisson workers. (Lister and Gomez, 1898; Almour, 1942.) The evidence is not convincing however as in many cases no check is made for deafness before employing the men and the use of noisy tools is far more likely to be a cause. Schilling and Everley (1942) examined a large number of submarine personnel and found deafness due to noise from diesel engines. More recently Coles and Knight (1960) carried out a careful audiometric examination of 62 divers and underwater instructors. Their conclusions were that there was no evidence that repeated minor barotraumatic incidents produced chronic deafness and that deafness was not a complication of normal diving.

Mention should also be made of noise in pressure chambers. Coles (1963 and 1964) has shown that in many chambers the noise of inrushing air is above acceptable limits and silencers should be fitted to the inlets.

CARE OF THE EARS UNDER WATER

The ear is a delicate and valuable organ and it is only right that everything should be done to protect it under water. It has already been stated that the potential diver should be free from any catarrhal condition and able to clear his ears without difficulty. A common cold, catarrh or upper respiratory tract infection should preclude the sufferer from going under water. Not only may such conditions cause ear pain but there is always the risk of producing a middle ear infection. Various decongestive sprays and drops have been recommended to make ear clearing possible under such conditions but it is much safer and more satisfactory, unless it is essential to go under water, to wait until the condition has resolved.

Where actual damage to the ear has been caused, as may be indicated by hyperaemia of the drum or haemorrhage, the condition should be allowed to recover completely before re-entering the water. This may take six weeks to three months and the advice of the expert should be sought.

The external ear too needs some attention. Excessive wax must be removed and on no account must plugs of wool or ear defenders be used. These may be forced further into the ear with increasing pressure, cause damage, and be difficult to remove. The danger of a tight-fitting helmet as a cause of 'reversed ears' has already been mentioned (Chapter V).

In some parts of the world, particularly in the tropics, the sea may contain fine particles of sand or coral which may irritate the outer ear. This may be followed by infection particularly if the ear has been vigorously poked with a dirty finger or the twisted corner of a grubby towel. Such infections are often difficult to treat and amateur applications of various antiseptic drops and wicks are rarely successful. The help of the expert must be sought when frequent careful cleansing with sterile swabs and specific treatment of the infection will produce the cure.

Ears need not be a problem under water provided common sense is used in understanding and countering the risks together with a strict observance of the basic principles of hygiene.

THE SENSE OF POSITION

In water there is no effort required to maintain posture, righting reflexes do not exist and muscles which normally are responsible for posture and balance are relaxed. When blindfolded and still, the sense of position is soon lost and a sense of disorientation not unlike that experienced in extremely high-altitude flying develops.

The underwater swimmer is largely dependent upon visual sensations for his navigation. The lighter water above him indicates the position of the surface and ascending streams of bubbles give him a vertical. Take away these and he is soon lost, he may swim round in circles, he may unwittingly increase his depth or even turn over. Many occasions have been reported, especially in the dark, where a swimmer, even an experienced one, presuming to be travelling along an even course has found himself on the bottom very many feet below his intended depth. Such loss of direction could be dangerous especially if an oxygen set were in use, in that it would be easily possible accidentally to exceed a safe depth.

For safety and accuracy the swimmer must rely on artificial aids such as the depth gauge and compass or from time to time break surface in order to get a bearing. Wherever possible the divers should maintain contact with surface craft either by a life-line or by themselves carrying a line with a surface float attached which will at least give them a known depth and allow them to be followed above. It is better that they should work in groups or pairs even linked together by a 'buddy' line. Currents too, may easily deflect the swimmer's course.

TASTE

Little can be said about taste; there is no evidence that it is altered by pressure other than possibly some loss of keenness with nitrogen narcosis.

There have been occasional accidents when sea water has been introduced into a self-contained breathing set and fouled the carbon dioxide absorbing canister. It is then possible to draw such water into the mouth when a very unpleasant burning taste results. This 'soda-lime cocktail' as it is called by the divers can indeed produce an alkaline burn of the lips and mouth.

Case and Haldane (1942) whilst carrying out a series of trials with air and oxygen at high pressure found that some subjects were able to taste both oxygen and nitrogen. Oxygen breathed at 6–7 atmospheres had a peculiar taste 'like dilute ginger beer' or 'dilute ink with a little sugar'.

Other subjects breathing air at 8–10 atmospheres complained of a harsh metallic taste. A mixture of helium and oxygen at this pressure did not have this taste which was therefore attributed to the nitrogen.

Though unimportant the sense of taste may be useful in recognizing an impurity in a breathing mixture such as oil vapour from a compressor but it cannot of course give any indication of the presence of carbon monoxide.

READING AND REFERENCES

Almour, R. (1942). 'Industrial Otology in Caisson Workers.' *New York State J. Med. 42*, 779.

Barnard, E. E. P. (1961). 'Underwater Visual Problems.' *Proc. Roy. Soc. Med. 54*, 755.

Case, E. M. and J. B. S. Haldane. (1942). 'Tastes of Oxygen and Nitrogen at High Pressures.' *Nature. 148*, 84.

Coles, R. R. A. (1963 and 1964). 'Noise Hazards in and Silencing of Pressure Chambers.' R.N. Medical School Reports 5/63 and 5/65.

Coles, R. R. A. and J. J. Knight (1960). 'Report on an Aural and Audio-metric Survey of Qualified Divers and Submarine Escape Training Tank Instructors.' *M.R.C. (RNPRC) Report He.S.* 29.

Glass, A. (1958). 'Trials of a Modified Underwater Contact Lens.' *M.R.C. (RNPRC) Report U.P.S.* 36.

Kinney, J. A. S., S. M. Luria and D. O. Weitzman (1967). 'The Visibility of Colours Underwater'. U.S. Naval Submarine Medical Center, Groton. Report No. 503.

Lister, J. C. and V. Gomez. (1898). 'Observations made in the Caisson of the New East River Bridge as to the effects of Compressed Air upon the Human Ear.' *Arch. Otol. N.Y. 27,* 1.

Luria, S. M. (1968). 'Stereoscopic Acuity Underwater'. U.S. Naval Submarine Medical Center, Groton. Report No. 510.

Schilling, C. W. and I. A. Everley (1942). 'Auditory Acuity among Submarine Personnel.' *Nav. Med. Bull. 40, Wash.* 664.

Sergeant, R. L. (1968). 'Improving the Intelligibility of Helium Speech'. U.S. Naval Submarine Medical Center, Groton. Memorandum No. 68–1.

CHAPTER XI

Decompression

M AN cannot go under water without experiencing increase in his environmental pressure. He cannot return to the surface without undergoing decompression. The processes by which he becomes adapted to depth must be reversed. Within modest limits of depth and time this can be achieved without difficulty, discomfort or damage. Unfortunately useful diving usually exceeds these limits and, unless precautions are taken on completion of the dive, the distressing condition of Decompression Sickness will occur.

As pressure increases during descent the respiratory gases are absorbed by the blood in increasing quantities and distributed throughout the tissues of the body in which they accumulate. This route taken by the gases, lungs–blood–tissue, is a simple and direct adjustment to their increased alveolar partial pressures. When the falling pressure of the ascent occurs the gases are carried from the tissues by the blood back to the lungs. This reversed route, tissue–blood–lungs, may not always be able to carry away quickly enough the gases liberated in the tissues.

With prolonged stay under pressure the rate at which gases diffuse into the tissues slowly decreases as the partial pressures of the already dissolved gases increase thus narrowing the pressure differences between lungs, blood and tissues. In time these pressures will become virtually equal so that no further gases will be absorbed. When this state of equilibrium has been reached the tissues are said to be 'saturated' for that particular pressure, just as on the surface the tissues are 'saturated' at atmospheric pressure. Saturation at increased pressure is sometimes referred to as 'Super-saturation'.

The time taken to achieve super-saturation will depend on the pressure applied. As the rate of absorption of excess gases is directly proportional to the pressure difference it follows that the transfer is rapid at first and finally becomes very much slowed down. Theoretically it never actually reaches 100%. For this reason it is convenient in calculations to consider 'half-times' for saturation, i.e. the time taken at a given pressure to achieve 50% saturation.

In practice several hours are required to reach acceptable saturation. Once this is achieved return to atmospheric pressure, though it may need a considerable period of decompression, is not affected by further even prolonged stay at pressure. This is the fundamental principle of the new technique of saturation diving.

If tissues have taken up a heavy load of excess gas this may on release of pressure come out of solution before it can be carried away and actually form bubbles. Such bubble formation, which may occur in many sites, at different rates and to various extents, is basically the cause of Decompression Sickness.

DECOMPRESSION SICKNESS

In its broadest sense decompression sickness must include any abnormality which is the direct result of reduction of environmental pressure. It can vary from the acute effects of explosive decompression in aviators to the chronic disabilities of caisson workers. It includes the burst lung of free ascent, the frightening paralysis of spinal bends and the transient itches and rashes of ill-timed dives. Burst lung has already been considered and the decompression illnesses and accidents in aviation medicine, having no true parallel under water, may for the time being be dismissed. What remains then is the Decompression Sickness which is the major occupational hazard of the diver and the caisson worker.

HISTORICAL

Over a hundred years ago Bucquoy (1861) published what was probably the first full account of the hazards of working in compressed air and the need for slow decompression. During the years which followed a large number of major engineering projects involving the use of caissons gave physiologists and physicians an opportunity to study the condition. (Oliver, 1904; Hill, 1912; Keays, 1912; Schilling, 1941; and Rainsford, 1942.) Little being known of the cause in these early days, many cases of decompression sickness occurred. Pain was the common manifestation, often severe, usually in joints and frequently shifting. Workers were rarely subjected to more than 35 lb. per sq. inch pressure ($3\frac{1}{2}$ atmospheres absolute) and symptoms usually occurred quite soon after release of pressure though occasionally they were delayed several hours. As well as pains, a wide range of nervous disorders occurred, paralyses, motor disturbances, anaesthesia and occasionally signs of cerebral irritation. The greater the working depths the more severe were the decompression effects. It was found by experience that a return to pressure would relieve the pain and in more recent high-pressure construction work compression chambers are provided for this treatment. In diving a similar picture was found, though divers on the whole were exposed to much greater pressures for shorter times. Symptoms were usually more severe and involvement of the central nervous system more frequent.

Paul Bert (1878) carried out experiments with animals, subjecting them to decompression after long periods under pressure and concluded that compressed air illness was due to the liberation of nitrogen in the form of bubbles in the blood and tissues. Boycott and Damant (1908) showed that fat animals were more liable to decompression sickness than thin ones and concluded that fat acted as a reservoir for nitrogen. Nitrogen was in fact known to be five times more soluble in oil than water. Haldane and Priestley (1935) also reported the presence of bubbles of gas in the mesentery of a goat after rapid decompression. Haldane (1922) had previously recommended to the Admiralty a method of decompression by stages and his 'tables', which came to be widely accepted, have stood the test of time very well. Present day diving tables do not differ greatly from them through some modifications have been made especially for prolonged deep dives.

In recent years investigations into the problem of decompression have continued. In 1952, Hempleman, Crocker and Taylor put forward new ideas for calculating decompression tables and in 1955 Rashbass also published new tables. These showed too high an incidence of decompression sickness during the sea trials and revised tables were later produced by Crocker (1957) which are in use today though for very long deep dives further tests are needed.

As deep diving becomes big business and helium is used in increasing amounts there is a growing demand for more efficient decompression schedules. Divers being human beings are prepared on occasions to take personal risks for greater gain and resulting attacks of decompression sickness place an unwelcome strain on the limited number of therapeutic treatment centres.

In the parallel field on land of compressed air engineering, research is becoming highly organized (Golding, Campbell, Griffiths, Hempleman, Paton and Walder (1960). An international working party met in London in 1965 to study decompression problems in Compressed Air Workers. It was apparent that, in this somewhat hazardous occupation, there was a need for greater care with decompression schedules and medical follow ups. The Proceedings have been edited by McCullum (1965) and published.

DECOMPRESSION SICKNESS — THE CLINICAL PICTURE

Any complaint however vague or unusual following exposure to pressure should be regarded and indeed treated as Decompression Sickness until proved otherwise. In practice however the term is used only for those conditions which result from the effect of reduced environmental pressure on blood, body fluids and tissues. It is generally presumed that these are caused by the liberation of excess gas with bubble formation. This definition thus does not, strictly speaking, include the condition of Pulmonary Barotrauma which is caused primarily by the physical effect of expanding gas which though within the respiratory system is outside, e.g. not dissolved in, any tissue. It is usual therefore to consider this condition quite separately.

ACUTE DECOMPRESSION SICKNESS

The early signs and symptoms of decompression sickness are commonly divided into Type I and Type II. This somewhat artificial separation has a practical advantage with regard to choice of treatment. The first represents the illness when presenting peripherally and the second the central and potentially more dangerous condition.

TYPE I.

(a) *Pain* is the most common feature being present in almost 90% of all cases of decompression sickness. It may vary from very mild pain in the limbs 'NIGGLES' to a very severe joint pain 'BENDS'. The pain usually takes the form of a slowly developing dull ache in or near a joint. It may be preceded by tenderness or numbness in the area and a pallor of overlying skin. Frequently there is also a general feeling of exhaustion sometimes with chill, sweating or fever.

(b) *Skin Involvement.* Quite commonly in decompression sickness, the first indication of the condition may be a localized burning or tingling itch which may spread over quite large areas though it usually becomes localized again. Such localization may be followed by the pain of a 'bend'. As well as the itching, a blotchy marbling rash may be present. These symptoms are common after short deep dives and rare after long shallow ones and may be the only evidence of decompression sickness indicating no more than a too rapid decompression.

The pathology of the condition is somewhat obscure but is most likely due to bubble formation in skin capillaries with rupture, haemorrhage and direct stimulation of sensory nerve endings. It has its parallel in the irritation of the lungs with 'chokes'. It is even possible that air may have entered the subcutaneous tissues by direct penetration of the skin under pressure and dissolved in the fat of sebaceous glands.

TYPE II

The onset of this type of decompression sickness is often more vague including all manner of subjective sensations,—epigastric pain, headache, angina, vertigo or actual signs of organic malfunction. By and large however most of the cases fall into either Central Nervous System or Pulmonary effects.

(a) *Paralyses.* Fortunately the involvement of the central nervous system is much rarer, usually occurring after grossly inadequate decompression from the deeper dives. The overall incidence is not more than 5% and even this includes a large proportion of cases where the only manifestation is giddiness, transient deafness or a visual disturbance. Paralysis more commonly occurs in one or both legs, is spastic in type and usually transitory. The picture is generally one suggesting a local involvement of the spinal cord but occasional cerebral symptoms may occur such as convulsions, aphasia or visual disturbances. Permanent brain damage is rare but degeneration in the cord may be permanent. It is not easy to give a finite picture of the effects of decompression on the cerebral nervous system, for the greater the number of cases studied the longer becomes the list of symptoms. Almost every possibility has been described, including changes in mood, sensory effects, anaesthesias and word blindness.

The effect on the legs and consequently the gait which may occur has resulted in this condition being called the 'STAGGERS'.

(b) *Pulmonary Effects.* Acute shortness of breath, substernal pain especially on inspiration and paroxysms of coughing may herald collapse, shock, and asphyxia. With the increasing dyspnoea the pulse, at first rapid, becomes feeble and an ashen grey pallor or cyanosis may develop. Unconsciousness may follow. This acute and serious happening may occur in conjunction with other symptoms in a severe attack of decompression sickness or it may be delayed in cases where a decompression routine has been inadequate. It may appear where other manifestations have not occurred or have been ignored. In such cases, which do not exceed 2%, there has been an accumulation of gas bubbles in the capillaries of the pulmonary circulation. This condition has been described in aviation in high-altitude selection tests where candidates are rapidly exposed in a decompression chamber, to an equivalent altitude of 37,000 ft. (Parsons, 1958). In both Aviation Medicine and Underwater Medicine this picture is known as the 'CHOKES'.

CHRONIC DECOMPRESSION SICKNESS

The more serious cases which involve various degrees of hemiplegia or paraplegia invariably condemn the patient to years of disability. Response to prolonged physiotherapy and rehabilitation is extremely rewarding, recovery often exceeding earlier expectations. Psychiatric changes may also occur but these are difficult to assess.

In recent years, largely as a result of increasing medical care of caisson workers, attention has been directed to the very real complication of Aseptic Necrosis of Bone found on routine examination of joints and long bones. This may in time cause joint deformity and arthritic changes. The present incidence is causing some concern. For example at the Clyde Tunnel Workings the lesions were found in 20% of men on completion of contract though only 4% were likely to have resulting disability (McCullum—1968). It is usually assumed that this condition, like other lesions of decompression sickness results from bubbles of nitrogen producing infacts in bones. There is no proof of this and it may well be that other mechanisms are involved.

Though of great interest today aseptic bone necrosis was described by James (1945) in three survivors from a submarine disaster who were exposed to rapid decompression and severe bends. They developed bone necrosis twelve years later. The condition is far more common in tunnel workers than divers though recently the discovery of a few cases among the latter (Fig. 44) has led to a much more careful radiological screening of professional divers. It is generally believed that inadequate or delayed treatment of a case of 'bends' is a predisposing factor.

THE TIME FACTOR

Generally speaking the signs of onset of decompression sickness occur shortly after completion of the decompression, the majority (85%) within the hour and half within 30 minutes. A few may even show signs during the actual decompression. Only 1% are delayed beyond six hours.

DIAGNOSIS

In commercial and naval diving or caisson work there is usually experienced medical advice available and diagnosis is not difficult. Nevertheless any complaint or abnormal behaviour observed after exposure to pressure, should be seriously considered. Details of the exposure and the decompression should be recorded for this may well give an immediate indication as to whether the patient has been at risk or not. It will be seen later that there is quite an extensive range of time and depth which can be accomplished without need for controlled decompression.

Itches, rashes, pains, respiratory distress, visual defects, paralyses, and signs of cerebro-spinal irritation are all strongly indicative of decompression illness.

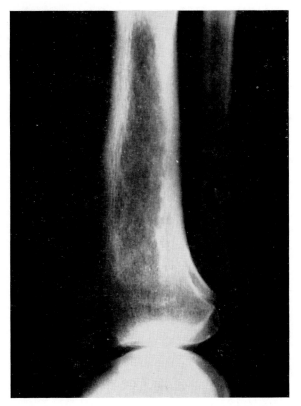

Fig. 44. Aseptic bone necroses in tibia of a diver.

The diagnosis may only satisfactorily be confirmed by subjecting the patient once more to an increase in pressure when the signs and symptoms should disappear. This is best done in a pressure chamber but if one is not available the diver can be lowered under water again. The rationale of this diagnosis is that since decompression allowed bubble formation, recompression should reduce the size of these bubbles, aid

12

their re-absorption so removing their local affect. If the signs and symptoms do not disappear after adequate recompression they are unlikely to be due to decompression sickness.

TREATMENT OF DECOMPRESSION SICKNESS

Itches and rashes alone need no special treatment and will soon disappear. All other signs and symptoms should be recompressed. An exception may be made sometimes of mild pains which will respond to rest, hot baths and aspirin. The decision to take this course can only be made by a medical attendant with experience of the condition but it does have the advantage of saving many hours of tedious treatment.

The possibility that, in the long run, inadequate treatment may lead to aseptic bone necrosis should however always be considered.

Where recompression is needed special Therapeutic Decompression Tables are used as will be explained. Briefly however the technique depends on firstly whether pain is the only symptom or whether in addition there are more serious indications such as unconsciousness, convulsions, paralyses, air embolism, motor or sensory disturbances, severe breathlessness or pain occurring whilst still under pressure. This gives two groups (i) Pain only (Type I) and (ii) Serious symptoms (Type II). In both cases the patient is put in the chamber and rapidly recompressed.

The pressure applied does not exceed an equivalent of 165 ft. but the pattern of subsequent decompression is dictated by the effect of the re-pressurization on the clinical picture. It may be for as little as $6\frac{1}{4}$ hours or as long as 38 hours. These may seem very long periods in a pressure chamber but it takes much longer to get rid of a bubble than to prevent it forming. Also if things do not go well during treatment even longer may be needed. Golding and his colleagues (1960) describe a case of decompression sickness where it was necessary to keep the patient in the pressure chamber for $9\frac{1}{2}$ days.

PREVENTION

Wherever men must work under pressure it is necessary to protect them from the risk of decompression sickness. They must be decompressed in such a manner that excess gases may escape from tissues without forming bubbles. For deep and prolonged exposures this can be a time-consuming practice but at present there seems to be no alternative though attempts are continually being made to shorten the times involved. Today decompression tables are available to meet the requirements of both caisson work and diving. If they are followed accurately decompression sickness should be very rare. Severe cases are very rarely seen and the incidence in diving is about 1% and in the Dartford Tunnel project only 0·6%.

The decompression routine is one in which the diver ascends through the water by steps, or pauses 10 ft. apart and increasing in time as he nears the surface. A large proportion of diving time would thus be spent in the water but many ways are being developed to lessen this. After deep dives for example the diver may be met by a diving bell or submersible decompression chamber (Fig. 16) which he can enter at the equivalent pressure of his depth. The chamber is then closed and hoisted on board ship without further reduction in pressure. The diver can then be stage decompressed within the bell or transferred directly under pressure to a larger chamber. By these means the process of decompression can be completed in relative comfort.

Another method which is showing great promise is Surface Decompression in which a diver having finished his work surfaces directly and, as quickly as possible, is placed in a chamber for immediate recompression followed by decompression to a pre-arranged schedule. This is of especial value to the self-contained diver for whom the endurance of the breathing apparatus is limited and on which prolonged underwater decompression makes a heavy demand.

The caisson worker who is normally under dry conditions throughout has a similar decompression schedule which he completes in an air lock between his working environment and the surface.

These various routines will be further described but before this is done it is necessary to study the theory and investigation which has led to the development of the decompression tables.

THE DECOMPRESSION TABLES

There is ample evidence that decompression sickness is due to the formation of gas bubbles in the tissues during decompression and the decompression tables represent an attempt to provide routines by which a diver or caisson worker may, on completion of his work, be decompressed in such a manner that excess dissolved gases may be got rid of without this bubble formation.

To appreciate how these tables work it is necessary to follow the disposal of excess gases as they are dissolved. The whole heart-breaking problem of decompression stems from the simple fact that the way the respiratory gases leave the body on decompression is by no means the reverse of the way they enter during compression.

When pressure is increased all the gases in the lung, and nitrogen in particular, will dissolve in greater quantity in the blood to be carried amongst the tissues and diffuse into them until a new equilibrium is reached. When the pressure drops the excess gases leave the blood as it passes through the lungs. That in the tissues returns to the blood-stream and is similarly lost. If there is a rapid drop in pressure the excess gas in the tissues may not escape quickly enough to reach the blood and consequently form bubbles within the tissues. This situation can be conveniently compared with the soda-water siphon which is charged from a small cylinder. The container is filled with water and the pressure of carbon dioxide released above it causes an excess of gas to dissolve in the water. The gas can only enter the water through its surface just as the pressurized respiratory gases can only enter the body through the lungs. When the pressure in the siphon is released by pressing the lever the excess carbon dioxide forms bubbles in the water before it can es-cape at the surface. In man though gases can only reach tissues via lung and blood they may be able on sudden release of pressure to form bubbles within the blood or tissues.

It is simpler at this stage to consider nitrogen alone, though both carbon dioxide and oxygen will be seen to play their part in the final picture.

THE DISTRIBUTION OF NITROGEN

At atmospheric pressure there is an equilibrium between the partial pressure of nitrogen in the lungs, the amount dissolved in the circulating blood and that contained in the tissues.

The whole object of the circulation is to bring oxygen into intimate contact with the tissues and remove carbon dioxide therefrom. Thus any nitrogen increase will be equally widely distributed and have oppor-tunity quite quickly to re-establish equilibrium throughout the vas-cular tissues. In tissues where metabolism takes place in an aqueous medium there will be a relatively rapid response in nitrogen absorption to changes in the blood. This will also equally reflect changes in alveolar partial pressures. There are however the non-aqueous or fatty tissues in which actual globules of fat with no respiratory requirement lie inert, either as minute intra-cellular fragments or as large interstitial masses. The extent to which they are exposed to excess nitrogen will depend upon the richness of the adjacent capillary network. Extra nitrogen will of course enter the fat in which it is indeed more soluble, but because it lacks the intimate aqueous transport it will be slow to penetrate. In time however the quantity absorbed may be great. At normal atmo-spheric pressure there is just about 1 ml. of nitrogen dissolved in every

100 ml. of blood and aqueous tissue and 5 ml. in the same amount of fat. In the whole body there is almost 1 litre of dissolved nitrogen of which 35% is in the fat.

In considering the distribution of nitrogen in the body therefore two kinds of tissue must be considered, aqueous tissue and fatty tissue. This is unfortunately not a simple division owing to the extreme differences in the way the fat is distributed. Haldane (1922) who pioneered this work suggested that many types of tissue should be considered and graded according to the speed at which they became saturated with nitrogen. The present tendency is however to limit consideration to the two tissues whilst appreciating the complication imposed by the irregular distribution of the fat.

Hempleman (1952) in a valiant attempt to simplify the problem takes as his basis the example of a blood vessel entering the centre of a globule of fat to which it quickly brings additional nitrogen following increase in alveolar partial pressure. This additional head of pressure causes nitrogen to enter the immediately adjacent fat and diffuse radially.

The rate at which the nitrogen diffuses through tissue is inversely proportional to the square root of the time which means that at any given time t the quantity of nitrogen in the tissue Q is proportional to the square root of the time t.

$$Q = K\sqrt{t} \qquad\qquad (K = \text{constant})$$

This formula should only be applied to the larger areas of fat because it does not take into account the slowing up effect of approaching saturation. It is however a simple and useful approach to the problem.

It is perhaps more easy to represent this graphically. In Figure 45 the large squares represent a unit of fatty tissue which, if the body was exposed to a pressure of 4 atmospheres, would take 8 hours to reach equilibrium with the blood, represented by the column on the left. The shaded area corresponds to the tension of nitrogen. It will be noticed that half the saturation is reached in a much shorter time of 2 hours as calculated by the formula. Similarly when pressure is released, excluding the possibility of bubble formation, a reverse in pattern would be expected with half the nitrogen being returned in the 2 hours followed by a falling off in rate of elimination.

The difficulty in applying such a simple formula to the human problem will be appreciated if a second source of blood supply is imagined on the opposite side of each tissue unit so that nitrogen would diffuse in from both directions. In such a case the new equilibrium would be expected to be complete in 2 hours. It is quite apparent therefore that small collections of fat will saturate quicker than large ones and local vascularity will play a big part. Fat distribution may be fairly constant for any individual but vascularity will vary with muscular exercise, metabolic activity and physical or even emotional changes.

The time factor is very important in the distribution of nitrogen and greatly influences the type of decompression sickness. It is even possible for diffusion into a fatty tissue to continue after the external pressure has been reduced. If, in the example given in Figure 45, the pressure was reduced to normal after 2 hours only, the saturated fat near the blood flow would quickly give up its nitrogen whilst the deeper concentration would continue to diffuse in all directions (Fig. 46a). Similarly if at this stage the external pressure was only partially reduced the tissue could still go on gaining nitrogen (Fig. 46b).

THE DISTRIBUTION OF NITROGEN UNDER PRESSURE

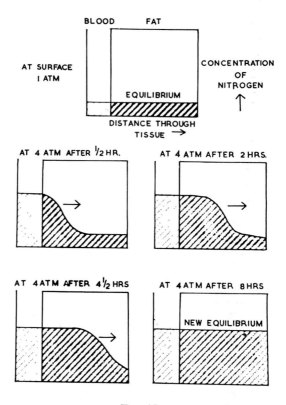

FIG. 45

REDISTRIBUTION OF NITROGEN IN PARTLY SATURATED TISSUE AFTER REDUCTION OF PRESSURE

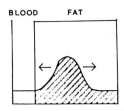

a) SITUATION IN TISSUE SHORTLY AFTER RETURN
TO NORMAL PRESSURE

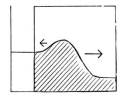

b) SITUATION AFTER PARTIAL REDUCTION IN
EXTERNAL PRESSURE
(TISSUE STILL GAINING NITROGEN)

FIG. 46

If decompression sickness is due to bubble formation, and there is no reason to doubt this, many clues are obtained by studying variations in time, depth and decompression. If very rapid decompression occurs even the aqueous tissues may show bubble formation. Blood samples taken immediately on rapid surfacing from depths are at first frothy and aviation medicine experts talk of 'boiling blood' in men exposed to rapid and extreme decompression. Very deep short dives are more likely to produce serious effects than prolonged shallow ones. Evidence of spinal involvement is commoner in the former and joint pains in the latter. Fat in the nervous system, e.g. in a myelin sheath, is likely to saturate more quickly than that in diffuse depots and on decompression will more easily produce bubbles. With the short deep dives also there is a smaller margin of safety than with less deep and longer ones.

THE CALCULATION OF DECOMPRESSION TABLES

Tables produced by Haldane have only recently been revised and the modifications made are not great. Haldane worked on the assumption that bubbles would not form with rapid decompression if this did not exceed a drop from $2\frac{1}{4}$ atmospheres to the surface pressure of 1 atmosphere. Thus it would be safe to drop from 2 to 1 atmospheres, i.e. come up from 33 ft. to the surface however long had been the exposure. Since tissues do not change volume with depth, halving the pressure at any depth would lead to the liberation of the same volume of nitrogen in that tissue. Thus if a decompression from 2 atmospheres to 1 atmosphere is safe so is one from 4 to 2 atmospheres, or from 6 to 3 atmospheres. This was in fact confirmed in practice using goats and later men. Assuming further that the parts of the body where bends could form would become half saturated in $1\frac{1}{4}$ hours it was possible to calculate the rate of loss during stops in decompression. Since, for convenience, stops every 10 ft. after the first one are used until reaching the surface, it was necessary to estimate the time, at each stop, required to lose sufficient nitrogen to make it safe to come up the next 10 ft. This time of course depends on the time spent on the bottom and the depth but the first stop is usually a short one. For a dive to 200 ft. it would be 3 minutes for half an hour or 15 minutes for an hour. At subsequent stops as they near the surface the rate of nitrogen elimination decreases progressively so that the stops must be proportionately lengthened. For a 200-ft. dive of 30 minutes the 3-minute stop at 80 ft. would be followed by one of 3 minutes at 70 ft., 5 at 60 ft., then 10, 15, 20, 30 and finally 35 at 10 ft.

Full details of Haldane's Decompression Tables have been widely published and used with much success (Haldane and Priestley, 1935).

In practice, dives using the Haldane tables have proved to be unnecessarily prolonged in the shallower dives and somewhat dangerous with the deeper ones. Because of this attempts have been made recently to improve them.

The most valuable starting point in the calculating of decompression tables is the knowledge of just how much time man can remain at various pressures and undergo rapid and complete decompression without symptoms. Figure 47 shows these times for depths down to 300 ft. Allowance must of course be made for the time the diver actually takes in descending and a good working rule is to add to the time on the bottom half the time it takes to get there. In general divers go down at a rate of 2 ft. per second and are brought up at 1 ft. per second.

The tolerance curve has been found quite reliable as a large series of trials carried out by Crocker and Taylor (1952) using both goats and men as subjects have shown. It may in fact be taken to represent the

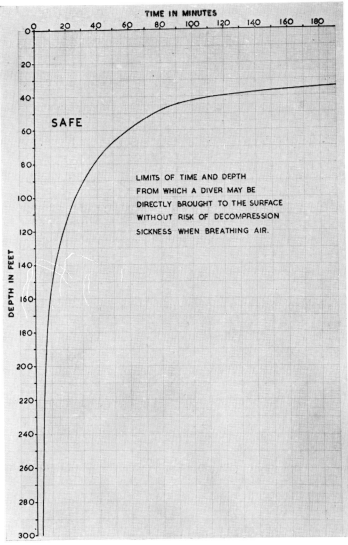

LIMITS OF TIME AND DEPTH
FROM WHICH A DIVER MAY BE
DIRECTLY BROUGHT TO THE SURFACE
WITHOUT RISK OF DECOMPRESSION
SICKNESS WHEN BREATHING AIR.

FIG. 47

maximum safe load of excess nitrogen which the tissues will carry. This can be put into arbitrary units if Hempleman's formula

$$Q = \text{Depth } \sqrt{\text{time}}$$

is used. Taking a known safe dive of 90 ft. for 30 minutes,

$$Q = 90 \sqrt{30}$$
$$= 493, \text{ say } 490 \text{ units.}$$

If 490 units is accepted as the tolerable excess nitrogen a simple table can be made with depth against safe time thus:

Depth in feet	Safe time in minutes
300	2·6
180	7·4
120	16·6
60	66·6
30	265·0

With this formula the shallower depths will have a finite time, e.g. for 30 ft. there is a limit of 4½ hours whereas it is known from experience that a diver may remain at 30 ft. indefinitely and still surface directly with safety. The formula however refers to a tissue through which the gas is diffusing freely and not one which fills up and diffusion ceases. The close approximation between these figures and what was in practice known to be safe encouraged Crocker and Taylor (1952) to calculate new tables on the basis of Hempleman's formula. Trials of these tables unfortunately showed them to be unsafe for dives deeper than 120 ft. though safe and time saving for shorter and shallower ones.

Soon after this work Rashbass (1954 and 1955) approached the problem from a different angle using as his basis the fact that a diver could remain at 30 ft. indefinitely. From this he assumed that a man could tolerate '30 foots' worth' of nitrogen at any level. On this basis he was able graphically to produce a promising series of decompression tables with considerable saving of time at all levels. Unfortunately these tables also, when tested at sea, did not meet the requirements of safety. The method of calculation nevertheless was certainly promising (Crocker 1957 a).

It was quite obvious that, though no satisfactory formula could be evolved which was applicable to the complicated tissue structure of man, a vast amount of practical experience was available. The need for reliable and economic tables was urgent and Crocker (1957 b) whose practical experience was second to none in this field, attempted, by studying the weaknesses in previous attempts, to produce a satisfactory answer. With commendable honesty and an appreciation of practical requirements he admitted that, since there was no ready-made quantitative solution, an empirical, trial and error, approach was necessary. Practical application was to be the criterion and any theoretical justification was to be a secondary consideration. In the ironing-out process all times were for convenience made multiples of five minutes. Successive stops were increased in time to give a balanced result. Crocker's tables when tested proved satisfactory for the normal range of diving and as safe as any others for exceptional dives. They were therefore generally adopted and produced, as customary, in two forms: Table I to cover the general requirements of diving and Table II for exceptionally prolonged dives. A depth of 200 ft. was accepted as a desirable limit for air diving.

It is interesting to compare the decompression times used in the different tables and as an example a dive to between 120 ft. and 130 ft. for 30 minutes may be taken:

Table	Depth ft.	Duration mins.	Time at Stops mins. 30 ft.	20 ft.	10 ft.	Total Time mins.
HALDANE	120–132	15–30		10	15	33
RASHBASS	130	20–30		4	9	13
CROCKER	120–130	25–30		5	20	25
U.S. NAVY	130	30		4·8	18	22·8
FRENCH	125	30			27	27

(In the above the time of ascent to stop is included in time at stop.)

U.S. Navy diving tables do not differ greatly from the British tables of Crocker especially in the deeper dives though they do give a shorter total time. The U.S. practice of timing to the nearest minute for the stops and fractions of minutes in ascent time to the first stop is a little unrealistic. Crocker's five-minute grading is simpler and less liable to error. Decompression tables can be found in most standard diving manuals. A simple form however has been produced from Crocker's tables covering the general requirements of divers. In this the time given at each stop includes the time taken to get there from the bottom or the previous stop (Fig. 48).

The Table I of this simple presentation has been issued by the British Sub Aqua Club for all qualified amateur divers as a 'Diver's Emergency Card'. The table is on one side the other giving an outline of the symptoms of decompression sickness with directions, including telephone numbers, of where and how treatment may be obtained.

TOTAL DECOMPRESSION TIME IN MINUTES.

MAXIMUM DEPTH IN FEET

MAXIMUM TIMES ON BOTTOM IN MINUTES	30	40	50	60	70	80	90	100	110	120	130	140	150	160	170	180	190	200
10												5	5	10b	10b	10b	10b	15
15				NO STOPS						5	5	10b	10b	15	15	20b	25b	25b
20									5	5	10b	15	20a	25b	30c	35b	40	45b
25								5	10b	10b	15	20a	30b	35b	45b	50d	55c	70c
30							5	10b	15	20a	25a	30b	45b	50c	65c	70c	80d	95b
35						5	10b	15	20a	25a	30b	45a	60a	70c	85c	95b	100c	120b
40						5	10b	20a	25a	35a	45a	60b	75b	85c	100b	115b	125b	145
45					5	10b	15	25a	30b	45a	60b	75b	95b	105b	120b	135b	150	170
50					5	10b	20a	30b	45a	60b	75b	90b	110	120a				
55					5	15	25a	35a	55b	70b	85b	105a	125a	135a				
60					10b	20a	30b	50b	65b	80c	100b	120a	140	155				
65				5	15	25a	35a	60a	75b	90b								
70				5	15	25a	55b	70b	85b	105a								
75				10b	20a	30a	65b	75b	95a	115a								
80				10b	25a	50a	70b	85b										
85				15	25a	55a	80b	90b										
90			5	15	30a	60a	85a	100a										
95			5	20a	35a	65a												
100			5	20a	50a	70a												
105			5	25a	55a	75a												
110			10a	25a	60a	80a												
115			10a	30a	65a	85a												
120			10a	30a	70a	90a												
130																		
135																		
	NO LIMIT																	

A B C

STEPPED LINES
AB = NO STOP LIMIT
AC = NORMAL WORKING LIMIT
(TABLE I)

KEY FOR STOPS FOR DECOMPRESSION TIMES

DECOMPRESSION TIME IN MINUTES	STOPS (MINS) 40′	30′	20′	10′
5	—	—	—	5
10a	—	—	—	10
b	—	—	5	5
15	—	—	5	10
20a	—	—	5	15
b	—	5	5	10
25a	—	—	5	20
b	—	5	5	15
30a	—	—	5	25
b	—	5	5	20
c	—	5	10	15
35a	—	5	5	25
b	—	5	10	20
40	5	5	10	20
45a	—	5	10	30
b	5	5	10	25
50a	—	5	10	35
b	—	5	15	30
c	5	5	10	30
d	5	5	15	25
55a	—	5	10	40
b	—	5	15	35
c	5	5	15	30
60a	—	5	15	40
b	5	5	15	35
c	5	10	15	30
65a	—	5	20	40
b	5	5	20	35
c	5	10	15	35
70a	—	5	25	40
b	5	5	20	40
c	5	10	20	35
75a	—	5	30	40
b	5	10	20	40

DECOMPRESSION TIME IN MINUTES	STOPS (MINS) 60′	50′	40′	30′	20′	10′
80a	—	—	—	5	30	45
b	—	—	5	5	30	40
c	—	—	5	10	25	40
d	—	5	5	15	20	35
85a	—	—	5	5	30	45
b	—	—	5	15	25	40
c	—	5	5	15	25	35
90a	—	—	5	10	30	45
b	—	—	5	15	25	45
95a	—	—	5	15	30	45
b	—	5	5	15	25	45
100a	—	—	5	20	30	45
b	—	5	5	15	30	45
c	—	5	10	20	25	40
105a	—	5	10	20	25	45
b	—	5	10	20	30	40
110	—	5	10	20	30	45
115a	—	5	10	20	30	50
b	—	5	10	20	35	45
120a	—	5	10	25	35	45
b	5	5	10	20	35	45
125a	—	5	10	25	35	50
b	5	5	10	25	35	45
135a	—	5	15	25	40	50
b	5	5	15	25	40	45
140	—	5	15	30	40	50
145	5	5	15	30	40	50
150	5	5	20	30	40	50
155	5	5	20	30	45	50
170	5	10	25	35	45	50

TIMES AT STOPS INCLUDE TIME OF ASCENT FROM BOTTOM OR PREVIOUS STOP.

RATE OF ASCENT = 1 FOOT PER SECOND

FIG. 48. Decompression Tables I and II

As deep and prolonged diving progresses decompression schedules will become increasingly complicated. Much work on tables continues and the mathematical approach is extremely difficult to understand. Interested readers are referred to the reports by Workman (1965), Hempleman (1967) and Keller and Buhlmann (1965).

It must not be forgotten that divers show profound individual differences in their reactions to working conditions. It is unlikely therefore that any table will be found to meet all requirements until the more personal psysiological variables such as weight, build, breathing patterns, etc. are taken into account. Perhaps the development of computers will enable such factors to be considered.

THE USE OF COMPUTERS

It may seem a little odd that a major break through in underwater medicine should come from the Institute of Aviation Medicine in Toronto. Nevertheless, no doubt due to one of the two workers having considerable underwater experience this was so. The Pneumatic Analogue Decompression Computor (Stubbs, R. A. and O. I. Kidd,— 1965) co-ordinates time and depth underwater with the theoretical nitrogen absorption ratios for four tissues using 'half-time' figures. By using the computer it should be possible to ascend from any dives on the safe side of the 'bends' threshold by continuous decompression. This as would be expected to start at a rapid rate on leaving the bottom slowing down and flattening out as the surface is approached.

The major advantage of this method is that it will cope satisfactorily with a random dive. The depths and times underwater, however irregular they may be are totted up and integrated by the computer to give a final ascent curve. This of course is of profound value in the case of multiple dives.

In spite of certain scepticism the computer shows great promise and many other workers are now following the lead given by Stubbs and Kidd. Robertson and Moeller (1968) for example, are considering a computer for both continuous and stage ascent working out its programme from estimates of inert gas tensions in nine tissues.

THERAPEUTIC DECOMPRESSION TABLES

As has already been stated the treatment for an established case of decompression sickness (except for the rashes and itches without pain) is recompression. For this a standard procedure based on the successful treatment of many cases by Van Der Aue, Duffner and Behnke (1947) has been widely adopted. The first essential in treatment is a differentiation between an uncomplicated bend or pain and other symptoms which might be indicative of cerebro-spinal involvement or air embolism. The routine for treatment of decompression sickness is as follows:

All cases are placed in the pressure chamber and if there is any suggestion of cerebral involvement this should be done with the utmost speed. Pressure should be increased at a rate equivalent to a descent of 25 ft. per minute and further action should depend on the patient's condition, viz.:

(i) If pain is the only complaint it may either
    (a) disappear before the pressure is equivalent to 66 ft.
    (b) disappear at a greater depth; or
    (c) persist for more than 30 minutes at 165 ft. which is the maximum depth used in therapeutic decompression.

(ii) If more serious symptoms are present, unconsciousness, paralyses, sensory disturbances, visual changes, dizziness, convulsions, chest pain or breathlessness, pressure should be continued until the 165 ft. equivalent is reached when either—
    (a) there will be relief within 30 minutes; or
    (b) there is no relief in 30 minutes.

According to whichever of the above categories the patient falls into so will subsequent decompression be dictated.

(i) (a)—requires Table 1.

(i) (b)—requires Table 2.

(i) (c)—is most unlikely to be decompression sickness and an alternative cause should be sought. If found, decompression can be carried out as for a normal dive to 165 ft. for the time involved.

(ii) (a)—requires Table 3.

(ii) (b)—requires Table 4.

When the ascent is taking place, a rate of not less than 1 minute between stops should be used. In some cases a longer interval of 5 minutes may be desirable. In the later stages oxygen may be used with advantage as indicated. (See table on facing page 191).

These tables though they have served very well in treatment are rather complicated and time consuming. In American practice a greater use of oxygen is made saving almost 4 hours on Tables 1 and 2. The advantage of oxygen is that it ensures that no atmospheric nitrogen enters the lungs and therefore lowers alveolar nitrogen partial pressure so hastening its liberation from the blood. It cannot be used at depth for fear of oxygen poisoning nor for long periods at the surface lest lung tissue be damaged.

Mackay (1966) emphasises the importance of treating divers with decompression sickness as human beings. The tables themselves are designed to give the best chance of success for any given set of signs or symptoms. An understanding doctor experienced in underwater medicine should have no hesitation, when treating unresponsive cases of decompression sickness, in taking the patient to greater pressures than normally prescribed, using oxy-helium mixtures during decompression and exercising personal judgement concerning the use of pure oxygen in the later stages.

It is furthermore of the utmost importance to pay careful attention to the comfort and personal needs of the patient, making sure that in prolonged treatment he is kept warm, allowed sleep, feed and above all kept interested. Much can and must be done to improve the amenities of therapeutic pressure chambers.

THERAPEUTIC DECOMPRESSION TABLES (AIR)

Equivalent Depth of Stops ft.	Times in minutes (unless otherwise stated)			
	TABLE 1	TABLES 2 AND 3		TABLE 4
165		30		30–120
140		12		30
120		12		30
100	30	12		30
		TABLES 1, 2 AND 3		
80		12		30
60		30		6 hours
50		30		6 hours
40		30		6 hours
	TABLE 1	TABLE 2	TABLE 3	
30	1 hour	2 hours	12 hours	12 hours*
20	1 hour	2 hours		2 hours*
20	2 hours (air or oxygen)			2 hours*

TOTAL TIME: 6h. 12m.   8h. 48m.   18h. 48m.   36½–38 hours

(*Oxygen may be used for final hour at each stop.)

VERY DEEP DIVING

It is unusual to descend beyond 200 ft. though tables are available for use down to 300 ft. in exceptional circumstances. For very deep diving beyond 300 ft. some mixture, which will do away with both the risk of oxygen poisoning and nitrogen narcosis which would be present with air, must be used. Density too, becomes a problem necessitating a lighter mixture. Helium is therefore used as a substitute for nitrogen and the oxygen content of the mixture reduced to a safe percentage according to the proposed depth of dive. Two mixtures are generally used, 13% oxygen in helium for depths down to 400 ft. and 9% oxygen in helium down to 600 ft. Since these mixtures are too weak in oxygen to be breathed at the surface it is necessary to start with air and then change over to the mixture between 100 ft. and 200 ft.

Helium also presents a rather different picture from nitrogen in that fatty tissues will absorb about one-third as much of it as nitrogen. Diffusion however is more rapid so that saturation is reached sooner and the gas leaves the tissues more quickly. This rapid release of helium makes bubbles in the blood more likely and therefore ascent should not exceed 30 ft. per minute. Because many divers find themselves more susceptible to cold when breathing helium plenty of warm clothing should be worn.

Decompression tables for helium take into account the fact that as the oxygen content is reduced so the partial pressure of helium is increased and a longer decompression schedule is needed. Decompression in the later stages, from 60 ft. to the surface, can be hastened by using oxygen, but even so the overall decompression time is somewhat longer comparatively than with nitrogen mixtures.

An example of what may be achieved with helium diving and some indication of the time-consuming decompression required may be found in the planning and achievement of a world record dive.

A WORLD RECORD DIVE

Lieutenant George Wookey, R.N., made diving history when in October, 1956, wearing standard diving equipment he descended to a depth of 600 ft. in a Norwegian Fjord and was able at depth to complete four minutes of useful work. Crocker and Hempleman (1957) were given the very difficult task of formulating his routine from experience of previous dives and the work they had been doing on new methods of calculating decompression tables.

Wookey left the surface breathing air and stopped at 40 ft. for two minutes to change to a breathing mixture of 9% oxygen and 91% helium. He then continued his descent arriving on the bottom at 600 ft., eight minutes after leaving the surface. Here he completed a simple task involving some manual dexterity and physical effort. After four minutes of this he was brought up to his calculated first stops of 1 minute at 260 ft. and 10 minutes at 220 ft. Meanwhile a submersible decompression chamber (Fig. 16) containing an attendant had been sent down to meet him, which it did at 220 ft. where the diver entered it and was able to take off his helmet and relax. In the chamber, now sealed, he breathed air as it was hoisted on board the parent ship. During raising the door of the chamber was closed and its pressure maintained to simulate further stops under water so that after 10 minutes at 220 ft. Wookey spent a further 10 minutes at an equivalent depth of 210 ft. in the chamber. Stops continued every 10 ft. as pressure in the chamber was reduced, being about 6 minutes each to 150 ft. then 12 minutes each to 80 ft., 30 minutes at 70 ft., 40 at 60 ft., 45 at 50, 50 at 40 and finally 60 minutes at 30 ft. Two minutes later he was released which was 6 hours and 33 minutes after he first left the surface to begin his dive. Of this 6 hours 21 minutes had been spent in decompression.

Unfortunately during the final stages of decompression this diver developed pains in both shoulders which gradually worsened. He was therefore transferred on reaching surface pressure to a standard compression chamber where at an equivalent depth of 50 ft. all his pain disappeared. He was kept for 30 minutes at this depth after which he had stops of 35 minutes at 40 ft., 65 at 30 ft. and 20 ft., and a final one of 125 minutes at 10 ft. before being released. Treatment of the decompression sickness therefore added a further $5\frac{1}{2}$ hours to the total time so that for 4 minutes on the bottom at 600 ft. the diver had spent $11\frac{1}{2}$ hours being decompressed.

Such deep dives as this certainly emphasize the limitations of present techniques. Very few underwater tasks could be imagined which would merit such expenditure of time. The one which the dive simulated was that of a diver assisting in a submarine rescue operation at this depth by shackling on a wire for rescue purposes.

Special mention is made of this dive because it in fact marks the end of the road for achievement with standard diving. It has shown that man can work at this depth but new methods will be needed to make this worthwhile. Standard diving enabled testing of decompression schedules in the water without risk to the diver whose welfare was controlled from above. The time has come when much of this responsibility can be transferred to the man underwater.

It is unlikely that 600 ft. will remain the record depth for a working dive. British Naval Divers are already progressing towards effective dives of up to 1,000 ft. and in 1962 Hannes Keller, a Swiss mathematician, actually reached a depth of 1,000 ft. in a diving bell, leaving it

13

for a few moments at this depth. This attempt cost the lives of two of his companions and Keller himself was rendered unconscious by nitrogen narcosis due to breathing the air in the chamber on re-entry. His life was saved only by the prompt raising of the bell. The dive was marred by over-enthusiasm and lack of adequate gas supply, and teaches a valuable lesson on the importance of careful preparation, experience and caution.

In spite of this unfortunate experience Keller has by no means given up his enthusiasm and is busily applying his mathematical skill to decompression schedules for deep diving (Keller and Buhlmann, 1965). He has become an accepted and respected worker in underwater physiology who is making a worthwhile contribution.

SURFACE DECOMPRESSION

Decompression following a dive, as so far described, has taken place either in the water or within a submersible decompression chamber sent down to meet the diver. Techniques are available too, whereby a man may be directly transferred from a submersible decompression chamber to a specially adapted pressure chamber without there being any change of pressure, thus enabling a decompression schedule to be completed in greater comfort.

Prolonged decompression in the sea may be undesirable or impossible for two reasons. The sea itself may be cold and intolerable for any great length of time and, with self-contained diving apparatus, cylinder endurance often imposes a great restriction on time in water making lengthy dives impossible.

Methods are available whereby the actual time in the water can be limited to the period of descent, time on bottom and direct ascent. Bubbles do not form quickly and if surfacing from depth is almost immediately followed by artificial recompression to the same depth, no ill-effects occur. This principle has been used as a method of 'surface decompression' which can be carried out if a compression chamber is available. Practice has shown that if a diver ascends from the bottom at 1 ft. per second and is in the chamber and under pressure within 5 minutes he can be returned to his original pressure and decompressed to schedule in the surface chamber. Methods of application are still under consideration for timing routines and the development of portable chambers is being studied.

When this method was first used divers spent their first ordinary stop in the water, were then rapidly surfaced and compressed again to the pressure of that stop. From this they completed a normal decompression routine in the chamber. Alternatively the diver could be brought straight up from the bottom, transferred to the chamber and recompressed to the equivalent depth of the bottom. Allowing extra time for his ascent and descent he was thereafter decompressed according to an appropriate routine.

More recently Crocker (1958) proposed that a diver should be brought directly to the surface and recompressed only to the equivalent depth of what would have been the first stop. In making his proposals Crocker was concerned that the recompression given should be dependent upon the degree of nitrogen saturation of tissue, that it should be sufficient to prevent further growth of or formation of bubbles and that allowance should be made for the fact that a potentially dangerous procedure had been carried out. He considered it particularly important, during decompression, to avoid sudden drops of pressure and also to limit the method to dives taking place within the normal working limit (i.e. Table I). The procedure recommended is therefore as follows:

(a) The diver should ascend at 1 ft. per second and be immediately transferred to the pressure chamber. This should not take more than 5 minutes which would allow time for attendants to remove heavy equipment, boots, diving apparatus, etc.

(b) He is then compressed to a pressure equivalent to a depth 30 ft. below what would have been his first stop where he remains for 5 minutes.

(c) From this he ascends to the equivalent of the first stop and is thereafter given a routine decompression for a dive of 10 minutes longer than the dive completed.

These proposals were later tried at sea (Mackay, 1958) and in 210 dives, all near the limits of normal (Table I) diving, an incidence of bends of 4·3% was found and considered acceptable. In practice this technique is proving very satisfactory for self-contained breathing apparatus and a convenient-sized chamber can be carried in quite a small attendant vessel. It certainly offers a very great improvement in economical use of cylinders of breathing mixtures with a considerable extension of time under water.

MULTIPLE DIVES

In a working day it is only natural that a diver might wish to go down more than once. This is certainly more likely with the self-contained diver whose duration for each dive is limited by the life of his cylinders and the depth of his dive. The need for surfacing to change cylinders may well present a need for two or three dives within the day.

Even when a normal decompression has been carried out after a dive the body still contains a surplus of nitrogen. It will be remembered that an equivalent to saturation at 30 ft. can be tolerated and decompression tables aim to bring the diver to the surface with such a load. Complete elimination of nitrogen will take many hours, six or even twelve. In fact it is usual in this country and America to modify the routine of a dive if it occurs within 12 hours of a previous one whereas the French practice is to make adjustments for the 6-hour period only.

Factors which must be considered are the depth of the first dive and the interval between the two. The simplest answer would be to add

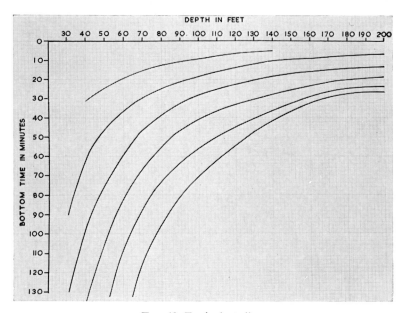

FIG. 49. Equivalent dives

together the times on the bottom for each dive and decompress after the second dive as if it had included this total time at the depth of the deeper dive. This is in fact the current practice in the Royal Navy.

Such practice would require much more decompression than necessary and takes no account of the interval between dives. Most methods for calculating a combined dive schedule make allowance for the depth and time of the first dive and the surface interval. It is convenient in the calculation to replace the first dive by one of the same depth as the second but with the time adjusted to give an equivalent nitrogen tension as in the first. Such an equivalent can be obtained from the graphs on Figure 49. If for example the first dive was 30 minutes at 100 ft. and the second

35 minutes at 140 ft. an equivalent time for the first dive at 140 ft. would, from the curves, be 20 minutes. The combined dives then require decompression for a dive of 140 ft. for 35 + 20 minutes = 55 minutes. Such a dive would require a total decompression time of 105 minutes (Figure 48.) As the interval between the dives increased so would this figure be less. To calculate this Crocker (1958) takes this figure less the decompression time of the second dive (105 − 45 minutes) as a 'basic loading' time, i.e. 60 minutes. From a further chart (Fig. 50) a reduced

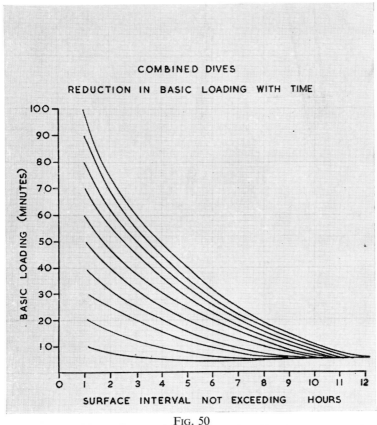

COMBINED DIVES

REDUCTION IN BASIC LOADING WITH TIME

BASIC LOADING (MINUTES)

SURFACE INTERVAL NOT EXCEEDING HOURS

FIG. 50

loading is obtained according to the interval. If the interval between these dives had been 3 hours the reduced loading would be 35 minutes. This means that with these two dives when the diver is ready to ascend at the end of the second one he should be decompressed as for a dive to 140 ft. for which the total decompression required would be 35 (the reduced loading) plus 45, the decompression time of the second dive, i.e. a total of 80 minutes. A dive to 140 ft. for 45 minutes requires a decompression of 75 minutes and one for 50 minutes needs 90 minutes decompression. The latter is therefore taken as being the safer and decompression is carried out accordingly thus: (Fig. 48.)

STOPS	40 ft.	30 ft.	20 ft.	10 ft.
TIME AT STOPS	5 mins.	15 mins.	25 mins.	45 mins. = 90 m.

This is still rather a tedious procedure and an urgent need for a simpler approach or presentation exists. The French diving schools go a good way towards this by using an adjustable card indicator. It will be seen (La Plongée, 1955), that the diving tables contain an additional column giving a coefficient for successive dives. Dives which have the same index have the same nitrogen tension. In the calculator there is a column for each index in which the depth of the second dive can be correlated with the time interval between the dives to give time in minutes which should be added to the bottom time of the second dive when looking up the decompression time.

By the French method the above dives would require a decompression routine as follows:

STOPS	9 m. (30 ft.)	6 m. (20 ft.)	3 m. (10 ft.)
TIME AT STOPS	15 mins.	27 mins.	34 mins. = 82 m.

A little less than the English routine and with the card obtainable without calculation.

BUBBLE FORMATION

If the way in which bubbles formed in tissues was fully known the problem of decompression sickness might be more easily understood. Under controlled conditions it is possible to saturate a solvent with a gas and then apply considerable reduction of pressure without bubble formation. To do this there must be no disturbance. Slight agitation quickly results in excessive bubble formation.

To form and grow a bubble starts as a gas nucleus which must overcome surface tension. This is very great while the bubble is small but decreases as it grows. Furthermore once a bubble has formed, no matter what gas originated it, a space has been produced into which all other dissolved gases will pass to establish an equilibrium. If the tension of the gases in the solution is great then the surface tension may be rapidly overcome and the bubble grow.

Newton Harvey (1955) describes a very simple and impressive experiment to demonstrate this effect. In a long upright tube a layer of water saturated with carbon dioxide is placed over a layer of water saturated with air, above the CO_2 layer is placed a further layer of water saturated with air. The top of the tube is attached to a vacuum pump and as pressure is reduced the bottom of the tube is tapped. Small bubbles form and ascend slowly; when they reach the CO_2 layer they suddenly increase in size and ascend more rapidly. They do however diminish in size and slow down as they pass through the upper 'air' layer.

It is quite certain therefore that where bubbles form in human aqueous tissues they will contain proportions of all other gases which are in solution. The same may well be true of the fatty tissues for all gases will diffuse into them and would take advantage of any bubble which formed.

Movement is known to promote bubble formation. In practice exercise is generally regarded as predisposing to 'bends' and although it theoretically should assist in the elimination of nitrogen it is for this reason discouraged.

The bubble will be more likely to form in the tissue which is most saturated when the decompression occurs. Cases have been described (Hickey and Stembridge, 1958) where as a result of sudden decompression bubbles have formed in fatty cells causing rupture of the cell membrane with liberation of fat into the bloodstream. Bends most commonly occur in the tissues surrounding joints where small fatty depots may exist in tight tissue so that bubble expansion may be restricted and cause pressure on sensory nerve endings. Similarly bubbles in the fatty deposits of the central nervous system may exert extreme local pressure on nerves whilst on the other hand there is no evidence of bubbles forming or at any rate producing symptoms in the large loosely packed fat masses of the subcutaneous and mesenteric areas.

It must be accepted that there will be, in the various sites and tissues, a threshold of bubble size which is necessary before symptoms occur. Wherever there is bubble formation in a tissue the pattern of nitrogen release from that tissue will be altered. Diffusion will take place into the bubble as well as to the circulating blood and it is possible in a fatty tissue that under certain circumstances a fairly stable and persistent bubble may form. All workers on the decompression problem have strong evidence that the way in which nitrogen leaves the body on decompression is very different from the way in which it enters during pressurization. It is certainly more difficult to get rid of than to absorb.

The presence of symptomless or 'silent' bubbles may well be the reason for the failure from time to time of simple schedules for multiple dives and the difficulty of getting rid of bubbles once formed is well shown in the lengthy procedure needed for therapeutic decompression.

The fact already mentioned that a bubble must contain all the gases in solution makes the use of multiple gases as means of decreasing the time needed for decompression disappointing. The actual degree of saturation of each of the gases would be correspondingly lower but the bubble forming effect would be additive.

Oxygen is not usually regarded as a bubble former since any excess in the tissues is rapidly metabolized. However from a purely physical point of view it must be a candidate and at least make some contribution to bubble content. Donald (1955) investigated this possibility using goats. (In diving research goats make a valuable substitute for men, their reactions being very similar and the presence of a 'bend' being shown when a leg is held off the ground and slightly flexed.) Exposures to pressures in a chamber equivalent to 150 ft. of sea water were used, with a breathing mixture containing 64% oxygen, maintained for one hour and followed by rapid decompression. A watch was kept for signs of oxygen poisoning and, of the 8 goats used, one was removed for this reason. Of the remaining seven, one was completely unaffected and six showed signs of severe decompression sickness within 5 minutes of surfacing, i.e. bends, restlessness, pulmonary rales, breathlessness and lying down. Five minutes later there was complete recovery without any treatment, a result which never occurs with the decompression sickness of such severity due to nitrogen. Furthermore control dives, in which the goats were given less oxygen but the same nitrogen exposure, were completed with no subsequent symptoms.

Though this work today is of more academic than practical importance it serves to show how complex the whole problem of decompression sickness can be.

What has so far been achieved results mostly from practical experience. New research techniques are needed for in their present form the decompression tables leave much to be desired. If the tables are to be streamlined consideration must be given to the effect of differences in sea temperature and work rates. Personal variation must be considered and some form of test is needed whereby an individual may have his nitrogen elimination rate and pattern assessed. The ultimate achievement may be that every diver will have his own decompression tables designed to meet his personal adaptation to the pressure changes. Alternatively perhaps a series of tables of varying pattern may be produced which might be assigned to divers according to their reactions.

THE DETECTION OF BUBBLES

The mechanics of bubble formation in decompression sickness is still a great mystery. It must depend on many factors such as the rate of pressure reduction, the presence or absence of nuclei on which bubbles may form and the degree of agitation at the time of pressure reduction. It is assumed that there is a threshold of bubble size to produce signs or symptoms or predispose to chronic changes. With therapeutic recompression, though a bubble may be rapidly reduced in size, its total re-absorption may be difficult.

Of the many attempts made to observe bubbles by both surgical and physical techniques, one of the most promising at present under investigation uses pulsed ultra sound to detect bubbles in living tissues. This technique has for many years been used in clinical medicine to pinpoint deep tumours in the brain or abdomen (Gordon 1965 and 1966). Recently Sutphen (1968) has shown the feasibility of using the method to detect bubbles of between 0·5 mm. and 1·00 mm. in diameter when artificial air emboli were produced in the circulation of dogs and rabbits. Admittedly, though this technique is very much in its infancy, at least a start has been made and future development with improved sensitivity is likely to produce valuable information about a most puzzling situation.

READING AND REFERENCES

Bert, Paul. (1878). *La Pression Barometrique*. G. Masson, Paris.

Boycott, A. E. and G. C. C. Damant (1908). 'Experiments on the Influence of Fatness on Susceptibility to Caisson Disease.' *J. Hyg. Camb. 8*, 445.

Bucquoy, E. (1861). '*Action de l'air Comprime sur l'economie Humaine.*' *M.D. Thesis*—Strasburg.

Crocker, W. E. and H. J. Taylor (1952). 'A method of Calculating Decompression Stages and the Formulation of New Diving Tables.' *M.R.C. (RNPRC) Report U.P.S.* 131B.

Crocker, W. E. (1957 a). 'Investigation into the Decompression Tables VII—Sea Trials.' *M.R.C. (RNPRC) Report U.P.S.* 162.

— (1957 b). 'Investigation into Decompression Tables IX. Revised Tables.' *M.R.C. (RNPRC) Report. U.P.S.* 171.

Crocker, W. E. and H. V. Hempleman (1957). 'The Decompression Problem of Diving to 100 ft.' *M.R.C. (RNPRC) Report. U.P.S.* 163.

Crocker, W. E. (1958). 'Proposals for Applying the New Standard Tables to Surface Decompression and Combined Dives.' *M.R.C. (RNPRC) Report U.P.S.* 175.

Donald, K. W. (1955) 'Oxygen Bends.' *J. Applied. Physiol.* 7, 639.

Golding, F. Campbell, P. Griffiths, H. V. Hempleman, W. D. M. Paton and D. N. Walder. (1960). 'Decompression Sickness During Construction of the Dartford Tunnel.' *Brit. J. Indus. Med.* 17, 167.

Gordon, D. (1965 and 1966). 'Ultrasonics in Diagnosis I and II'. *Biomedical Engineering.* Dec. 1965 and Jan. 1966.

Groupe D'Etudes et de Recherches Sous-marine (1955). *La Plongée.* B. Arthaud, Paris.

Haldane, J. S. (1922). *Respiration.* Yale University Press.

Haldane, J. S. and J. G. Priestley (1935). *Respiration.* Clarendon Press, Oxford.

Harvey, E. N. (1955). 'Bubble Formation.' Underwater Physiology Symposium. National Academy of Sciences—National Research Council. U.S.A. Report 337.

Hempleman, H. V. (1952). 'A New Theoretical Basis for the Calculation of Decompression Tables.' *M.R.C. (RNPRC) Report U.P.S.* 131A.

Hempleman, H. V. (1967). 'Decompression Procedures for Deep, Open Sea Operations'. Proc. 3rd Symp. Underwater Physiology (Lambertson) Williams and Wilkins Co., Baltimore.

Hickey, J. L. and V. A. Stembridge. (1958). 'Occurrence of Pulmonary Fat and Tissue Embolism in Aircraft Accident Fatalities.' *J. Av. Med.* 29, 787.

Hill, Leonard. (1912). *Caisson Sickness and the Physiology of work in Compressed Air.* Edward Arnold, London.

James, C. C. M. (1945). 'Late Bone Changes in Caisson Disease.' *Lancet II*, 249 (7 July 1945).

Keays, F. L. (1912). 'Compressed Air Illness.' *Am. Labour Legislative Rev.* 2, 192.

Keller, H. and A. A. Buhlmann (1965). 'Deep Diving and Short Decompression by Breathing Mixed Gases'. *J. Appl. Physiol.* 20, 1267.

Mackay, D. E. (1966). 'Decompression Sickness in Divers'. M.D. Thesis—University of Glasgow.

McCallum, R. I. (1965). *Decompression of Compressed Air Workers in Civil Engineering.* Oriel Press Ltd., Newcastle.

McCallum, R. I. (1968). 'Decompression Sickness—A Review'. *Britt. J. Indus. Med.* 25, 4.

Oliver, T. (1904). 'Discussion on Compressed Air Illness or Caisson Disease.' *Brit. Med. J.* 2, 317.

Parsons, V. (1958). 'A Brief Review of Aviators' Decompression Sickness and the High Altitude Selection Test.' *J. Roy. Nav. Med. Service.* 44, 2.

Rainsford, S. G. (1942). 'The more recent additions to our knowledge of the effects of compression and decompression on man.' *J. Roy. Nav. Med. Service.* 28, 326.

Rashbass, C. (1954). 'Investigation into the Decompression Tables V.' *M.R.C. (RNPRC) Report U.P.S.* 139.

— (1955). 'Investigation into Decompression Tables VI—New Tables.' *M.R.C. (RNPRC) Report U.P.S.* 151.

Robertson, J. S. and G. Moeller (1968). 'Computation of Continuous Decompression Schedules for Deep Sea Dives'. Brookhaven National Lab. Report. B.N.L. 50104.

The Royal Naval Diving Manual. B.R. 155C. Admiralty, London.

Schilling, C. W. (1941). 'Compressed Air Illness.' *Nav. Med. Bull. (U.S.A.).* 39, 367.

Stubbs, R. A. and D. I. Kidd (1965). 'A pneumatic Analogue Decompression Computer'. Canadian Forces Med. Serv. Int. Av. Med. Reports 65–RD–1.

Sutphen, J. H. (1968). 'The Feasibility of Using Pulsed Ultra sound to Detect the Presence of in Viro Tissue Gas Bubbles'. U.S. Navy Submarine Med. Center. Report No. 508.

U.S. Navy Diving Manual. U.S. Government Printing Office, Washington.

Van Der Aue, O. E., G. J. Duffner and A. R. Behnke (1947). 'The Treatment of Decompression Sickness.' *J. Indus. Hyg.* 29, 359.

Workman, R. D. (1965). 'Calculation of Decompression Schedules for Nitrogen, Oxygen and Helium Oxygen Dives'. U.S. Navy E.D.U. Report 6–65, Washington.

CHAPTER XII

Saturation Diving

MEN will not be satisfied until both depth and time on the sea-bed are increased to an economical level. The price which must be paid in decompression time for a very short period of time at depth would seem to be quite unacceptable. Eight hours of decompression for five minutes work on the sea-bed at 600 ft. is commercially unthinkable.

There is however a glimmer of light when one studies just what is happening to man on deep submergence. The secret lies in figure 45 in the previous chapter where after 8 hrs. at 4 atmospheres a 'new equilibrium' is established.

When the body is under pressure nitrogen and oxygen, or helium if this is used, will diffuse into the blood stream from the lungs and pass into all the various tissues of the body. The speed of this process will depend upon the difference in partial pressures of the gases breathed and that of the quantities already in solution. Thus as time passes and tissues become 'topped up' the difference in partial pressures will decrease rapidly at first and finally more slowly until for all intents and purposes the pressures become equal and the tissues are said to be saturated. When the saturation is reached no further transfer of respired gases into solution in the tissues take place. The natural processes of utilization of oxygen however will continue so that it is important to ensure that the partial pressure of oxygen in the environment atmosphere remains physiologically acceptable.

Having reached the stable state of 'saturation' for the new pressure or depth the simple fact remains that to return to atmospheric or surface pressure would require the same decompression schedule whether or not it took place immediately after reaching the state of saturation or after an indefinite period at that same depth or pressure. Thus when saturation is reached it is possible for man to remain at and work at 'saturation depth' for short or long periods with the same subsequent decompression schedule.

It would be unthinkable for divers to remain in the water for these long periods but if they can be accommodated in relative comfort in pressurized chambers either on the sea-bed or in a surface vessel and enter and leave the water without change in pressure they could perform useful periods of work on the sea-bed or underwater for weeks or even longer. To have the pressure chamber in a surface vessel would necessitate commuting to and from the working depth in a pressurized transfer capsule.

Pioneers in this work have been Captain George Bond of the U.S. Navy and Jacques Cousteau in France. Both were working out their plans as early as 1957 and since then others have joined them. The conquest of the continental shelves has been the common object with depth of 1,200 ft. in mind. It is not necessary to be saturated for this maximum depth since excursion dives of considerable degree can be made from saturation at a shallower depth without harm or delays. For example dives from saturation depths of 850 ft. to 1025 ft. and 600 ft. to 750 ft. and back to saturation depth with 'stops' have been made by American, French and British divers.

The most notable saturation dives made to date in the open sea are as follows:—

1962—Cousteau—'Conshelf 1'	7 days at 35 ft. (2 men.)	
1962—Link—'Man in Sea project'	24 hrs. at 200 ft. (1 man.)	
1963—Cousteau—'Conshelf 2'	1 month at 33 ft. (5 men.)	
	7 days at 85 ft. (2 men.)	
1964—Link—'Man in Sea Project'	49 hrs. at 432 ft. (2 men.)	
1964—U.S. Navy—'Sealab I'	11 days at 192 ft. (4 men.)	
1965—Cousteau—'Conshelf 3'	22 days at 330 ft. (6 men.)	
1965—U.S. Navy—'Sealab II'	15 days at 205 ft. (3 teams of 10 men).	
1969—U.S. Navy—'Sealab III'	12 days at 600 ft. (planned) (5 teams of 8 men).	

These memorable saturation dives in the sea have of course been preceded and tested by similar dives in 'wet' pressure chambers ashore in many countries. The British contribution has been considerable and U.S. teams have taken advantage of the excellence of British chambers and Royal Navy divers took part as members of the diving teams in Sealab III.

One of the most informative and successful of these 'trial dives' in the wet took place in December, 1968, at Duke University, North Carolina under the direction of Professors Saltzman and Kylstra. Five men, including one doctor, spent 77 hours at 1,000 ft., exercising regularly in the wet section of the chamber and carrying out physiological measurements. Even such difficult tests as blood gas analysis were completed in the chamber. A unique feature of this dive was that a slow compression of 24 hrs. was used. This may well be a factor in the absence of any adverse effects during the period under pressure.

Subsequent staged decompressions occupied a further seven days. An interesting finding was that maximum exercise in the water was accompanied by carbon dioxide retention. (Kylstra, 1968.)

A further well documented saturation dive 650 ft. was carried out by Ocean Systems Inc. in 1965. The descent was rapid, the bottom time 48 and the decompression a linear one over 6 days. Physiological findings are fully documented (Hamilton, MacInnis, Noble and Schreiner, 1966.)

GENERAL PROBLEMS IN SATURATION DIVING

Saturation diving provides an economical answer to the problem of prolonged post-dive decompression and all dives so far completed both in land chambers and at sea show that given controlled conditions the practice is physiologically acceptable.

The pressurized atmosphere in which the divers live between their excursions into the sea must be such that the risk of oxygen poisoning, nitrogen narcosis and carbon dioxide retention from increased density are removed or reduced as far as possible. Ideally the partial pressures of oxygen and nitrogen should remain the same as in the surface atmosphere and the additional pressure made up by adding helium. The mixture used in Sealab III was 1·6% oxygen, 6% nitrogen and 92·4% helium.

With such a small concentration of oxygen it is essential to maintain continuous and accurate atmospheric monitoring. Excess carbon dioxide can be removed with conventional scrubbers containing lithium hydroxide. Chamber temperature must be maintained within the comfort zone which bearing in mind the cooling effect on the body of helium should be about 92 F.

There is work here for both the engineer and the physiologist. So far the work has been largely experimental though an element of international competition seems to be creeping in. Now that the technique has been shown possible attention must be turned to the divers themselves to ensure that their environment is maintained as near as possible to their accustomed atmosphere. Food, clothing, privacy, activity and entertainment must be provided with great care. The psychological factors of isolation in an unfriendly environment may in the early days of adventure not yet be a deterrent but will need consideration when seabed living becomes a matter of routine.

The potential of saturation diving militarily, commercially and recreationally is immense and though much of the equipment is intricate and costly the problems of entry and return from the environment are negligible when contrasted with those of space.

The tendency so far has been to build underwater dwellings in the form of strong metal spheres of cylinders with few windows or scuttles. Provided it is always possible to maintain the pressure within the same as that without the construction need not be exceptionally robust. Recently the British Diving Magazine 'Triton' ran a competition for the design of an underwater 'house'. The winner is shown in Fig. 51. The door as far as entry into the sea is concerned must always be underneath but for transfer to pressurized mobile capsules a locking device on the upper surface may be necessary. There is no limit to the imagination when design for comfort and use of such accommodation is under consideration.

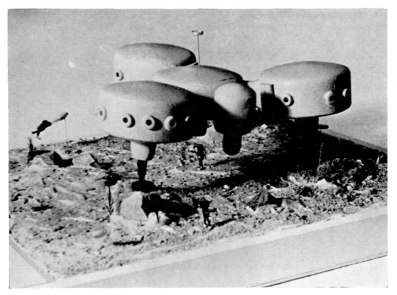

Fig. 51. An imaginary underwater 'house'—from Triton.

ALTERNATIVE TECHNIQUES

In recent years the accent has been largely on the underwater dwelling on a sea-bed site where divers may be required to function. This is essentially dependent on the presence of a large surface support vessel which is subject to the influence of bad weather and problems of deep, secure moorings.

An attractive alternative would be to construct a suite of pressurized chambers in a surface vessel itself in which the divers could live at the pressure of the sea bed on which they were required to work. A pressurized submersible capsule could be designed to lock onto the parent chamber to enable the 'duty watch' of divers to transfer under pressure and be lowered to their working depths where they could leave the capsule which would stand by to raise them back—still under pressure —when their underwater shift was completed.

This method has three major advantages.

(i) It is mobile and available for different areas of the sea-bed without major mooring problems for the parent vessel.

(ii) Though still under pressure the divers are when off duty in intimate contact with their surface support crew.

(iii) In bad weather they need not dive and the surface vessel can seek shelter if necessary.

No doubt there is a need for both these techniques according to underwater requirements.

Much is still speculation—but so was 'Sealab' ten years ago. On the recreational side in interesting and attractive waters one can imagine a series of pressurized hostels—with the comforts of a holiday camp at different levels. The deeper one would be for the experts with time to spare. They would saturate there and enjoy their prolonged decompression by appropriate stays at the shallower 'chalets'—enjoying their diving at decreasing depths until they were finally ready to surface. This would help to dispel the boredom which today mars the current techniques.

Finally—and again with imagination, it should be possible to design some underwater submarine with a pressurized section which would transport divers with close support, yet under pressure appropriate for work at any chosen depths. The submarine crew and maintenance staff would be at atmospheric pressure with a series of locks through which divers may pass with adequate compression and decompression as required. If such a vessel could be built with a series of pressure hulls one within the other, the innermost being pressurized to working depth and having suitable locks, great saving in hull thickness might be acceptable and very deep depths reached.

Saturation diving is very much in its infancy—it shows great promise and will certainly extend man's underwater influence both wide and deep which can only be to his lasting advantage.

It is well however to proceed with caution maintaining a careful watch on man's individual reaction at all times. There is always the risk that the enthusiasm of the divers and engineers may outpace the caution of the doctors and physiologists.

One very simple fact remains. However carefully controlled the high pressure environment there will be an excess of gas molecules, oxygen, nitrogen or helium dissolved in and diffusing through human tissues. Will this additional load have any effect on the delicately balanced biochemical process of human biology? If they reach, as some surely must, the intrically balanced intracellular structures they may effect or even displace other molecules or perhaps more important actual ionized radicles.

This is an abnormal situation to which in practice the human body seems able to adapt adequately. Only time will tell to what extent this adaptation is without adverse effect. Let it be emphasized therefore that however promising the results, however glamorous the achievement, man is in an unnatural environment which may or may not impose limitations or as yet unknown stresses. The physiologists have a great responsibility and must insist on controlled investigation prior to every step man takes to increase his exposure time under increasing pressure.

REFERENCES AND READING

Hamilton, R. W., J. B. MacInnis, A. D. Noble, and H. R. Schriner (1966). 'Saturation Diving to 650 ft.'. Tec. Memo. B.411 Ocean System Inc., New York.

Cousteau, J. (1964). 'At Home in the Sea'. *National Geographic, 125*, 465.

Link, E. (1965). 'Outpost under the Ocean'. *National Geographic*, April, 1965, p. 530.

Bond, G. F. (1967). 'Medical Problems of Mulliday Saturation Diving in Open Water'. Proc. 3rd Underwater Physiology Symposium, p. 81. William and Wilkins Co., Baltimore.

Kylstra, J. A. (1968). Personal communication.

CHAPTER XIII

Some Underwater Accidents

IN THE preceding chapters the many hazards which beset the underwater swimmer or diver have been considered and examples given. These are well-known dangers and the means of avoiding them are generally appreciated. Where underwater activity is carefully planned and experienced personnel are involved accidents from these causes are rare.

Compared with other pastimes and occupations, underwater accidents are fortunately not too common. They are certainly less common than road, domestic and industrial accidents but as more and more people venture into the new environment the total accident rate will increase.

In almost all aquatic accidents where death is the outcome, this is the result of drowning. The problem of drowning will be discussed in the next chapter. The present concern is the circumstances which lead up to the situation where drowning becomes inevitable.

In road, rail or air accidents there is often mutilation or destruction of the body as a result of impact which may make it very difficult to ascertain the true cause. Very often when there is an underwater accident the body is spared such ill-usage and may, if recovered, produce sufficient evidence to enable an accurate interpretation of the predisposing factors to be made.

That underwater accidents are not always fatal depends not so much upon the nature of the accident but on whether there is someone available at the time to effect a rescue. In non-fatal accidents on land the injured person could lie around until help arrived but in the water if help is not immediately to hand that victim may well drown. It must therefore be accepted from the outset that all mishaps in water are potentially dangerous. This must be emphasized during training and not until the trainee has achieved a high degree of confidence and efficiency should he be allowed to venture out of easy reach. Also it is most undesirable that even experienced underwater swimmers should ever be alone.

Some examples of this may be given.

(A) ACCIDENTS DUE TO LACK OF EXPERIENCE

(i) A party of experienced divers had just completed the demolition of a rocky obstruction on the bottom of a small harbour in a Mediterranean island. Conditions were ideal and when the job was done they just swam around underwater for the fun of it. Finally, as the last man left the water an envious onlooker, with a limited experience, borrowed a breathing set from a friend and jumped in, not bothering to check how much air was left in the cylinders. Just after he entered the water someone yelled from a nearby hut that tea was ready and everyone trooped off, leaving the one man in the water. When they returned he had disappeared. Many hours later his body was found on the bottom with the set exhausted.

(ii) An enthusiastic spear-fisherman taking part in a contest and using a Schnorkel tube was operating singly, well away from other swimmers and boats. He was last seen swimming 200 yards from shore against strong currents and offshore winds. When help arrived he had disappeared.

This again indicates the folly of being alone in the sea and as a result of this accident the organizers of the competition now insist on the contestants carrying a marker buoy.

(iii) Many underwater breathing sets have a mouth-piece within the face mask. It is not uncommon for the face mask to become flooded. An expert can blow excess water past the mouth-piece and out of the face mask. A number of fatal cases have occurred where inexperienced men have had this flooding and presumably panicked in the attempt to blow out the water and lost the mouth-piece. Beginners should come to the surface to carry out such a manœuvre.

(iv) An English underwater photographer, well trained in the use of an open circuit air breathing apparatus, was invited by an Italian frogman to try a closed circuit oxygen breathing set. Quite correctly and largely by signs the frogman ensured that the photographer washed out the nitrogen in his lungs by repeatedly breathing in from the set and out to air.

Having done this he set out accompanied by a colleague who was breathing air. They planned to swim out about a mile on the surface then dive to take pictures. On the outward swim the first photographer removed his mouth-piece to talk with his companion, a perfectly safe procedure with an air set. However, whilst talking, his lungs filled with air which he failed to appreciate when he replaced the mouth-piece without any attempt to wash out his lungs again with oxygen. Thus when he resumed the swim his closed circuit contained possibly three or more litres of nitrogen. When the spot for diving was reached the men separated and dived to take their photographs. The unfortunate man with the oxygen set, engrossed with his work, failed to realize that he was using up oxygen without replacement. The presence of nitrogen would prevent the re-breathing bag becoming empty which, with oxygen only in the circuit, would be a signal to refill it from the cylinder. When eventually this man was found he was lying peacefully on the bottom, with his mouth-piece still in position, with no evidence of struggle, but very dead, a typical example of death from dilution anoxia.

(B) ACCIDENTS DUE TO NEGLECT OF PRECAUTIONS

In organized diving many of the regulations and recommendations made to protect the individual are sometimes rather tedious. An expert may find them irksome and from time to time ignore them. It is surprising how many times this leads to trouble. Nobody wishes to put a damper on the enthusiasm of the underwater swimmer, but those who have, by experience, gained the wisdom to come to terms with the aquatic environment, owe it to their successors to point out the dangers and make recommendations for their avoidance.

(i) A most striking example of this occurred some years ago in a standard diver working on a wrecked vessel. The ship had rolled over about 60° and entry was made through hatches no longer uppermost on the vessel. In some compartments air had been trapped above the water on the surface of which was oil fuel which had leaked from nearby tanks. The diver in question was engaged mainly in a survey of the wreck but one morning he dived with two attendants and after a little while called for a cutting torch, presumably to cut away some obstruction. Shortly after this an explosion was felt in the attendant boat and when an attempt was made to raise the diver only his helmet which was grossly distorted came to the surface.

When the body was finally recovered it showed multiple fractures of long bones, many abrasions, a backward dislocation of the spine, internal haemorrhages and burst ear drums. Such a picture was in fact consistent with a close underwater explosion, the force of which had not only bent the diver backwards but damaged his suit and sprung the helmet completely off the breast plate.

The folly of using a cutting torch under such conditions as this, where a pocket of air under pressure may contain oil vapour, is well known. Diving regulations emphasize this danger and instruct that holes should be drilled in the uppermost surfaces of such compartments to let out trapped air before salvage continues. Failure to observe this cost the diver his life.

(ii) Two divers were swimming along, one above the other, the lower one following the sea-bed. Both were breathing pure oxygen and after 20 minutes the lower one was seen by his companion to stop swimming and begin to convulse violently. The unaffected diver tried to bring his struggling companion to the surface but failed to hold him. The convulsions dislodged the mouth-piece and the diver drowned.

When the accident was investigated it was found that the water was 84 ft. deep which meant that the lower swimmer was at about 80 feet whereas 25 ft. is the accepted safe depth for oxygen. Both the men should have known this but had in fact not been adequately instructed in this matter.

Failure to observe this depth limit for safe oxygen breathing has accounted for quite a few deaths. Unfortunately the very nature of the convulsion is such that the mouth-piece may easily become dislodged when drowning is almost inevitable. To use oxygen with safety, depth must at all times be accurately known either by using a float and line or a reliable depth gauge. It is not easy to swim along a level course and many divers have been surprised to find themselves hitting the bottom or breaking surface far below or above their estimated depth.

(ii) A very inexperienced diver had failed to appreciate the importance of being sensible about food and drink before diving and after a liberal ration of spirit and a very heavy meal set off on a long underwater swim. He was soon in trouble, vomited into his face mask, inhaled the vomit and died from asphyxia.

This man was notoriously a ravenous eater and the post-mortem showed whole unchewed potatoes in the stomach.

(c) ACCIDENTAL ACCIDENTS

Occasionally it is difficult to attribute an accident to ignorance or carelessness and it is put down to pure misfortune. One example of this is a diver who struck his head on an underwater projection, stunned himself and sank until he was overcome by the convulsions of oxygen poisoning and drowned.

Similarly another diver became entangled with the propeller shaft on which he was working, attempted to 'ditch' his set but became fouled up in the process and drowned.

A third diver swimming at a depth of 20 ft. off the Malayan Peninsula was attacked by a shark which inflicted a massive laceration of leg and buttock with haemorrhage shock and death. This accident caused great consternation in the diving world for most divers believe that if a dark underwater swimming dress is worn a shark will not attack. The report has it that this unfortunate man was wearing a suit but there are those who claim that this could not be so. Those who trust the shark insist that if the victim was wearing a suit the attacker was a Barracuda. This is a

thin excuse really because the bites were typically the mutilating laceration of a shark rather than the clean cut bite of the Barracuda. Similar
lacerations have been produced by the screws of motor boats striking
surfacing divers.

(D) ACCIDENTS DUE TO ILLNESS

In everyday life there are, from time to time, medical emergencies
which cause unconsciousness. On land help arrives sooner or later and
the patient is taken to hospital. In the water he usually drowns. The age
group of divers and the usual high standard of physical fitness required
usually eliminates many of the potentially acute illnesses. However on a
purely statistical basis, even though rare, some crises must occur with
the patient in or under water. One must always be prepared for the odd
surprise in underwater accidents and be ready to consider such conditions as epilepsy, coronary thrombosis or cerebral haemorrhage. Dia-
betics presumably would not continue aquatic activities and epileptics
certainly should not, though particularly with the latter there is a tendency to keep the complaint a secret.

Three quite dramatic cases will serve to illustrate this possibility.

(i) A very well-built active man of 22 years, who had regularly played
games and apparently been in first-class physical condition, left the
ladder of a ship one dark January night for a practice dive. Two or three
minutes after entering the water he returned to the ladder indicating he
was not well and was coming out of the water. As he was being helped
up the ladder he suddenly lost consciousness, fell back into the water,
and disappeared. He was incidentally still wearing and using his closed
circuit oxygen breathing apparatus when he sank out of sight.

Other divers were sent for and a search began. One of these, 1½ hours
after the accident, was swimming along the bottom at a depth of 40 ft.
when he heard groaning and discovered the victim still alive and breathing from his apparatus though apparently unconscious. He was quickly
brought on board ship and regained consciousness five minutes later.
His condition seemed fairly hopeful though he was coughing up blood-
stained mucus. He improved somewhat, recognized his friends and
spoke a little but three hours after being brought out of the water he had
a copious haemorrhage and died. This was a disappointing sequel to the
dramatic recovery and it was very difficult to imagine just what had been
the cause of the first illness and collapse.

The following day a post-mortem examination cleared away all
doubt. The lungs were congested and the lumen of the left coronary
artery was reduced to half its diameter by atheromatous infiltration and

completely blocked by a thrombus. Atheromatous patches were also seen on the aorta.

It was unexpected in such a young and seemingly healthy man to find such advanced atheromatous changes and coronary thrombosis. How much had the excitement and stress of the night dive and the cold water to do with the crisis? How much longer would he have lived had he not been diving? There is of course no answer to these questions and such events must be accepted as rare and due to chance. No economical medical screening can be recommended and it would be unreal to expect every would-be underwater swimmer to have an electro-cardiograph taken.

(ii) Another young man very keen to become an underwater swimmer spent the first part of a forenoon during his early training swimming about on the surface of an artificial lake. This was followed by an underwater swim at a depth on a submerged rope. After the swimmer had been traversing the bottom for ten minutes, a following swimmer noticed he was lagging behind and seemed in difficulties. He therefore helped him to the surface where he was grabbed by an attendant in a dinghy. By this time he was unconscious and obviously in serious trouble. He was then towed as quickly as possible to the lakeside where artificial respiration was given but with no success and by the time the doctor arrived the victim was dead.

Once more a death with no apparent cause! The breathing set when examined was in perfect working order and the diver had been given a careful medical examination three days before the accident. Again the post-mortem examination gave the answer for it revealed that both lungs were widely affected with an acute haemorrhagic, presumably virus, pneumonia. This was quite sufficient to account for the death but made one wonder just how ill the patient was before he went into the water. Probably he felt wretched but was determined not to miss his opportunity for the dive.

Pneumonia of this type can develop with amazing rapidness but it is almost incredible that a man should feel well enough to swim around in water at one moment and be dead fifteen minutes later. It may be that in some way the use of an oxygen breathing apparatus under pressure, even as little as $1\frac{1}{2}$ to $1\frac{3}{4}$ atmospheres, may in some way irritate an inflamed lung. It is quite possible too that if the gas was trapped in clusters of alveoli by inflammatory secretions in tiny broncholi, going under pressure would cause these pockets to contract drawing infected matter into alveoli. Decrease in pressure would have a reverse effect.

It certainly does seem as if spread of respiratory infection is enhanced in underwater swimming. A similar, though non-fatal, case occurred about the same time when a diver using air, who felt well enough to carry out a routine underwater swim, reported sick when he came out of the water.

The development of his symptoms was frightening to watch. Starting with some nausea and breathlessness he rapidly worsened and could only tolerate a sitting position, being acutely dyspnoeic with retrosternal pain, cyanosis and scattered rales in both lung fields. Radiographic examination showed a diffuse clouding of both lung fields. There seemed to be little doubt that some direct connection existed between the dive and the unusual spread of the infection.

Cases such as these should serve as a warning that, where there is even the slightest evidence of any respiratory tract infection and especially during an influenza epidemic, underwater swimming or exposure to increased pressure should be avoided.

(iii) The third fatal underwater accident attributed to illness is less convincing than the above cases. A group of fairly experienced underwater swimmers were undertaking a long underwater swim on oxygen. There is no reason to suspect that they exceeded a safe depth but as the swim continued they became scattered. One of them surfaced and was seen to be having what the observers described as a convulsion. Unfortunately before the boat could reach him he sank and was never recovered.

On this very slender piece of evidence it would be tempting to assume that the diver exceeded his safe oxygen depth and developed oxygen poisoning. He might even have had time to surface as a result of feeling unwell or having lip twitches and only developed the true convulsions on the surface, lost the mouth-piece and drowned.

In this case other evidence was available. A year before this same diver was about 30 ft. under water with oxygen but not exerting himself. He later reported that he remembered having some difficulty with breathing and then all was blank until he was on the way back to his diving school.

This time he was under constant observation by his instructor. He was seen to stop all movement and, apparently in trouble, was quickly removed from the water. He was unconscious with a gasping respiration. His diving apparatus was removed and he soon regained consciousness. His behaviour was very odd and he had to be restrained from dressing himself in diving gear and re-entering the water. Though conscious during this period he never remembered it. Even after his apparent full recovery for many hours he complained of headache and a state of strange sleepiness throughout which time he showed a rapid (120 per minute) pulse rate.

At the time this incident was provisionally diagnosed as an oxygen syncope, though without much confidence, for the picture, particularly the abnormal behaviour and amnesia, was most atypical.

When however this event and the circumstancs of his death were considered together the possibility of the episodes being of epileptic origin seemed quite possible. No other single diagnosis will fit both events and though the second may have been oxygen poisoning the first was not typical of any common diving mishap.

The answer in this case can never be known but on the evidence available it has been classified as death by drowning as a result of an epileptic fit.

SOME UNDERWATER ACCIDENTS

Of the authors series of 200 diving accidents 51 were fatal. (Miles, 1967.) This is a high proportion of deaths and points to the great need for care in all underwater activities where unconsciousness however brief invariably leads to drowning unless rescue is very prompt. On land unconsciousness may remain without help for long periods and still survive.

The following table gives a summary of these accidents:

Cause	Fatal	Non-fatal	Total
ASPHYXIA	22	11	33
ANOXIA	8	16	24
ILLNESS IN WATER (i) CORONARY THROMBOSIS	2	1	3
(ii) ACUTE PNEUMONIA	2	1	3
(iii) EPILEPSY	1	2	3
OXYGEN POISONING	5	5	10
SYNCOPE AND COLLAPSE	—	46	46
PULMONARY BAROTRAUMA	5	2	13
DECOMPRESSION SICKNESS	—	35	35
EARS AND VERTIGO	—	10	10
SHARK BITE	3	—	3
OTHER CAUSES	3	8	11
TOTAL	51	149	200

OXYGEN SYNCOPE AND COLLAPSE

This condition has already been described in Chapter VIII but amongst the symptoms which tended to summate in producing the oxygen syncope were the following:—

PANIC	4
ANXIETY AND HYPERVENTILATION	12
HYSTERIA	2
HANGOVER	2
LACK OF FOOD	7
POOR VASO-MOTOR TONE	4
INCREASED INTRA-PULMONARY PRESSURE	5
FATIGUE	3

Panic, anxiety and hyperventilation are not uncommon in beginners and in some are such that they must be regarded as temperamentally unsuitable for diving. In two of the more experienced divers the anxiety resulted from a personal domestic difficulty. In one there was a conflict between the pleasure of diving with its financial advantages and a desire to please a new wife who was afraid of her husband going under water. It was difficult for him to admit to his friends he would give up diving for this reason, so his subconscious came to the rescue and he became unable to retain a mouth-piece in position for any length of time. This became almost an obsession and when finally with apparent reluctance he gave up he was quite emphatic that there was nothing he would like to do better than continue diving if it wasn't for the 'objectionable' mouth-piece.

Both instances of hangover occurred in the experienced divers. One is of particular interest. He remembered being cold in the water with a very bad headache and extreme nausea. He was brought unconscious from the water looking flushed but quickly recovered. As a matter of course the breathing apparatus was examined and to everybody's surprise a concentration of 0·005% carbon monoxide was reported. As a result it was sent to analytical chemists for confirmation and there it was found that the carbon monoxide reaction was in fact due to the presence of a volatile reducing substance—possibly methane. On questioning the diver admitted that the previous night he had eaten a heavy meal which he washed down with several pints of very rough cider. It was from the metabolism of the cider that the volatile gases were produced to be exhaled from his lungs into the breathing bag.

Lack of food was a surprisingly common finding not only in these cases of syncope but amongst the population generally. Many people it seems will take a last meal between 6 and 7 p.m. in the evening and be content with a cup of tea and a cigarette for breakfast. Forenoon diving with such a routine is not to be recommended.

Poor vaso-motor tone is applied to the few cases who have a lowered syncope threshold, who faint easily in the dentist's chair, on seeing blood or when given an inoculation. Increased intra-pulmonary pressure may be quite severe when inexperienced swimmers try forcibly to clear their ears when suffering from a catarrhal infection. Fatigue in underwater activity is very common.

The mishaps due to ANOXIA might almost be called carelessness. In seven of the fourteen cases the wrong mixture had been put into the cylinders of the breathing apparatus and in three, where mixtures were being used with re-circulation, the wrong setting had been applied to the flow rate. The remaining four were underwater swimmers diving without apparatus who hyperventilated before entering the water to undertake a strenuous effort and lost consciousness as a result of latent anoxia.

Two of the three epileptics under the heading of ILLNESS IN THE WATER were pulled out during the fit and a diagnosis of epilepsy subsequently confirmed by clinical and electro-encephalographic examination. The third was not suspected at the time but when later he had a second attack in the water and drowned epilepsy was presumed. The other three who lost consciousness in the water were all found, on admission to hospital, to have developed pneumonia. The significance of the sudden onset, presuming the divers felt well enough to go under water, has already been mentioned.

Next on the list is ASPHYXIA which, in three cases, resulted from the underwater swimmers exhausting their supply cylinders. Such accidents are usually due to carelessness but there is some excuse for one of these victims, a professional diver who was doing an underwater 'stand in' during the filming of one of the post-war 'frogman' epics. Expecting a short appearance he took only one breathing set and no reserve breathing mixture. He just couldn't meet his commitment with his available resources and kept on going until he and the set were fully exhausted.

Of the remaining three cases of asphyxia one had a faulty mouthpiece which allowed water to enter with each inspiration, another lost his mouth-piece when trying to blow water out of the face mask and nearly drowned. The third was very nearly strangled by going into the water wearing a hood with a neck seal which was much too small. He was pulled out unconscious with an ashen face and black lips but recovered with artificial respiration and oxygen, though his neck was very sore for many days.

Four of the five instances of OXYGEN POISONING all occurred as a result of relatively long exposure with heavy work or hard swimming at depths beyond the safe limit of 25 ft. In fact periods of 25, 45, 40 and 37 minutes were spent at depths of 33 ft., 50 ft., 30 ft. and 33 ft. respectively. All convulsed but recovered when brought out of the water to breathe air at atmospheric pressure.

Three cases of BURST LUNG occurred in underwater swimmers. Retrosternal emphysema occurred in a diver practising 'ditching' his breathing set and ascending free from 50 ft. He had acute retro-sternal pain on surfacing but recovered in a pressure chamber. A second swimmer flooded his set at 20 ft. and surfaced without it with acute pain in the right side of the chest and coughed up blood. A right-sided pneumothorax was found which responded to normal hospital treatment. Finally an underwater swimmer some hours after surfacing from a dive of 25 ft. for 40 minutes reported with an aching pain in the left foot which was swollen, tender and hot to touch. Immediate relief was obtained by recompression and with therapeutic decompression there was complete recovery. This very unusual case was treated by Crocker whose experience in this field is such that his diagnosis of an air embolism of a small branch of the dorsalis pedis artery is most certainly correct.

Cases of burst lung are very rare, especially in underwater swimming. They do occasionally occur during training in submarine escape techniques and will be referred to under this heading.

Many of the cases described above have occurred with closed circuit breathing apparatus. Such apparatus is likely to become more used in underwater swimming as its sphere of activity increases. Generally however the open circuit air set is at present widely used and such accidents as oxygen syncope and latent anoxia will not occur. It will also perhaps be less likely for the wrong gas mixture to get into an air cylinder, though it has happened.

Decompression sickness is not usually regarded as an accident of diving (it rarely endangers life in the water) but rather as a complication. It has anyway been fully described, as have injuries to the ears.

The increasing use of the aqua-lung in commercial fishing, particularly by individuals who in order to increase their catch tend to spend more time at depth and less in decompressing, is producing an increasing number of cases of decompression sickness which in many countries is stretching to the limit treatment resources. When diving for profit the decompression tables seem lengthy. The temptation to shorten them must be resisted as adequate treatment may not always be available. Delayed symptoms are not always recognizable by doctors unfamiliar with the condition.

In order to lessen this risk the British Sub-Aqua Club has produced a tough plastic Divers Emergency Card 4 by $2\frac{1}{2}$ inches. On one side is a summary of Diving Table I as shown in fig. 48 and the other is as follows:

DIVERS' EMERGENCY CARD

DECOMPRESSION SICKNESS

'If the bearer should develop any symptoms after diving not directly attributable to some other cause, these should be suspected as being due to decompression sickness until proved otherwise. As a general rule, symptoms may be expected to develop within four hours of diving, but may be delayed for as long as twenty four hours.

COMMON SYMPTOMS OF DECOMPRESSION SICKNESS

1. PAIN—Usually in or near a joint.
2. DISTURBANCES OF THE NERVOUS SYSTEM—Giddiness, disturbances of vision, numbness and tingling of the limbs, paralysis of legs, difficulty with speech, convulsions or coma.
3. DISTURBANCES OF THE RESPIRATORY SYSTEM—Shortness of breath, pain in the chest, coughing or collapse.

AIR EMBOLISM may occur, usually immediately on leaving the water and produces severe symptoms in categories 2 and 3.

THE ONLY METHOD OF CONFIRMING THE DIAGNOSIS AND ONLY EFFECTIVE TREATMENT IS RECOMPRESSION. DELAY MAY LEAD TO PERMANENT DISABILITY.

In all cases where decompression sickness is suspected, the nearest recompression chamber should be contacted. A list of chambers which may be available in emergency is maintained at H.M.S. Vernon, Portsmouth. Phone calls in an emergency should be made to the Superintendent of Diving or his deputy (telephone OPO5—22351 ext. 72375) during working hours and to the Officer of the Watch (ext. 72588) outside of working hours. It is advisable to make long distance calls as a 'Personal Call', made via the telephone operator.

Where the nearest chamber is some distance away the Police may be able to assist with transport of cases.'

The final paragraph could be modified to suit availability of treatment resources in other countries.

THE INVESTIGATION OF UNDERWATER ACCIDENTS

Rarely are two underwater accidents alike and frequently by detailed examination and inquiry it is possible to reconstruct the events and obtain information which may lessen the chance of recurrence.

Underwater research is still very much in its infancy and every scrap of information is necessary. Most underwater organizations have well-planned safety regulations which their members respect. There is however a need for a common approach to the investigation of underwater accidents. Much more is needed than a coroner's verdict of death by drowning or misadventure.

A contribution which every underwater swimmer can make, which would be of personal interest and general value, would be the maintenance of a personal diving 'log' book. This should be continuous record of all his underwater activity with particulars of his training and medical tests as well as a detailed account of every dive. Location, weather conditions, depth time, types of apparatus and object of the dive should all be recorded. It should be a personal record primarily, with impressions of the environment and notes of any mishaps or mistakes however trivial.

For the investigation of accidents a more formal approach is needed although at present there is no universally accepted form of report. It should be emphasized that every underwater accident is worthy of investigation, not only the fatal ones. Something on the following lines is essential and the more complete the report the more valuable will it be.

(i) *Personal Report*

The conventional personal details of the victim should be listed, age, occupation, etc. with special reference to his underwater experience and competence.

Details of recent medical history or examinations should be included. The activities of the victim immediately before the dive should be described with special reference to food and drink taken.

(ii) *Incident Report*

If the victim recovers his own narrative is most important. In addition the observations of witnesses and experts should be recorded. This must include full details of the dive, local conditions, location, depth duration, water temperature, visibility, tides, currents, condition of bottom and the object of the dive. The incident must be fully described including personal feelings and general observations.

The type of apparatus used should be mentioned though it is

concerned in a separate section of the report. The sequence of events following the accident must also be included with details of rescue, resuscitation, treatment and results.

(iii) *The Breathing Apparatus*

This is a most important part of the investigation and it is essential to know whether or not the apparatus is responsible for the accident.

Where facilities for expert examination exist, the set, when removed from the victim, should be sealed, all taps turned off and with a brief account of the accident, sent along for investigation. Information usually given includes analysis of the gas in various parts of the set, the pressures in the cylinders and the efficiency of the absorbent if a closed circuit set is involved. Impurities such as carbon monoxide and oil vapour are also usually tested for. The integrity of the apparatus and the working efficiency of the valves, cocks, reducers, etc. must also be evaluated.

This may not always be possible but a well-trained diver can usually give a good opinion as to the efficiency of the apparatus. There have been many occasions when a second diver has used the set just to see if it is all right and there have been very nearly as many occasions when this second diver has become a second victim. This is not a practice to be encouraged though tempting to adopt. It should on no account be attempted unless precautions have been made for immediate recovery. On one occasion when a swimmer was pulled out unconscious his companion tried the set and he too was likewise removed from the water. Even so the instructor with the group also used the set and in a few minutes a third unconscious victim was removed from the water. This happened when the oxygen bottles of a closed circuit set had been filled with air.

(iv) *Medical Investigation*

A full report of the medical examination is very valuable and special attention should be paid to the cardio-vascular and respiratory systems.

Medical treatment should also be recorded especially the form of artificial respiration used and whether oxygen or drugs were administered.

Careful inquiry should be made for any information which might point to some latent or developing illness particularly of the respiratory system.

In fatal cases a summary of the pathologist's post-mortem report should be included.

Where there is recovery a summary of the investigation as well as an account of the accident should be entered in the victim's personal log book.

THE PREVENTION OF UNDERWATER ACCIDENTS

The primary purpose of this book is to make some contribution to the lessening of underwater accidents.

Underwater activity can be very safe provided the requirements of respiration are adequately met and provided the limitations set by the environment are appreciated, understood and respected.

Since the majority of accidents are due to human error the answer is largely in the hands of the men who dive and those who train them.

READING AND REFERENCES

Miles, S. (1964). 'One hundred and sixty-five Diving Accidents.' *J. Roy. Nav. Med. Service. 50*, 129.

Miles, S. (1967). 'Medical Hazards of Diving'. p. 111 in *The Effects of Abnormal Physical Conditions at Work*. Ed. Davies, Davies and Tyrer, E. S. Livingstone Ltd., London.

CHAPTER XIV

Drowning

FOR those who are impressed by statistics it is estimated that every year 140,000 persons drown. This is a rate of 5·6 deaths by drowning per 100,000 of the world's population per year. It is of course not evenly distributed between the various countries as the following four examples show:

Country	No. of Drownings per year	Rate per 100,000 Population per year
JAPAN	8,000	9·0
AUSTRALIA	500	5·5
U.S.A.	7,000	4·6
UNITED KINGDOM	2,000	4·0

It is not unexpected that Japan should have a high incidence being an overcrowded island community with a high proportion of fishermen and an enthusiasm for aquatic activity. In Australia at least 75% of the population live near the coast, there being no large inland industrial areas comparable with those found in Britain and America. For this reason Australia shows a somewhat higher incidence than those two countries.

Baker (1954) has studied the death rates from drowning in England and Wales and made some interesting comparison with other accidents and some diseases. For example she shows that under the age of 25 years drowning is second only to road accidents as a cause of death and about 25% of the total are children under 10 years of age.

Drowning is one of the more distressing causes of death since it so frequently occurs in young children at play and in adults whilst enjoying holidays or recreation. Swimming, diving and small boat sailing have greatly increased in popularity in recent years resulting in an increasing number of tragedies. Very fortunately, due to a growing awareness of the hazards, the increase in accident rate has not kept pace with the increase in the number at risk. Nevertheless drowning accidents are all too frequent and most could be avoided. It is surprising that a cause so high up on the list should, over the years, have received so little attention. Indeed few conditions have been so neglected. It is as if the fear of drowning, which is possibly the most dramatized way of dying, has in some way been reflected in a reluctance to probe too deeply into its mysteries. It still tends to be veiled with an aura of witchcraft as

15

instanced by the supposed immunity given if born with a 'caul' or the reluctance of many seamen to learn to swim lest they prolong the agony of drowning. All too frequently when tragedy occurs the event is dismissed as misadventure and drowning, with little or no inquiry into the type of drowning or the predisposing sequence of events.

TYPES OF DROWNING

Books of Forensic Medicine usually define drowning as an 'asphyxial death due to submersion in water' (Glaister, 1942; Smith and Fiddes, 1949), but this is by no means adequate. In addition to the asphyxia, changes result from the effects of any water inhaled into the lungs. This has been simply demonstrated by the fact that a minute and a half of complete submersion will kill a dog whereas recovery will occur in similar dogs after four minutes' complete deprivation of air by other means (Smith and Cook, 1948).

Not only must the question of water in the lungs be considered but also whether that water is fresh or salt. The difference here is very great for in the lungs inhaled water is brought into intimate contact with the circulating blood. Fresh water must be absorbed into the circulation in an attempt to establish osmotic equilibrium with the blood whilst sea water, on the contrary, having greater electrolyte concentration than the blood, will cause water to be drawn out of the circulation.

Three quite different types of drowning are therefore apparent—

(i) 'Dry' drowning in which little or no water enters the lungs, when death will be due to a straightforward asphyxia.

(ii) Fresh water drowning where there is haemodilution and haemolysis as well as asphyxia, and

(iii) Sea water drowning where the asphyxia is complicated by haemoconcentration.

(i) *Drowning without Inhalation of Water*

Generally speaking when people drown there is a period of apnoea and struggle at the end of which violent inspiratory efforts occur. In such cases entry of water into the lungs would seem inevitable though in some cases the water may be swallowed rather than inhaled.

If however consciousness is lost in the water as with anoxia due to some other cause or a person falls into the water after being stunned or whilst intoxicated it is possible for the respiratory centre to be so depressed that the violent inspiratory efforts do not take place.

Alternatively in persons with sensitive laryngeal reflexes the presence of water may cause reflex laryngeal spasm. This is presumably more likely to occur where there is no excessive exhaustion as with a non-swimmer falling into deep water. Swann (1956) estimates that in 20% of drownings, laryngeal spasm prevents entry of water into the lungs whereas Fainer, Martin and Ivy (1951) give a figure as high as 40%.

That water does not necessarily enter the lungs was observed as long ago as 1815 by James Curry in his admirable monograph on 'Apparent Death'. His remarks on this subject are best quoted in their original form:

'From considering that a drowning person is surrounded by water instead of air and that in this situation he makes strong and repeated efforts to breathe, we should expect, that the water would enter and completely fill the lungs. This opinion, indeed, was once very general and still continues to prevail among the common people. . . . Upon drowning kittens, puppies etc. in ink, or other coloured liquors, and afterwards examining their lungs, it is found that very little of the coloured liquor has gained admittance to them. To explain the reason why the lungs of Drowned Animals are so free from Water, it is necessary to observe, that the muscles which form the opening into the Wind-Pipe, are exquisitely sensitive and contract violently upon the least irritation. In the efforts made by a Drowning Person or Animal to draw in Air, the water rushes into the Mouth and Throat, and is applied to these muscles, which immediately contract in such a manner, as to shut up the passage into the Lungs.'

From these observations Curry concludes:

'It appears then, that in a case of drowning, no injury is done to the structure of any of the parts essential to life, so as to render it impossible to restore Animation.'

This last statement is true only of that type of drowning where water does not enter the lungs and consequently it is this type too which has the best chance of recovery when artificial respiration is used.

(ii) *Drowning with Inhalation of Fresh Water*

It is difficult to get useful information on the mechanics of drowning in man but a number of experiments have been carried out using dogs and other animals. It is not known however whether the results of such experiments are wholly applicable to man, though much valuable basic information is obtained.

One thing quite certain, is that any fresh water which enters the lungs will be largely absorbed. In animal experiments dry lungs are rare and if the amount of water is large, death may ensue before the bulk of it can be absorbed.

Swann (1956) using a radioactive tracer in the fresh water in which dogs were submerged showed that within three or four minutes the circulating blood had been diluted by half its own volume of inhaled water. In one case this amount of water absorbed actually exceeded the original blood volume in two or three minutes.

Such haemodilution cannot be without profound effect. The electrolyte concentration will be reduced and extensive haemolysis occur. In the presence of the anoxia this electrolyte reduction rapidly causes ventricular fibrillation.

There is, however, no convincing evidence that man, drowning in fresh water, will develop this profuse haemolysis and ventricular fibrillation although Gordon, Raymon and Ivy (1948) have shown it to occur in cows, pigs and horses. It would therefore seem most likely to occur in man, at least to some extent.

More recently Halmagyi and Colebatch (1960) found that instilling very small amounts (5 ounces) of fresh or salt water into the lungs of sheep caused rapid death. A very considerable increase in the elastic resistance of the lung was found with changes in surface tension causing some alveoli to collapse and blood to be shunted through unoxygenated areas. No change was found in the mortality between the fresh and salt water drownings in these sheep. Swann (1956) however has pointed out that sheep are less likely to develop ventricular fibrillation than dogs and larger animals.

It has been generally assumed that the sequence of events of man drowning in fresh water is first a short period of struggling and apnoea followed by inhalation of a copious draught of water. Water is absorbed and the change in electrolyte balance in the blood, in the presence of the developing anoxia, precipitates within one to three minutes a ventricular fibrillation and death. If laryngeal spasm prevents this then death will be delayed and recovery more likely.

There is a danger however in applying too closely the results of animal experiments to man. In many cases of fresh water drowning there is the reaction of pulmonary irritation (particularly if the water is dirty) and the presence of the fine froth so typical of sea water drowning. Fuller (1963) in a study of 3,000 cases finds no record of ventricular fibrillation in man. The onset of this however in the true situation is likely to be so sudden and effective as to produce death before being seen by a physician. Furthermore the significance of the lipoprotein lining of the alveolae described by Pattle (1963) in the pathology of drowning is not yet understood. It may well lessen the differences in electrolyte transfer in sea and fresh water drowning.

(iii) *Drowning with Inhalation of Sea Water*

The electrolyte concentration of sea water is greater than that in the blood so that when it is inhaled water will pass from the circulating blood into the lungs and to some extent, salt into the blood. This results in a haemoconcentration but there is no haemolysis and no ventricular fibrillation. The heart action just slowly fades away as a result of a myocardial anoxia, taking up to eight minutes to do so. Donald (1955) suggests however that this haemoconcentration may not be so marked in man as some animals. A high systolic blood pressure with a falling diastolic and a final terminal drop in systolic is typical.

The sequence of events is similar to that in fresh water but cardiac failure may take a few minutes longer to develop and man's increased buoyancy in salt water may delay slightly the final inhalation of water.

POST-MORTEM APPEARANCES IN DROWNING

It is important when a body is taken from water to be sure that the cause of death is in fact due to drowning. In most cases the circumstances of the accident will confirm this but when there is doubt post-mortem examinations should remove it.

It is essential, particularly in diving accidents, that the examination should be complete as drowning may only be the sequel to some other condition. Special attention should therefore be paid to the lungs, not only for signs of drowning, but with regard to inflammatory processes, obstructions to bronchi and bronchioles and emphysematous bullae. The heart and its vessels, and the brain, should also be carefully examined and special note taken of any injury which could have caused unconsciousness.

Where burst lung or decompression sickness is suspected the presence of air bubbles in the circulation or loose tissues may be seen. The lungs should be removed with exceptional care to avoid damage and examined under water for obvious leaks.

Where water has entered the lungs, salt or fresh, a little may be drained off. This is likely to be slightly more in cases of salt water drowning. The lungs themselves are distended having lost their elasticity, pit on pressure and show rib compressions.

The presence of water plus the mucous exudate from the tissue and what little air may have been trapped in the alveoli results in the production of a very fine white stable foam. This foam or froth which occasionally may be pink, tinted with blood, is characteristic of drowning. It forms an obstruction to aeration and, though generally more abundant in the smaller passages, frequently extends into the nose and mouth from which it may exude.

The stomach contents are also of importance and may contain copious amounts of the water in which the victim drowned. The presence of large quantities of food and alcohol may have a significant bearing on the case, especially if there is also evidence of vomit in the respiratory passages.

Examination of the blood for electrolyte changes may be important but unless the sample is collected very soon after death it is sometimes difficult to interpret the findings as being solely due to the accident.

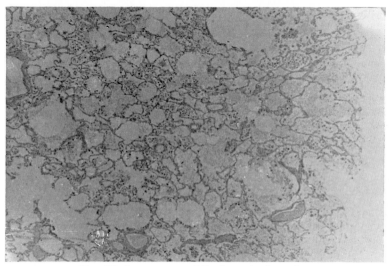

FIG. 52. Appearance of the lungs in drowning

The general signs of an asphyxial death too will be present such as congestion and petechial haemorrhages, especially in the nervous system.

SECONDARY DROWNING

There have been a number of cases with apparent recovery from drowning where death has occurred very much later. In animal experiments small quantities of water introduced into the lungs have produced death. In man pulmonary oedema may develop. A mild form is actually quite common and a chest X-ray taken soon after rescue frequently shows diffuse mottling. Deaths have occurred from this as the following example very well illustrates (Jack, 1959).

A Naval Artificer, carrying a tool chest, was boarding a submarine across a narrow plank. He lost his balance and fell, possibly about six feet, and landed on the 'saddle tank' of the submarine with his head under water. He was recovered still breathing strongly in less than one minute and regained consciousness a few minutes later. He was restless and vomited but respiratory effort remained very good. He had no recollection of the accident. When examined he had a good colour, reflexes were sluggish and crepitations were heard all over the chest. He died two and a half hours later.

A post-mortem examination showed that the lungs were heavy and waterlogged with only the lower marginal parts being aerated. A pink froth was present in the bronchi. The brain and other tissues showed moderate congestion. There was no bone injury.

It would appear that this man fell and struck his head causing concussion. The head being under water for a little while would allow inhalation of sea water but he was rescued before either the immersion or inhalation could cause asphyxia. Subsequently the salt water would draw fluid from the blood extending the waterlogging of the lungs and producing a pulmonary oedema of sufficient extent to cause death (Fig. 52.)

This is a recent case but Curry (1815) knew too that some cases of recovered drowning later died for he writes:

'Either owing to the distension which the arteries of the Lungs have suffered, to the sudden change from great coldness to considerable Warmth, or to the general commotion that attends returning circulation, it now and then happens, that the patient is attacked, soon after recovery, with Inflammation of some of the parts within the Chest. This occurrence is pointed out by pain in the Breast or Side, increased on inspiration and accompanied with frequent and full or hard Pulse, and sometimes with Cough.'

THE IMMERSION SYNDROME

There are occasional reports of immediate fatal collapse following jumping into cold water by young adults.

DROWNING—THE OVERALL PICTURE

Too often drowning is considered solely as the terminal event in accidental immersion whereas it is undoubtedly a condition which is greatly influenced by the circumstances in which it occurs. Every study of drowning should therefore embrace all relative circumstances and not just the momentary and terminal event. It should be regarded as a sequence of events which may start with the donning of the bathing trunks or 'bikini' and end on the cold slab in the post-mortem room. Predisposing factors may be ill-health, ignorance, carelessness, bravado, overindulgence in food and drink or sheer misfortune. In some cases even foul play may be involved.

The condition of the victim at the time of drowning may be of great importance in determining whether or not excessive volumes of water will enter the lungs. Deaths in the water from anoxia, a medical crisis, where a breathing set is found in position should not be classified as drowning. 'Drowning' is as vague a definition as 'poisoning' which without reference to circumstances is meaningless. It might be worth while considering the abandonment of the term altogether and replacing it by such terms as 'Asphyxia due to immersion' when no water is inhaled or 'Asphyxia with pulmonary flooding' when this occurs making special reference to ventricular fibrillation or cardiac anoxia if present. Only by such differentiation can any reasonable correlation be obtained between the circumstances and effects of drowning, the results of which may well influence subsequent methods of treatment and suggest ways and means of prevention.

In cases of near drowning too, much may be learnt from the circumstances though the drama of the event may have caused much attention to be focused on the sensations of the victim in the final moments. Rarely does the narrative cover the events immediately before the catastrophe though sometimes cramp is blamed. This, which may incapacitate a good swimmer in the water, is often attributed to cold, and especially to cold prior to entering the water.

The fortunate cases who have been saved in the final moments before drowning have occasionally on recovery related their experiences. Some have sounded convincing whilst others would seem to be influenced by vivid imagination. One of the most quoted as reliable is that of Lowson (1903) a medical man who, about to drown, found that when his apnoea became intolerable and he was forced to breathe he did in fact take water into his mouth, and immediately swallow it. This occurred ten times and gave him some relief which he suggested might have been due rather to the sedative effects of a carbon dioxide build-up. He lost consciousness but recovered on the surface and struggled to the shore where he vomited large quantities of water. Later there was no clinical evidence that water had in fact been inhaled and he no doubt owes his survival to a brisk laryngeal reflex. What is difficult to understand is that, having lost consciousness in water, he should regain it.

An authentic account which is convincingly written appeared in the editorial column of the *British Medical Journal* of 1894 (a) where a youth who nearly drowned in Portsmouth Harbour described his experiences as follows:

'From the moment that all exertion had ceased a calm feeling of the most perfect tranquillity superseded the previous tumultuous sensations . . . drowning no longer appeared to be an evil. I no longer thought of being rescued, nor was I in any bodily pain.'

He then went on to describe how the outstanding events of his life were presented to him as a 'panoramic view'. When rescued he 'found his return to life much less pleasant than drowning'.

This published report led to many more in which victims reported having 'been to heaven', having 'seen relatives and friends around them with tears in their eyes' and experiencing the 'ringing of bells and vivid colours'. All reported that when the struggling stage was over their experiences were pleasurable and painless.

Nevertheless in a later number of the same Journal a Dr Cullen (1894) attended a lady who nearly drowned and recorded her account. This is lacking in any colourful imagery and is so convincing that it is worthy of repeating:

'Accompanied by my husband and sister I went into the sea at 7.15 a.m. for our usual plunge. As the water was very cold and there was a thick mist we agreed to keep near the land; so on entering the water I commenced to swim along the shore. After a few minutes my breath failed me, and I put down my feet expecting to feel the solid ground, as I was not more than 50 yards or so from the shore. To my surprise I felt my feet and legs sucked under by a strong current, and I sank in a fairly deep hole that the swirl of the water at this point had scooped out of the loose gravelly bed of the sea. I swallowed a considerable quantity of water, and with difficulty got my mouth above the surface. So strong was the "swirl" that I found it beyond my strength either to swim out of it or to turn on my back and float. Finding I was in serious trouble I glanced round to see where the others were, and to my horror saw them quietly swimming away in the other direction quite unconscious of my distress. Up to this point I had not felt any great fear, as I imagined my husband had seen my difficulty, and I expected every moment to feel him grasp me. But when I found that my struggle was unobserved the dread seized me that I should drown unnoticed, that my husband and sister would never know where I had disappeared, or what had happened to me. I expended all my remaining breath in an effort to call my husband's name, but I felt as if my voice had died in my throat, and I was conscious of making no sound. As I sank again I gasped involuntarily, and immediately all other sensations were overpowered by the agonizing, scorching pain which followed the rush of salt water into my lungs. From that moment I was conscious only of that burning suffocation and the intense desire that the others might know what had become of me. Except for that one thought my brain was dulled. I had no vision of my past life, such as I have always believed a drowning person to experience. I was conscious of no fear of death, and no special desire to be saved. I had no thought of my children. There was a roaring in my ears, and a red mist before my eyes; but I neither saw nor dreamed dreams—I only suffered. Not more than three minutes elapsed from the moment when I first sank until my husband (who *had* heard my cry) rescued me.'

When this lady was brought ashore she was quite unconscious and vigorous means were needed to revive her.

It would seem that this account may well be accurate but the occasions previously reported must also have some factual basis. There are too many of them to ignore. If in fact these 'panoramic views' of past life do occur it is interesting to speculate on their origin.

An interesting and possibly relevant point in the last report is the 'agonizing scorching pain which followed the rush of water into the lungs'. Similar sensations though infinitely less severe occur if a pipe smoker who normally does not inhale his smoke inadvertently does so. It is therefore very probable that the unfortunate lady did in fact inhale water while still conscious.

Possibly, and this can only be speculation, it is those fortunate near-drowners, prevented from inhaling water by swallowing and glottic spasm, who, due to a rising of tissue carbon dioxide tension and anoxia, experience the flash backs of memory. Indeed, it may well be that these persons make up the bulk of those who recover after rescue. Where any quantity of water enters the lung chances of survival, however efficient subsequent treatment, may well be quite remote. When drowning is complete there is almost invariably post-mortem evidence of water entering the lungs. Where recovery has taken place it is often so complete that it can be assumed that no water entered. Furthermore the adverse effects of inhaled water are well shown in those instances where in spite of maintained respiratory activity death occurs later from pulmonary oedema.

INVESTIGATIONS OF DROWNING ACCIDENTS

It is almost impossible to carry out a scientific study of the effects of drowning on man, and animal work on this subject does not necessarily present the human picture. Physiologists are however showing some interest and at present some most promising work is being done in Australia by Halmagyi and Colebatch (1961) whose further findings are awaited with interest.

There is one way in which the general practitioner, the life-saving organizations and even the general public can help and that is to make sure that every case of drowning is investigated as fully as circumstances permit. Large organizations might do well to form accident investigation units.

The investigation should not be limited to the immediate incident but should include the victim's past history, aquatic experience and general background.

Information should be collected from:

  (i)   The victim if he survives.
 (ii)   Companions of the victim, and if he has died, his relatives.
 (iii) The rescuers and witnesses.
 (iv)   Any who gave immediate first aid.
  (v)   The ambulance personnel who transported the patient to hospital.
 (vi)   Any attending medical practitioner or hospital officer if the patient survives.
(vii)   The pathologist who conducted any post-mortem examination.

The report should be completed as soon as possible after the accident and sent to whatever local authority has accepted the responsibility for the investigation.

For convenience, the form of report could be in two parts, an incident report and a hospital or medical report.

PART I—INCIDENT REPORT

As well as the personal particulars of the victim (sex, age, nationality, occupation, swimming experience and any known medical condition), the time and location of the accident should be recorded with special note of weather and water conditions (including temperature and whether salt or fresh). The activity of the victim in the 24 hours before the incident should if possible be summarized, how long he was in the water and what he was doing immediately before going in. His activity in the water should be stated, the cause of his distress and how this was noticed.

Details of the rescue should include the time from distress signal to rescue, method of rescue, condition when reached in the water, any obvious injury, resuscitation given in water and condition during rescue and resuscitation. A note should be made of general appearance, colour.

particulars and quantity of any vomit, consciousness or otherwise, whether breathing and if so whether noisy bubbling or frothy. Full details of continuing resuscitation, its duration, difficulties and the victim's reactions throughout should follow with comments of any witnesses, especially medical ones.

If a breathing apparatus has been used this needs special attention and the inquiry should follow the lines given in the preceding chapter.

PART II—HOSPITAL AND MEDICAL REPORT

If the patient lives, an early chest X-ray is most valuable. In fact this should be a routine in all cases of near drowning whether or not they are admitted to hospital.

Special attention should be paid to the clinical condition of the lungs and upper respiratory tract.

A blood sample should be taken as early as possible after leaving the water for a 'packed cell volume' and electrolyte balance estimation. This should be carried out if possible in fatal cases also.

In fatal cases a summary of the full post-mortem report should be included with special comment on appearance of the lungs, stomach contents and any evidence of injury or illness which may have been a prelude to the drowning.

If the investigation of drowning accidents could be established on a large scale there would be no difficulty in introducing some standard questionnaire to include whatever of the above suggestions are considered desirable in a simple and convenient form.

THE URGENCY

Over the years progress in the understanding of drowning in men and its treatment has been almost negligible, yet it remains a vital and growing problem deserving of the most full and urgent consideration.

In support of this rather discouraging statement, pronunciations by four eminent persons covering a span of almost one hundred and fifty years are quoted. There is very little difference in their messages.

(i) *In 1815*. Curry in his 'Observations on Apparent Death from Drowning, etc.' wrote:

'It need scarcely be said, that whatever concerns the preservation of human life cannot be too generally known. On no branch connected with the Science of Medicine, however, is knowledge, less generally diffused, than upon that which makes the subject of the following pages.'

(ii) In the summer of *1894* (b) the *British Medical Journal* opened its editorial columns with a note on 'Drowning' which contained the following statements:

'The public is taking an increasing interest in the treatment of the apparently drowned; this is not surprising at a season when so many fatalities from this cause are registered and attention is now more and more attracted to the subject by the rapid increase of swimming boating and skating clubs. . . .

Dr Bowles has for many years pressed these points (the need for a satisfactory method of resuscitation) on the attention of the profession and there has been a committee of the Royal Medical and Chirurgical Society now for a long time at work in the hope of settling authoritatively the relative merits of the three best known methods of resuscitation.'

(iii) In the summer of *1955* Donald wrote:

'Despite the great interest taken in drowning by various lay organizations in this country, there has been a truly astonishing neglect of this subject by physiologists and medical men. Another bathing season has begun and the usual crop of drowning accidents may be expected.'

(iv) And in *1960* at the opening of the International Conference on Life Saving, Judge Curlewis, President of the Life Saving Association of Australia, pointed out that:

'There was a great need to improve techniques to reduce deaths from drowning and asphyxia in all its forms. . . . The tragedy of this is that most of these lives were lost while the victims were taking their recreation.'

(v) Finally much work has been done in recent years particularly on the physiology, pathology and treatment of drowning, largely as a result of the growing interest in aquatic sports (Miles, 1968).

READING AND REFERENCES

Baker, Audrey Z. (1954). 'Drowning and Swimming.' *The Practitioner.* *172*, 655.
Curry, J. (1815). *Observations on Apparent Death.* E. Cox & Son, London.
Cullen. (1894). 'What Drowning Feels Like.' *Brit. Med. J. 2*, 941.
Donald, K. W. (1955). 'Drowning.' *Brit. Med. J. 2*, 155.
Editorial. (1894 a). 'What Drowning Feels Like.' *Brit. Med. J. 2*, 823.
— (1894 b). 'Drowning.' *Brit. Med. J. 2*, 373.
Fainer, D. C., C. G. Martin and A. C. Ivy (1951). 'Resuscitation of Dogs from Fresh Water Drowning.' *J. Applied Physiol. 3*, 417.

Fuller, R. H. (1963). 'Drowning and the Post-immersion Syndrome.' *Military Medicine. 128*, 22.

Glaister, J. (1942). *Medical Jurisprudence and Toxicology.* E. & S. Livingston, London.

Halmagyi, D. F. J. and H. J. H. Colebatch. (1960). 'Mechanics Involved in Drowning.' International Conference on Life Saving Techniques, Sydney (Report in Press).

— (1961). 'Ventilation and Circulation after fluid aspiration.' *J. Applied. Physiol. 16*, 35.

Jack, D. B. (1959). 'Immersion followed by Acute Pulmonary Oedema.' *J. Roy. Nav. Med. Service. 45*, 228.

Lowson, J. A. (1903). 'Sensations in Drowning.' *Edin. Med. J. 13*, 41.

Miles, S. (1968). 'Drowning'. Brit. Med. J., *3*, 597.

Pattle, R. E. (1963). 'Lining Layer of Alveoli.' *Brit. Med. Bull. 19*, 41.

Smith, S. and W. G. H. Cook (1949). *Taylor's Principles and Practice of Medical Jurisprudence. Vol. 1.* p. 537. J. & A. Churchill, London.

Smith, S. and F. S. Fiddes (1949). *Forensic Medicine.* J. & A. Churchill, London.

Swann, H. G. (1956). 'Mechanics of Circulatory Failure in Fresh and Sea Water Drowning.' *Circulation Research. 4*, 241.

PART III

Coming to Terms with the Environment

CHAPTER XV

The Treatment of the Apparently Drowned

THE RESCUE

The rescue of a person in difficulty in the water has a three-fold aim:

(i) To support the victim, prevent inhalation of water and thus prevent drowning,

(ii) To bring the victim to a place of safety as quickly as possible, and

(iii) To ensure that treatment is commenced at the earliest possible moment.

Much thought and practice has gone into the important question of life-saving techniques and there can be no doubt whatever that such planning and repeated training is the only sure way of achieving the essential combination of speed and efficiency.

The rescue of a person drowning is the means by which he is removed from a position of peril to one of safety where urgent treatment can be commenced at once. To be effective this treatment must be initiated in that brief interval between the failure of respiration and the cessation of the heart's activity, which is only a matter of minutes; five at the most but, in fresh water, possibly as little as two.

Insisting, first, that rescue must be swift, it is of the greatest importance to consider in detail the treatment of drowning.

TREATMENT OF THE APPARENTLY DROWNED

Everything possible must be done to prevent the development of anoxia, in the presence of which changes in blood chemistry, brought about by inhalation of water, are most effective.

The first requirement is the immediate establishment of some efficient form of artificial respiration. No time must be wasted in draining the patient of excess fluids, for the structure of the lungs is such that little or no water will drain out from their depths, even when the patient is up-ended.

If the rescuer is able, whilst the victim is being brought ashore, to inflate the lungs, even just a few times, this will be of far more value than more complete methods which cannot start till later. This can be achieved with an expired air method.

16

If the heart is not beating, no amount of air or oxygen pumped into the lungs will be of any use for, without a circulation of blood, oxygen cannot be transported from the lungs to vital tissues. Artificial respiration MUST be started before the heart fails and therefore SECONDS COUNT. Not only must no time be wasted in vigorous attempts at drainage but there is not time either for choosing a convenient site, searching for gadgets or examining the patient. Nothing must, under any circumstances, delay the onset of artificial respiration. Where there is obvious obstruction in the mouth, weed, froth, vomit, etc. it should be rapidly scooped out with a finger, handkerchief or suchlike.

Artificial respiration must be continued, uninterrupted, for 15 minutes when a short pause may be taken to assess the position and re-arrange the patient if necessary. Usually by this time the outcome has been established but attempts at resuscitation should continue until medical opinion has pronounced death or there is no possible doubt about it. In the absence of such opinion it is usual to continue the arti-ficial respiration for an hour or more with operators working in relays. There may in fact be no justification for this other than the presence of friends or relatives who refuse to give up hope. There are many cases re-ported in which this time has been extended, though not with success. Curry (1815) even recommended that it be 'repeated, in a regular and steady manner, either until natural respiration begins, or until this and the other measures recommended, have been persisted in for at least six hours, without any appearance of returning life'.

While artificial respiration is being administered other bystanders can be employed in summoning professional assistance, gently removing wet clothing and covering with dry coats, blankets or whatever is avail-able. The habit of rubbing the limbs and applying heat should be dis-couraged. Heat and friction cause dilation of the skin vessels which puts additional strain on the heart which may already be embarrassed. Sufficient covering is needed to prevent shivering and no more.

If signs of returning natural respiration appear these should be care-fully watched and the artificial respiration adjusted so that its rhythm is in phase with the patient's efforts and continued until the natural breath-ing is fully established and continuous.

At all times the victim must be handled with the utmost gentleness. No unnecessary movement should be made for, in this critical period, rough treatment will prejudice recovery and may cause vomiting.

If after six or eight inflations by exhaled air resuscitation (or other method) there is no improvement, if no pulse can be felt in the neck or wrist and there is an over-all appearance of impending death, closed chest cardiac massage should be commenced. Exhaled air resuscitation should also be continued with one inflation after every six or eight compressions.

Wherever possible, and with minimum delay, the patient should be transferred to hospital where further investigations, including a chest X-ray, may be done and more intensive treatment initiated which might include oxygen, intravenous plasma or even treatment by hypothermia which is believed to give the brain some protection from the effects of anoxia.

It is most exceptional in cases of apparent drowning for expert treatment to be immediately to hand and the situation may have to be faced by a person with little or no experience or, at the best, some first-aid training. The least that can be done is some attempt at artificial respiration and it is the duty of every citizen to have some knowledge of one method so that if the occasion arises he can at least try to help.

METHODS OF RESUSCITATION

Much controversy has developed and still continues, as to which method is best and there is a risk that, in the arguments over detail, a sober view on fundamental requirements may be clouded.

The requirement is simple. A universal method is needed which is easy to teach and practical. It must produce an adequate ventilation of the lungs, need no additional equipment whatever, be simple enough to be carried out by a child of 12 years or so on a large adult and not be too exhausting to maintain.

For organized rescue and life-saving personnel, who may regularly be called upon to administer resuscitation and who are from time to time standing by to do so, additional equipment and refinements in technique may well be available.

Methods at present used may be divided into two groups: (i) Negative pressure methods and (ii) Positive pressure methods. Each of these may be further subdivided as follows:

(i) *Negative Pressure*
    (*a*) Manual
    (*b*) Rocking
    (*c*) Mechanical
and (ii) *Positive Pressure*
    (*a*) Expired air
    (*b*) Bellows and bags
    (*c*) Mechanical

In each of these groups the first subdivision (*a*) can be carried out without additional apparatus and with the minimum of training. All the remainder need special apparatus and additional training.

(i) *Negative Pressure Methods*

These methods depend on air being drawn into the chest by artificial enlargement of its volume and offer a somewhat similar condition to normal breathing.

In apparent drowning when there is respiratory paralysis the chest is at rest containing about 40% of the vital capacity. Normal respiration would increase the chest volume from this level. In conventional methods of manual artificial respiration an attempt is made to increase lung volume by extending the arms upwards and outwards in the supine position (Sylvester) or raising the elbows backwards and forwards in the prone position (Holger Neilsen). Unfortunately in this manœuvre the arm movements are transferred to the chest through muscular attachments which themselves, especially in the unconscious person, are somewhat elastic. Thus much of the effort is lost in stretching these muscles and the volume of air drawn into the lungs is disappointing. It is however also possible to supplement this intake by pressing on the chest wall to decrease its volume so that when pressure is released the return to the original relaxed position draws in air. In the Schaefer method this is the sole means of ventilation. This too is not entirely satisfactory because it only utilizes chest movement on the expiratory side of the resting position, e.g. a part of the expiratory reserve. This gives only limited expansion of the lungs so that the alveoli are not stretched and the field for gaseous exchange is small. When both routines are used together a reasonable exchange is obtained in many cases, though this varies very much with circumstances.

Alternative movements to arm lifting such as raising or rolling the hips may give better ventilation but are more tiring to perform.

EFFICIENCY OF MANUAL METHODS

Three methods are at present taught which are (i) 'SCHAEFER' in which with the victim prone pressure is exerted on the back of the thorax, and released.

(ii) 'HOLGER NEILSEN' where, again in the prone position back pressure is alternated with a forward raising of the arms usually holding them at the elbows; and (iii) 'SYLVESTER' in which with the patient supine the chest is compressed and the arms raised upwards and outwards.

In a more recent modification of this method (SYLVESTER-BROSCH) a fairly solid pillow, pad, or roll of clothing is placed well back beneath the shoulders to raise the chest and allow the head to fall back allowing a greater chest expansion and better air-way. This is probably the most efficient of the manual methods.

Many reports have been made on the efficiency of these methods. Gordon and a group of workers (1951) measured tidal volumes by various methods in volunteers who had been anaesthetized with thiopentone and rendered apnoeic with d-tubocurarine. When relaxed a cuffed endotracheal tube was introduced. Karpovitch, Hale and Bailey (1951) used subjects who were relaxed and breathing quietly into a spirometer. The manual methods were then superimposed on the natural respiratory movements. The results of these two groups of workers are quite similar.

Method	Tidal volume c.c.		
	Gordon	Karpovitch	
	Mean	Mean	Range
PRONE PRESSURE (SCHAEFER)	378	451	275– 593
ARM LIFT BACK PRESSURE (HOLGER NEILSEN)	975	938	445–1183
ARM LIFT CHEST PRESSURE (SYLVESTER)	—	1068	591–1835

These figures have since been strongly criticized, particularly by Safar (1958), who claims that the use of an endotracheal tube greatly facilitates ventilation. The superimposition of an artificial method upon natural breathing furthermore is hardly realistic.

The manual methods in most cases will give good ventilation only if an adequate air-way is present and this is quite often difficult to achieve except by artificial means. This was shown by Gordon and his co-workers in a later report (1958) when he made a special note of the cases which were actually ventilated successfully when no tube was used.

Method	With cuffed tube	With mouth-piece and nose clip	
	Tidal vol. c.c.	Tidal vol. c.c.	% Successful ventilated
ARM LIFT CHEST PRESSURE	920	450	50
ARM LIFT BACK PRESSURE	950	580	63
HIP LIFT BACK PRESSURE	1090	650	75

These figures showed that without the endotracheal tube, not only was there a considerable reduction in ventilation, but also in an unacceptably high number it was impossible to give adequate ventilation.

Safar (1958) in a similar investigation used a group of 167 trained rescuers and, as a criterion of success, demanded a tidal volume of 500 c.c. to be reached within one minute. The percentage of success for the methods tried was as follows:

Method	Percentage Success	
	With artificial air-way	*No air-way*
ARM LIFT BACK PRESSURE	39	14
ARM LIFT CHEST PRESSURE	50	31

These figures are not very encouraging and success seems to be particularly dependent upon an adequate air-way. When using these manual methods single-handed it is not always easy to control the position of the head. With the arm-lift-back-pressure method of Holger Neilsen (and also the prone pressure of Schaefer) the head is generally turned to one side which in itself tends to produce obstruction. In the prone position the head must be fully extended with the occiput towards the back bone. The chin may be conveniently rested on the victim's hands. When the arm-lift-chest-pressure of Sylvester is used a pad or pillow beneath the shoulder blades will allow the head to fall back into the fully extended position.

In all forms of artificial respiration the head, neck and body should be in the positions as used by sword swallowers.

(i) b. Rocking Methods

Reminiscent of earlier methods of resuscitation where victims were rolled to and fro on barrels or lashed to the backs of galloping horses, Eve's Rocking method has developed as a tidy adaptation for any stretcher or plank to rock the victim between 45° head up and 45° head down. With such movement the heavy abdominal contents, e.g. liver and spleen are like a piston below the diaphragm. Though with this method tidal volumes of 600 c.c. or so may be obtained, there is little to commend it as a routine, for the equipment is bulky and rarely to hand where needed. An advantage sometimes claimed is that one operator could in the case of multiple casualties carry out resuscitation on two or more victims if the stretchers or planks are lashed together. This may be so but such a situation can hardly be visualized.

(i) c. Mechanical Methods

Mechanical methods which simulate the normal action of breathing are usually limited to hospitals. By the time a drowning victim reaches one he is either dead or breathing naturally. The best known is the Drinker's Apparatus or 'Iron Lung' where the patient, all but head and neck, is enclosed in an air-tight box. A pump continually withdraws and replaces a set volume of air out and into the box so causing the same volume to pass in and out of the patient's lungs.

Small mechanical breathing devices working on a similar principle have also been designed which enclose the thorax only.

These mechanical methods are rarely if at all available for resuscitation of the apparently drowned and require the most skilful and experienced personnel to control them.

POSITIVE PRESSURE METHODS

During the past few years there has been a growing awareness of the general inefficiency of manual methods of artificial respiration and a tendency to adopt positive pressure methods. One of these which qualifies as generally acceptable because of its simplicity and lack of gadgetry, is the 'expired air' method.

Unfortunately the propaganda used to popularize this undoubtedly efficient method has left much to be desired. Many experts have made different recommendations and there is a clash of opinion as to whether mouth to nose, mouth to mouth or mouth to air-way should be taught; and if the last what sort of air-way. Teaching has been presented as a major obstacle because of the need for expensive dummies or training films, the scrapping of established handbooks and the overcoming of some fears and prejudices. The multiplicity of names given to the method has not helped, e.g. Exhaled Air Resuscitation, Mouth to Mouth, Mouth to Nose, Mouth to Air-way, Face to Face, Lung to Lung, Rescue Breathing, the 'Elisha Method' or the Kiss of Life.

The 1960 International Conference in Australia used the term 'Expired Air Resuscitation' being, quite rightly, unable to come to a decision to recommend mouth to mouth to the exclusion of mouth to nose or vice versa. Unfortunately the man in the street will not accept such terminology and it is the man in the street who must try to save the lives. Let the medical men and professional life-savers haggle over the refinements, details and nomenclature, but give the ordinary citizen something simple and easy to remember. All that is needed is:

EXHALED AIR RESUSCITATION

(i) With a finger or cloth very quickly wipe out any obvious debris from the victim's mouth.

(ii) Extend the head fully backwards so that the mouth and throat are as near in a straight line as possible.

(iii) With your own breath repeatedly inflate the victim's chest through the nose or mouth (or both in children).

In an emergency confidence will come once the chest is seen to move. Where possible instruction should be given by experienced teachers who will point out the reasons for extension of the head and other refinements such as placing padding under the back. In most subjects when the head is fully extended the mouth will open naturally. If a good airway is not immediately obtained—and this too will be obvious—then adjustments to the position of the head will usually put things right. In a very small percentage of cases it may be necessary to pull the jaw forward. Whether to use the nose or mouth will depend largely on the preference or training of the individual and the appearance of the victim. As far as the rate of inflation is concerned this rather takes care of itself for after each blow the operator will raise his head and look at the chest as he himself breathes in again. When the extended chest subsides and movement ceases it is ready for the next inflation. When the mouth is used the nose may be closed by the cheek or with the thumb and fingers of a free hand. Similarly when the nose is used the cheek may cover the mouth or it may be held shut.

All this is very very simple. It must be so and it is better that the mass of people know these simple actions than a select few have complete training. As enthusiasm for the method grows so will more people wish to become proficient and seek instruction. Finally rescuers should be reminded that whereas in adults strong blows may be needed, for children gentle puffs only are needed, and for infants even gentler. Chest movement is the guide in all cases.

Exhaled Air Resuscitation is the most satisfactory name though, even today, in organized training classes it is generally referred to as the 'mouth to mouth method'. Many societies teach only mouth to nose.

One word of warning must be given to the enthusiastic advocates of this routine regarding its success. With cases of apparent drowning it would be wrong to expect a dramatic reduction in the incidence of fatalities for in the majority of cases the outcome is decided before the victim is brought out of the water. Where face to face methods may be particularly successful is in those instances where they can be administered earlier than the conventional methods, e.g. whilst still in the water or whilst being carried through shallows by other helpers.

THE ADVANTAGES AND DISADVANTAGES OF
EXHALED AIR RESUSCITATION

(i) *Aesthetic Objections*

There are still many unenlightened people who believe that the act of breathing into an apparent corpse would be repugnant and impossible. They add to the supposed horror of the situation with ill-conceived clichés such as 'kissing moribund strangers' and emphasize the risks of contracting communicable diseases.

Yet in spite of such objection when the moment of decision arises it is quite inconceivable that any person however prejudiced originally would deny an unfortunate victim a possible chance of life through selfish prudery. The method has been used time and time again by persons from all walks of life sometimes when blood-stained froth and vomit have been present. The face of the victim has in most cases been washed clean by the water and in any case a quick wipe with the hand or convenient cloth will render it tolerable. It must never be forgotten that the victim is not a 'moribund stranger' but a fellow human being, in dire need of help.

Stories indeed come from South Africa where the most vehement supporters of *apartheid* have not hesitated to use these means in attempts to save a person of a different colour.

The question of 'aesthetic objection' must not be allowed to influence teaching. It is doubtful if it really exists at all. It is best forgotten.

(ii) *The Danger of Infection*

This again has been raised as an objection but, although it may be justifiable to refrain from training with methods which involve direct personal contact, this very small risk must be accepted when the real occasion arises.

It must be remembered that there is only contact between the operator's mouth and the victim's face during the former's period of expiration and nothing is inhaled from the patient. This is a point well to remember when treating cases of respiratory paralysis from gassing or chemical poison.

The risk of infection can be no greater than the accepted practice of kissing, particularly as used in courtship. It is salutary to observe that in Australia in 1959 the New South Wales branch of the Royal Life Saving Society knowingly took the risk of practising on living persons 'for the sake of progress' (Buchanan, 1960). No medical book could condone such a practice if applied to large sections of the population, but the enthusiasm of this particular group cannot but be admired. No objection however can be raised against practice by members of a family on each other.

(iii) *Training Difficulties*

This has been put forward as the major objection to accepting any expired air method assuming, as one must, that direct contact for training purposes should not be encouraged.

The next best thing for training is the life-size dummy or manikin which can only be inflated with the head in the correct position. Many of these are now in the market but the cost is often prohibitive for small organizations. Buchanan (1960) has developed a light-weight transparent mask which can be placed over a volunteer's face and having a separate side outlet can be used for training without direct contact. A similar apparatus now available is the Cheshire Wilson Trainer.

A simple and inexpensive home-made training aid which can be assembled from a half-gallon tin, some tubing and a plastic bag, has been described by the author (Miles, 1963).

A number of very good teaching films have been produced all of which should enable a relatively intelligent observer to carry out the technique satisfactorily. Safar (1958) found that after watching one demonstration 131 out of 145 untrained laymen (i.e. 90%) were able to perform mouth to mouth resuscitation satisfactorily on anaesthetized curarized subjects. This is a very significant result in the light of the poor success achieved by trained rescuers using manual methods and would indicate that single demonstrations are well worth while and should be widely given. In 1963 the Royal Navy produced a series of excellent films on Exhaled Air Resuscitation and Closed Chest Cardiac Massage which have achieved world wide acclaim and distribution. They are available for general showing and suitable for both school children and adults.

It is a great pity that there should be any hesitancy in recommending some simple training technique when the aim must be, in any country, to teach the whole population.

(iv) *Mouth to Mouth or Mouth to Nose*

Expert opinion is still divided on which of these two methods is the more effective. This however must not be allowed to cloud the issue. As long as the reviving air gets into the lungs the route is immaterial.

The disciples of 'mouth to nose' claim that it is easier to perform, is more likely to have a clear air-way, is less objectionable, has less danger of over-distension of the lung and inflation of the stomach is less likely.

Those who advocate 'mouth to mouth' claim that better inflation is possible, it is more natural and nasal obstruction may be an obstacle if 'mouth to nose' is used. It has been estimated that nasal obstruction is not likely to be found in more than 2% of cases.

When children are the victims it is frequently possible for the operator to inflate the lungs by enclosing both the nose and mouth in his own mouth.

In all cases the mouth must be wide open to cover the victim's mouth or nose (or both) and to ensure a good air-tight seal.

(v) *Effect on Circulation*

In natural breathing where air is drawn into the lungs by increase in chest volume there must also be an effect on the pulmonary circulation so that during inspiration blood will be drawn into the pulmonary circulation and aid cardiac filling.

When the lungs are inflated by positive pressure this circulatory benefit is lost and there is some tendency for the pulmonary blood flow to be diminished. Colebatch (1960) however, pointed out that the effects on the circulation were dependent upon the mean pressure throughout the respiratory cycle, and therefore infrequent large inflations were less detrimental than frequent less powerful ones. The former may be achieved more easily with the mouth to mouth methods.

The crucial test however is the degree of oxygenation of the blood and Clifton (1960) measured arterial oxygen saturation in anaesthetized curarized volunteers undergoing mouth-to-mouth and mouth-to-nose artificial ventilation and found in each case it remained between 95% and 98% for the whole operating period of 30 minutes. Under similar conditions Elam (1959) and his colleagues were able to maintain, by this method, an arterial blood oxygen saturation between 87% and 100% in a group of 25 subjects.

(vi) *Application of Exhaled Air Resuscitation*

Without doubt the greatest advantage offered by face to face methods is that they can be performed in the most awkward positions, in water, up electric pylons, in small boats, during transport, in cramped positions, in fact in any situation where the rescuer can bring his face into contact with that of the victim's.

It must not be forgotten that drowning is only one condition demanding artificial respiration and it is also perhaps the least likely to give a satisfactory response. Electrocution, gas poisoning and asphyxia from various causes may need similar treatment and it is in these conditions that the expired air methods will be more likely to prove themselves superior or otherwise.

There is little risk in using expired air technique with gas or chemical poisons as the patient's expired air is not inhaled by the operator. If there is a possibility of contamination of the victim's face a lightly woven cloth can be used as a cover. This is sometimes recommended for aesthetic reasons also. In special cases where the respiratory paralysis is a result of contamination with an anti-cholinesterase insecticide or similar substance the risk to whoever administers resuscitation is too great to permit any close contact and alternative methods, manual or mechanical, should be used. This is possibly the only situation where an exhaled air method is contra-indicated and as this occurs under circumstances where the hazard is known, local arrangements can be made available to give the necessary service in the event of accident. The special nature and rarity of such incidents is such that they give no justification for the universal teaching of more than one method of artificial respiration.

(vii) *The Risk of Over-inflation*

This is of greater importance when bellows or similar apparatus is used. It is virtually impossible for one adult to over-inflate the lung of another with expired air. It takes a pressure of 60 to 80 mm.Hg to produce a burst lung in dogs. Data for man is lacking though burst lung has occurred in ascent through as little as 7 ft. of water which would produce an excess pressure of 160 mm.Hg.

With adults it may be assumed that no risk from this exists but when children and infants are being resuscitated special care is needed. This is so obvious that it would seem quite unnecessary to remind anyone of average intelligence of the necessity for gentle inflation of small chests. Nothing further is needed than that there should be obvious movement of the chest without over-distension.

(viii) *Inflation of the Stomach*

Inflation of the stomach during exhaled air resuscitation usually means that the head is not correctly positioned. With full extension and a good air-way the stomach should not receive any air. If it does it will be seen to be distended in which case firm pressure over the epigastrium will usually expel the excess air. Gentleness however is needed to avoid causing vomiting.

Inflation of the stomach is more common in children but it is also more easy to deal with.

(ix) *The Position of the Patient*

Exhaled air resuscitation is normally carried out with the victim in the supine position and often with the shoulders raised. This has been strongly criticized for not allowing drainage of the lungs and that any vomit is more likely to be inhaled. When an apparently drowned person is brought out of the water any gross amounts of water in the larger upper respiratory passages will run out with tilting but little or nothing escapes from the smaller passages and alveolae. If he is then placed on his back little is lost in this respect and head positioning is much simpler. The Sylvester method was once criticized because it used a supine position but now with the back raised this is considered the best of the manual methods. Vomiting is less likely to occur if the shoulders are raised above the stomach and in any case the risk tends to be exaggerated. When unconsciousness is deep, vomiting is unlikely. It is in fact unlikely to occur before respiration is restored and usually a protective cough reflex also has become re-established. Where large quantities of sea water have been swallowed, vomiting is likely and therefore once natural breathing has restarted the patient should be turned gently on to one side and the attendants warned to watch for vomiting and ensure that it is voided freely.

A very real objection to the prone position is that when natural respiration begins to return a large proportion of body weight must be lifted with each breath.

Whatever the chosen position of the body that of the head is vital. In an unconscious person with the head in the normal position the tongue falls back, completely obliterating the air passage behind it. Hyperextension of the head draws away the tongue from the posterior pharyngeal wall and gives a clear air-way. This extreme backward bending of the head is the secret of all these methods and must be maintained throughout. In most cases with the head in this position the mouth falls slightly open. In those very few instances where inflation of the lungs is still difficult it may be necessary to grasp the jaw and pull it forward.

THE USE OF TUBES AND AIR-WAYS

There has been much propaganda for the use of tubes and air-ways as an adjunct to expired air resuscitation and to overcome any aesthetic objection (Safar and McMahon, 1958). Though the tube has some advantages, it cannot be accepted for general use because the requirement is a method which can be performed with NO additional equipment whatever. Nor is it desirable for a relatively inexperienced person to insert an air-way into the mouth of an unconscious victim. On the other hand, ambulance workers and professional medical auxiliaries, who might repeatedly be called upon to give artificial respiration, could well be trained in the use of air-ways, which they then could keep to hand when on duty. Training however is important and a variety of sizes of tube is really needed. Safar's tube has the advantage in that one way round it is suitable for an adult and the other way for a child. Tubes specially designed for the purpose, though desirable, are by no means essential. Anaesthetic oro-nasal masks, short bits of hose-pipe or similar alternatives may be used.

(i) *Bellows and Bags*

Though these can never replace the person to person methods they are always welcome if they happen to be handy when required. The idea is by no means new for Curry (1815) after describing the use of a box-wood tube as an air-way goes on to say—'there are few cases where the lungs cannot be inflated by a person of ordinary strength, blowing through this tube with his mouth: and should he become fatigued, another may take his place; or instead of that a pair of common kitchen or parlour bellows may be employed for the purpose only wrapping a strip of linen, or a piece of broad tape, ribbon or garter round the nozzle so as to make it fit the tube accurately.'

Bellows are of particular value in situations where there is a possibility of asphyxia from chemical agents which would make direct methods unsafe for the operator.

It is most important to make it impossible to exceed a safe pressure. Bellows pump into the victim's lung leaving natural chest elasticity to ensure exhalation. They are usually fitted with a relief valve which will prevent too great a pressure being applied. A good working rule is that for inflation of the chest the pressure should not exceed 30 mm.Hg and for deflation a negative pressure of not more than 20 mm.Hg.

A convenient form of bellows complete with relief valve and oro-nasal mask has been described by Lucas and Whitcher (1958). It is compact, easy to use, safe and efficient but there is still the need as with all other methods of maintaining an adequate air-way.

Simpler perhaps than the bellows is the self-inflating bag, or balloon resuscitator which has a bag with a foam rubber type wall such that after squeezing it refills with air and regains its shape. From the bag a corrugated connecting tube leads to an oro-nasal mask or mouth-piece. For use the bag is squeezed to inflate the lungs with the mask or mouth-piece held in position by a rubber strap. The head as before must be hyperextended.

(ii) *Intermittent Positive Pressure Resuscitators*

Manufacturers of breathing apparatus have produced some very attractive portable automatic resuscitators. These usually supply oxygen and are so constructed that this is alternately introduced into and withdrawn from the lungs whilst making sure that pressures in either direction are kept well within the safe limits. They have many refinements such as suction aspirators and can be used for more than one patient at a time. They are very useful for well-organized casualty units, ambulances, fire brigades and the like but they are inevitably expensive.

These are rarely available at the site of the casualty, particularly in drowning incidents, and if it is only required to give oxygen there are simpler ways of doing so.

ADDITIONAL TREATMENT

Though aeration of the lungs is of the greatest importance and essential in cases of apparent drowning there are other steps which may be taken which will increase chances of survival. The artificial respiration will only provide oxygen to the blood and have no effect on the action of fluid within the lungs. It may in some cases be of little use.

Fainer, Martin and Ivy (1951) used a large series of dogs, which were submerged in fresh water under general anaesthesia, until terminal gasps were observed. No difference in survival rate was found between those who were given artificial respiration at this stage and those which were not. Death in all cases was presumed due to ventricular fibrillation. It must not however be implied that the same would happen in man.

Redding, Voigt and Safar (1960) asphyxiated lightly anaesthetized dogs and, when breathing ceased, flooded the lungs with sea water. Three types of treatment were then given as follows.

(i)   Intermittent positive pressure resuscitation with air.

(ii)   The same but using oxygen.

(iii)   As in (ii) but ten minutes after start of resuscitation they were given 50 ml./kg. of dog plasma intravenously.

Though those given oxygen were better oxygenated than those on air, the only dogs to survive were four out of five who were given the intravenous plasma. The remainder died later with pulmonary oedema.

Colebatch and Halmagyi, in some work as yet unpublished, obtained very good results in saving anaesthetized curarized sheep who had sea water instilled into the lungs, by using pure oxygen under pressure. Air was not satisfactory.

This work indicates that more treatment than artificial respiration is needed. It is difficult with present knowledge to give hopeful advice in cases of fresh water drowning but with sea water the early introduction of positive pressure oxygen administration and an intravenous injection of plasma would seem greatly to improve the survival chances. This will not be easy under practical conditions but with more research and thought some formula may be evolved whereby, in the more populous areas, at least, improved treatment might become available.

Efficient artificial respiration however must still remain the most important and immediate requirement, being maintained until more elaborate facilities arrive.

THE ADMINISTRATION OF OXYGEN

When oxygen is available it should be administered if this can be done efficiently. There are many ways it can be given apart from the expensive and complicated resuscitators. Bellows and self-inflating bags can be quickly adapted and, provided a pressure reducing valve is used, direct inflation through a mask from a cylinder with push button valve is simplest of all if used by an experienced person. Underwater swimming organizations may possess oxygen cylinders and demand valves. A rescuer practising expired air resuscitation may well fill his own lungs with oxygen for each breath. Australian life-savers use a life-line for rescue which is a flexible pipe carrying oxygen to a demand mouth-piece. Such an arrangement enables oxygen to be administered to a drowning man whilst still in the water.

Oxygen administration should not be continued for long periods once normal respiration is re-established owing to its irritant properties, unless there are definite indications for its use, such as cyanosis or evidence of pulmonary oedema. Mixtures containing carbon dioxide should on no account be used (Donald and Paton, 1955) because of the risk that there may already be some increase in carbon dioxide tension in the tissues and further increase may prejudice the recovery of the respiratory centre.

A further and quite simple aid in the treatment of drowning which may well be made available in ambulances and first-aid posts is the mechanical sucker or aspirator. This can be a simple foot-operated apparatus or be driven from some power source. With a fine catheter on the end of its suction tube it can be used to remove water, froth and mucus from the upper respiratory passages without interfering with the progress of continued artificial resuscitation.

All cases of apparent drowning *must* be taken to hospital and there treated as acute medical emergencies, special efforts being made to prevent secondary drowning. Positive pressure oxygen should be available and intravenous plasma given immediately. Electrolyte disturbance should be corrected even, in extreme cases, to the extent of a complete replacement transfusion.

Other supplementary therapy may include hypothermia to reduce damage to cerebral tissues, tracheotomy for improved ventilation, pulmonary washout if there is gross contamination and possibly hyperbaric oxygen. An X-ray on admission is well worth-while and all patients should be kept under close observation for at least 24 hours. Where ventricular fibrillation persists the use of a defibrillator is indicated. This is, however, not a 'first aid' measure and would be dangerous on a wet victim at the water's edge. Closed chest cardiac massage will maintain a circulation even when the heart is fibrillating.

In hospital the lungs should be further protected by anti-biotic therapy and consideration be given to the use of steroids. If the delay in restoring circulation is prolonged the possibility of cerebral oedema should also be considered and protective treatment given e.g. intravenous urea or bicarbonate solution. This is a controversial matter best left to the attendant consulting physicians. Recovery even after cerebral damage is usually good. Some psychological care may also be needed as a person who has experienced 'near drowning' will need a great deal of help and encouragement before he can once more enjoy swimming or other aquatic activities.

CLOSED CHEST CARDIAC MASSAGE

When any new technique is introduced there are always those who take great pains to prove it to be as old as the hills. The Bible is usually quoted for reference. Exhaled Air Resuscitation has been attributed to Elisha, and God breathed into the nostrils of Adam. Closed Chest Cardiac Massage is the modern equivalent of the raising of the dead by the 'laying on of hands'.

The parallel acceptance in recent years of both Exhaled Air Resuscitation and Closed Chest Cardiac Massage is more than coincidence. Many of the physical methods of artificial respiration, rocking, rolling over barrels, strapping to the backs of galloping horses or oxen, and the more recent techniques of Schaefer, Sylvester and Holger-Nielsen, will produce some limited cardiac compression. Exhaled Air Resuscitation on the other hand, though extremely effective, is solely ventilatory.

The technique as known today was first described in July, 1960, by Kouwenhoven and his colleagues in Baltimore (Kouwenhoven, Ing, Jude and Knickerbocker, 1960) following a series of careful experiments on dogs and trials on human patients. Their paper contains an observation which deserves a place amongst the foremost of great statements in the history of medicine 'Anyone, anywhere, can now initiate cardiac resuscitative procedures. All that is needed are two hands'.

17

This team during a period of ten months treated twenty patients between the ages of two and eighty years of whom fourteen made complete recovery. Their report stimulated world-wide interest and the method they described is now universally accepted and practised as recommended in this first paper.

Many studies of the effectiveness of Closed Chest Cardiac Massage have been made in the last five years and these are summarized in Table I. Kouwenhoven's (1960) first claim of a 70 per cent recovery rate was exceptional, the reason for this being no doubt careful selection of patients. The figures of subsequent workers are more realistic and the average of 18 per cent full recovery is in keeping with present day experience. This of course includes cases treated both in the hospital and elsewhere, and it is to be expected that the higher recovery rate will be found in the former. This is certainly confirmed in Wilder's (1964) cases resuscitated in ambulance with a 10 per cent full recovery rate.

TABLE I—Effectiveness of closed chest cardiac massage

Authority		Cases Total	Restored Beat No.	%	Full Recovery No.	%	Comment
Kouwenhoven	1960	20	14	(70	14	(70)	
Jude	1961	118	107	(91)	28	(24)	76 outside O.T.
Rivkin	1962	70	30	(43)	15	(21)	
Johnson	1963	49	18	(37)	5	(10)	
Klassen	1963	126	42	(33)	17	(13)	
Semple	1964	29	20	(69)	11	(38)	
Wilder	1964	153	52	(34)	15	(10)	All in ambulance
Smith	1965	254	80	(32)	40	(16)	
Total		819	363	(44)	145	(18)	

Available figures for open chest cardiac massage show a full recovery rate of about 20 per cent, in other words, very little difference. It must be remembered, however, that with very few exceptions this technique is limited to the operating table. Closed Chest Cardiac Massage, therefore, though not producing a greater recovery rate, extends the application to a very much greater variety of situations and can be practised by trained lay persons. Though the recovery rate is not high, the fact remains that but for the technique, death would have been inevitable.

Closed chest cardiac massage demands a considerable degree of pressure upon the sternum and cases are reported from time to time of broken ribs and damage to underlying tissues. When such cases are investigated it is often found that the technique has been carried out incorrectly. Few comprehensive reports of these injuries are available but two are given in Table II. These at least give some indication of the risk which is seen to be by no means high and is indeed a small price to pay for the saving of many lives.

The method employed is an indirect one and a considerable loss in cardiac efficiency is inevitable. Success is usually signified by the presence of a palpable pulse in peripheral arteries or a blood pressure of 90 mm. of mercury or more. Mackenzie, Taylor, McDonald (1964), were able in three patients to compare the actual cardiac output with recorded blood during normal heart actions and in closed chest cardiac massage. They show that although the method undoubtedly produced a flow of blood, this was of the order of 50 per cent less than from the normal heart and pointed out that the blood pressure recorded, not a forward flow, but a pressure pulse. This fair warning is timely and would support those who still believe that internal cardiac massage should be performed where circumstances permit, e.g. when the patient is already in the operating theatre. These findings, however, detract in no way from the value of external massage which is widely supported by growing experience and observations.

Observations on the marked improvement in colour and in blood flow from wounds of patients during resuscitation is ample evidence of this.

TABLE II—Injury following closed chest cardiac massage.

Authority		Cases-total No.	Fractured ribs or sternum No.	%	Viscereal damage No.	%
Klassen	1963	126	25	(20)	5	(4)
Smith	1965	254	19	(7)	3	(0·5)
Total		380	44	(9)	8	(2)

It is most important that closed chest cardiac massage is carried out correctly. The technique depends on compression of the heart between the sternum and the vertebral column and over-lying tissues. Sufficient pressure over the cardiac area, to the left of the mid-line, cannot be achieved without damage to the ribs. The following points are essential.

1. The patient must be on his back on a hard surface.

2. Pressure must be applied to the lower half of the sternum and be absolutely vertical.

3. This is best achieved by kneeling at the side of the patient and placing the 'heel' of one hand on the lower half of the sternum with the other hand over it. During pressure the arms should be straight and the shoulders above the mid-line of the body.

4. A depression of the sternum of $1-1\frac{1}{2}$ inches should be achieved in adults and correspondingly less in children. (This is usually possible in the unconscious patient but should not be attempted when practicing on a conscious individual.)

5. A rate of sixty compressions a minute (one per second) is recommended.

6. With children, one hand only should be used and with infants and babies, two or three fingers.

7. The pressure required is equivalent to about half the body weight of the patient.

In all training classes the method is taught in conjunction with exhaled air resuscitation. It is scarcely, if at all, used by itself. The location of the pressure area and the direction of pressure can be demonstrated on the conscious volunteer and the rhythm and feel can be practised quite simply on a set of bathroom scales, the pointer being forced every second to the six stone mark for an adult and smaller amounts to stimulate children (e.g. half body weight). When combined with E.A.R. the lungs are inflated after each 6–8 cardiac compressions, the hands being withdrawn for this.

The combined resuscitation is quite exacting for a single operator but relatively easy for two to perform.

Opinions differ greatly on this, some limiting the method to medical personnel and the other including the whole adult population.

In all cases where closed chest cardiac massage is indicated, it should be remembered that failure to apply it must result in death. Thus it should be as widely taught as possible. It should certainly be included in all organized first-aid training. Indeed any person with the intelligence to learn it should do so. Although correct application of the technique is essential for maximum success, it would be impossible to condemn the uninitiated individual who, having a vague notion of the method, made some attempt at cardiac resuscitation when faced with a moribund casualty. It is thus only possible in this paper to present the method and make recommendations. The ultimate decision as to whom should be taught must be with the administrators.

The diagnosis of cardiac arrest is not easy and must depend upon inability to feel a pulse, widely dilated pupils, no improvement in colour after six or eight inflations of the lungs by exhaled air resuscitation or other methods and an overall appearance of impending death.

The success of cardiac resuscitation is indicated by the return of a palpable pulse, improvement in colour, contraction of pupils and a re-appearance of haemorrhage from any wounds if present.

The limitations of closed chest cardiac massage must be fully appreciated. It is no more than a single process in the complicated procedure of resuscitation, invariably combined with exhaled air resuscitation. These two processes do not more than maintain a limited circulation and an acceptable degree of pulmonary ventilation. They are essentially first-aid measures (a 'do-it-yourself' heart lung machine) but since, both asphyxia and cardiac arrest will produce death in a few minutes, their main contribution towards survival is that of time. Together they provide the necessary period during which transport to hospital can be achieved and the more elegant processes of resuscitation initiated.

Attention to detail in carrying out the technique is of paramount importance and provided that this can be assured the method should be widely taught in conjunction with that of exhaled air resuscitation.

Cardio-respiratory resuscitation is, however, an interim measure to postpone the onset of death. It must be followed by more strenuous emergency hospital treatment and a period of 'intensive care'.

READING AND REFERENCES

Buchanan, L. (1960). 'Rescue Breathing for the Partly Drowned.' *Med J. Australia*. 12 March, 1960.

Clifton, B. (1960). 'The Comparative Efficiency of the Various Methods of Artificial Respiration.' International Conference on Life Saving Techniques, Sydney.

Colebatch, H. J. H. (1960). 'The Physiological Basis of Artificial Respiration.' International Conference on Life Saving Techniques, Sydney.

Curry, J. (1815). *Observations on Apparent Death*. E. Cox & Son, London.

Donald, K. W. and W. M. D. Paton (1955). 'Gases Administered in Artificial Respiration.' *Brit. Med. J. 1*, 313.

Elam, J. O., D. G. Green, E. S. Brown and S. A. Clements (1958). 'Oxygen and Carbon dioxide exchange and energy cost of expired air resuscitation.' *J. Am. Med. Ass. 167*, 329.

Fainer, D. C., C. G. Martin and A. C. Ivy (1951). 'Resuscitation of Dogs from Fresh Water Drowning.' *J. Applied Physiol. 3*, 417.

Gordon, A. S., J. E. Affeldt, M. Sadove, F. Raymon, J. L. Whittenberger and A. C. Ivy (1951). 'Air-Flow Patterns and Pulmonary Ventilation During Manual Artificial Respiration on Apnoeic Normal Adults.' *J. Applied Physiol. 4*, 403.

Gordon, A. S., C. W. Frye, L. Gittelson, M. Sadove and E. S. Beattie, Jnr. (1958). 'Mouth to Mouth versus Manual Artificial Respiration for Children and Adults.' *J. Am. Med. Assoc. 167*, 320.

Johnson, J. D. (1963). *J. Amer. Med. Assoc. 186*, 468.

Jude, J. R., Kouwenhoven, W. B. Ing, D., and Knickerbocker, G. G. (1961). *J. Amer. med. Assoc. 178*, 1063.

Karpovitch, P. V., C. J. Hale and T. L. Bailey (1951). 'Pulmonary Ventilation in Manual Artificial Respiration.' *J. Applied Physiol. 4*, 458.

Manual Artificial Respiration. *J. Applied Physiol. 4*, 458.

Klassen, G. A., Broadhurst C. Peretz and Johnson, Al. (1963). Lancet *1*, 1290.

Kouwenhoven, W. B., Ingd. Jude J. R., and Knickerbocker, G. G. (1960). *J. Amer. med. Assoc. 173*, 1064.

Lucas, B. G. B. and H. W. Whitcher (1958). 'Artificial Respiration.' *Brit. Med. Jour. 2*, 887.

Mackenzie, C. J., Taylor, S. H., McDonald, A. H. and Donald, K. W. (1964). *Lancet 1*, 1342.

Miles, S. (1963). 'Exhaled Air Resuscitation.' *Family Doctor*. June 1963.

Redding, J. S., G. C. Voigt and P. Safar (1960). 'Treatment of Sea Water Aspiration.' *J. Applied Physiol. 15*, 113.

Rivkin, L. M., Roe, B. B. and Gardner, R. E. (1962). *Amer. J. Surg. 104*, 283.

Safar, P. (1958). 'Ventilatory Efficacy of Mouth to Mouth Artificial Resuscitation.' *J. Am. Med. Assoc. 167*, 335.

Safar, P. and M. McMahon (1958). 'Mouth to Airway Emergency Artificial Respiration.' *J. Am. Med. Assoc. 166*, 1459.

Semple, T. (1964). 'Practical Results of Cardiac Resuscitation'. Resuscitation and Cardiac Pacing (p. 152) (1965) Cassell, London.

Smith, H. J. and Anthonison, N. R. (1965). *Lancet 1*, 1027.

Symposium on Emergency Resuscitation (1961). *Acta Anaesthesiologica Scandinavica*. Supplement IX.

Wilder, R. J., Jude, J. W. Kouwenhoven, W. B. and McMahon, J. H. C. (1964). *J. Amer. med. Assoc. 190*, 581.

CHAPTER XVI

Water Safety

I T IS quite remarkable how little attention is paid to 'water safety' as compared with 'road safety', industrial accident prevention, safety in the home and the safety methods applied to other forms of transport, even though as a killer drowning holds a very high position.

The reasons for this are to be found in the unique character of aquatic accidents as compared with those on land. The rare events of shipwreck and submarine disaster are of course not at the moment under consideration as they are special problems not directly concerned with the present context.

Possibly the most important factor which removes drowning from the full attention of public interest is its exclusiveness. In all other forms of accidents there is, in addition to the fatal cases, a far greater number of non-fatal injuries with all degrees of mutilation and disability. It is these which are noticed and their impact on the casualty departments, the hospital wards and the compensation courts is far greater than the smaller group who are killed. Accidents in water are rarely spectacular and most often affect one person only. If a group is affected it is done so collectively and one person is not usually directly responsible for the misfortune of the others. There is very little dramatic appeal, and quite frequently no body. No grim evidence of the accident remains to hold the curious crowd and the majority will have occurred where few witnesses are present for the more people there are about the less likely is there to be a drowning accident. There is invariably death or complete recovery.

It is important to appreciate these subtle differences in the background of aquatic accidents for they greatly influence the application of any safety organization. Man quite naturally loathes restrictions but will accept them if they are for the obvious advantage of the community. Where only himself is at risk he resents being taken care of by impersonal appeals. There have indeed been many tragedies where warning notices or advice have been wilfully disregarded. In some cases it would seem that the warning itself stimulates a spirit of foolhardy challenge.

The approach to the problem is particularly difficult and most success is obtained in professional and private organizations where a team spirit and a desire for a good record of safety prevails. Public enlightenment would seem to be the most profitable aid to Water Safety especially

263

in ensuring that young persons develop water consciousness early in life.

The responsibility for water safety must be shared between state or municipality, professional bodies, voluntary organizations and the individual; and the closer the co-operation between these the more effective will be the outcome.

STATE OR MUNICIPAL RESPONSIBILITIES

Local governments of areas where there are facilities for surface and underwater activities are usually alive to their responsibilities and make some attempt to assess the dangers of local waters and where necessary place warning notices. They can however do much more in the way of propaganda and encouraging the formation of local aquatic clubs. Once such a club is established the way is easy.

If a state can provide facilities whereby every child can become a proficient swimmer it will have made a major contribution. This should be accompanied by the provision of swimming baths and, in shark infested waters, netted bathing beaches. A good example of this comes from Australia—a country very conscious of Water Safety—where a nation-wide 'Learn to Swim' campaign is most successful. Its aim is to train, free of charge, every child in the country to become an efficient swimmer and it is well on the way to doing so. The Australian is very proud of his association with the water and it is the boast of many that their children can swim before they can walk. They certainly have much in their favour in the way of climate and coastline of which they take full advantage, as the high standards reached by their competitive swimmers show. They are undoubtedly masters in the art of what can only be called 'beachmanship'.

Learning to swim is without any doubt the most important contribution to water safety but a good standard should be reached and confidence gained. Methods by which non-swimmers may remain afloat in deep water have from time to time been demonstrated (Lanoue, 1964). They depend on the majority of human beings being slightly buoyant and demand little expenditure of energy. It is however doubtful if a person who has not had an opportunity to learn to swim would in an emergency have the presence of mind to carry out even these simple movements especially if negatively buoyant. Such teaching must not therefore be allowed to replace instruction in swimming.

A further and valuable contribution to safety often provided by local authorities in dangerous areas is life-saving equipment such as life-lines, buoys and winches.

RESPONSIBILITIES OF VOLUNTARY ORGANIZATIONS

Accepted with a high degree of pride by voluntary organizations, safety precautions, invariably of the highest standard, are issued in the form of manuals and frequently practised. Although groups directly associated with underwater swimming and diving will of necessity produce safety regulations to meet their own requirements, other general associations will be more directly concerned with accident prevention, rescue and revival.

On appropriate organizations will fall the responsibility of training the individual to appreciate the hazards, to master any apparatus he may use and to come to terms with the environment. Useful information will be collected and distributed concerning tides, dangerous currents, location of underwater obstacles, particulars of the sea-bed and anything else of possible value. In some parts of the world special precautions must be taken to meet the problem of dangerous marine animals which may vary from the destructive shark to the less obvious but deadly poisonous sea wasp.

Those bodies whose primary object is life-saving tend to confine their services to safeguarding the general public and are most active in the more popular resorts keeping an eye open not only for persons in trouble but for dangerous surf conditions or sharks. Those directly concerned with underwater activities tend to be more mobile and, though willing to help wherever required, confine their activities more to their own interests.

Whatever the object, organization is the keynote of such service and again typical examples are to be found in the water-conscious continent of Australia where there are thriving associations of Surf Life Savers, Beach Life Guards, Spear Fishermen, Underwater Researchers, branches of the Royal Life-Saving Society and many others, bursting with enthusiasm, entirely voluntary and attracting the best young men and women to their ranks. All are strong swimmers, passionately devoted to the sea, whose success over the years in rescue and life-saving has been a splendid reward. Their activities are associated with a great deal of pageantry and their techniques are practised with military precision under a colourful background of banners and uniforms. Their method of doing everything by numbers pays hands down in an emergency when seconds count and everything is done at the rush. Each member of the team knows his job and whatever is needed is carried out with efficiency and no time is lost.

In many cases, in addition to the first-class training, modern equipment is available which includes surf boats, life-lines, belts and winches and inflated life buoys designed to be pulled out by the rescuer and so shaped as to offer practically no resistance in the water and yet fasten easily round the victim. Also available may be hollow life-lines carrying oxygen, breathing apparatus and underwater towing machines.

All this costs money which is generally obtained from membership fees, competitions, aquatic sports, displays and various social activities. Very very rarely is a donation ever received from one of the many persons rescued. In fact so rare is this that one club when it received a cheque in recognition of a life saved regarded it as such a novelty that it was not cashed but framed and displayed in the club-house as a curio. There is something very strange in the behaviour of a person rescued from the sea, a kind of furtive shame which is quite different from that of someone rescued from danger on a mountain or an overturned sailing dinghy. Once more the mysterious influence of the sea on human behaviour is apparent. Few persons in trouble in water will, even when life guards are patrolling, just give the raised arm signal for help and tread water until help arrives. Most will panic and after rescue and revival there is sometimes almost indignation or at the best begrudgingly mumbled thanks before the lucky individual slinks away into obscurity.

THE RESPONSIBILITY OF THE INDIVIDUAL

Since drowning is a very individual occurrence the success or otherwise of any water safety instruction depends finally on the application of the individual. His best safeguards are training and discipline which can only be achieved by becoming a member of the group. Any person who wishes to enjoy the adventure and excitement of the underwater environment must have adequate instruction and the benefit of belonging to a team. In no other recreational or professional activity is this so absolutely essential. On land there are few things which cannot be achieved by trial and error but in and under water the errors invariably have a fatal result.

Even when trained and efficient the temptation to exceed discretion is always present. Underwater activity demands an exceptionally calculated approach to every situation. There is no room for emotional influence. Discretion is not the better part of valour, it is all the valour. Many a spear-fisherman has been lost through being carried away by the enthusiasm of the chase and quite a few divers enthralled by the wonder of their surroundings have lost touch with reality—and life.

The underwater swimmer is quite often the proud owner of his breathing apparatus and if it fails him under water he may be very reluctant to let it go and surface without it, lest he lose it for ever. On the other hand a pilot in trouble will not hesitate to eject himself and abandon the plane. In each case a moment's hesitation may cost a life.

It has been stated that training is essential for the underwater swimmer and in general this is accepted. It is however possible for anyone to purchase a breathing apparatus without producing any evidence of proficiency. Also in this present day and age, when the 'do-it-yourself' enthusiasts are building almost anything, a few will attempt the assembly of a breathing set on the absolute integrity of which their life will depend. Sets can be built but only with expert knowledge and facilities for satisfactory trial and test.

Breathing apparatus purchased and used by the ignorant or built by the inexperienced may well lead to disaster but even more frightening is a facility which exists in some waterside communities where a stranger can hire a breathing apparatus for a few hours and no questions asked.

Until the individual joins an organization it might be said that he only has himself to blame if he gets into difficulties. This is true enough up to a point but such is human nature that a man in difficulties must be rescued however inexperienced the rescuer and many a life has been lost in trying to save one whose thoughtlessness, ignorance, or bravado alone was responsible for the disaster.

Propaganda must persist and sub-aqua clubs and the vendors of the underwater breathing apparatus must be loud in their insistence that would-be underwater swimmers and divers take the safe path to proficiency and enjoyment by enrolling as a member of a recognized association.

There is no danger that by so doing individuality may be lost. There are few people in the world more individualistic than the professional diver or the experienced amateur. However organized and grouped the community up top, down below, in the enveloping waters, every swimmer is in his own exclusive world though in fact he is still dependent on the team for his safety.

To put it into a nutshell the responsibility of the individual in contributing to water safety is to join a club, achieve proficiency and stick to the rules.

THE RESPONSIBILITY OF THE PROFESSIONALS

Since the men who spend far more hours working underwater are the divers engaged in naval or commercial practice it is to them that others must naturally look for guidance. In professional diving, even more so than recreational diving, the safety of the individual is of paramount importance. Any accident however trivial is investigated in the greatest detail to find any flaw in the safeguards and every step is taken to prevent recurrence. At the same time a realistic view is taken of safety and the requirements of the work considered. A well-balanced compromise is reached which allows unrestricted work with minimal risk.

The balance is naturally achieved by experience but is founded essentially on good training, supervision and a high standard of equipment. It is thus only to be expected that the professional organizations will set safety standards for the rest but as the requirement expands these will be modified to meet special needs. The safety rules are promulgated in Service Diving Manuals (1964) and many non-professional organizations (British Sub Aqua Club (1968)) also produce well-informed publications specially directed to their own interests. Manufacturers of diving apparatus also issue handbooks which include useful advice on safe usage of their products.

The importance of water safety cannot be over-emphasized and therefore some of the more important factors will be brought together with special regard to the underwater swimmers. The training of the individual is of the greatest importance and will therefore be considered separately in the next chapter.

SAFETY PRECAUTIONS FOR THE UNDERWATER SWIMMER AND DIVER

(i) *Training*

Adequate training by qualified and experienced instructors is essential. All candidates should already be swimmers.

(ii) *Health*

Medical standards must be reached (Chapter XVII) before training. Subsequently any evidence of illness, especially that of the respiratory tract, should prevent entry into the water. Diving should not be resumed until there is complete recovery.

(iii) *Conditions*

Conditions of weather and water should be taken into account before diving. No chances should be taken.

(iv) *Companions*

The most important of all the water safety rules is that under no circumstances should the swimmer or diver be alone. He should have companions with him in the water or be on the end of a life-line from shore or a boat.

(v) *Breathing*

Techniques of breathing will have been taught during training but it is most important not to indulge in the practice of overbreathing or hyperventilation in an attempt to prolong breath-holding time.

(vi) *Life-lines*

The life-line is a very real safety device and should be used wherever possible. It is essential for beginners, and for those working in dark or dirty water.

In clear shallow water it may be dispensed with provided there are a number of swimmers operating within sight of one another.

A useful alternative is the 'buddy line' by which two swimmers, operating as a pair, may be joined together for mutual safety by a thin line. This should not exceed 15 ft. in length.

Independent divers may also tow a float to give their position on the surface.

The life-line is also available as a means of signalling between the diver and his attendant and an agreed system of pulls can be arranged. Usually the signalling system is adopted and standardized throughout the organization.

(vii) *The Knife*

A sharp sheath knife should be a standard part of the equipment for, though the life-line is an important safety device, it can become snagged on underwater obstacles and then must be cut. The knife has of course many other obvious uses.

(viii) *Food and Drink*

Underwater swimming being a highly social activity may be associated with a fair amount of conviviality. It is important that diving should not follow any over indulgence in food or alcohol. This has caused many accidents. On the other hand diving on an empty stomach is equally undesirable. Good sense and moderation is required. Professional divers who are doing a day's work will be content with frequent cups of tea, soup and snacks, avoiding the conventional heavy midday meal and keeping off alcohol until work is done.

It has not been possible to find out how the popular belief originated that one should not enter water until one hour after a meal. It may possibly have been made in the days of the Victorian 'blow outs'. It is certainly not observed today and provided the intake has been moderate there is no obvious physiological objection to a quiet post-prandial dip.

(ix) *Apparatus*

The swimmer's apparatus is his link with survival. It must never fail and therefore careful maintenance and repeated inspection is essential. At the beginning of every dive a quick test in the water for leaks and working efficiency should be carried out whilst it is still possible to receive immediate help. A few minutes' quiet breathing from the set before entering the water while valves and cocks, etc. are being checked is also a wise precaution.

(x) *The Dive*

It is as well to have the dive planned and times worked out before entering the water. It is essential to keep well within the limits of endurance of the apparatus making due allowance for increased consumption at greater depths and with work.

The precautions taken to avoid the specific hazards of diving, decompression sickness, narcosis, oxygen poisoning, burst lung, etc. have all been fully discussed and means to avoid them are included in the regulations of the diving organizations. Apparatus at present available for the amateur is unlikely to introduce much danger from these conditions but future developments may demand much greater care in depth and timing of the dive.

(xi) *Attendants*

When a man is in the water somebody else should know that he is under water and roughly where he is. If a life-line is used occasional signals should be exchanged to check the diver's welfare.

A safety boat too should be present with facilities for recovering swimmers in trouble. In a recent accident when a man surfaced in trouble the only attendant was one man in a dinghy. The diver lost consciousness and had to be supported on the surface. The attendant was thus completely immobilized, being unable to drag the victim into the boat or row to the shore. Careful planning and foresight is necessary if such situations are to be avoided.

In most cases where diving is in progress the limitation of time in the water by apparatus endurance or decompression limits is such that invariably there are more men out of the water than in it and an adequate system of control can be maintained.

(xii) *Action in an Emergency*

(*a*) *'Ditching Drill.'* An individual whose breathing set has failed should not hesitate to abandon it and most have a quick release mechanism. A last breath should be taken if possible but in any case ascent to the surface should be made as calmly and as quickly as possible with the muscles relaxed and the lips pursed to blow out expanding air from the chest.

If positive buoyancy can be achieved without abandoning the set, e.g. by shedding weights and inflating a breathing bag or swim-suit this is to be preferred, as it gives buoyancy when the surface is reached.

(*b*) *Action by Others.* Whenever there is any sign that a diver may be in trouble however trivial a further diver should go down without delay. He may be able to follow the victim's life-line or indicator line. It is in fact desirable that at all times while swimmers are under water a 'stand by' diver should be dressed and ready to enter the water immediately if required.

In all group diving operations one man, essentially one with adequate experience, should be in overall charge and responsible for the conduct of the operation and its safety organization.

(*c*) *Emergency Signals.* Signals by life-line between diver and attendants have been mentioned. In well-equipped professional teams underwater telephonic or equivalent voice communication may be available.

There are however times when the surface attendants need to call the swimmers quickly out of the water, e.g. for an abrupt change in the weather. The most efficient way of doing this is by a small underwater detonation. A detonator or thunderflash is a convenient size of charge which should be thrown into the water well clear of any diver.

Underwater there is a great opportunity for progress. The possibilities are only just beginning to be exploited. It is however imperative that the progress should be tempered with reasonable caution and that the experience of those who have come to terms with the environment should be available for their successors. In no other field is an efficient accident prevention effort so important, for as has been repeatedly said there are no half measures. ALL ACCIDENTS IN WATER ARE POTENTIALLY FATAL.

It is therefore the responsibility of every person in any way connected with aquatic activity to play his part in the dissemination of knowledge and the establishment of true WATER SAFETY.

READING AND REFERENCES

Lanoue, F. (1964). 'Drown-proofing.' Herbert Jenkins, London.

Royal Naval Diving Manual (1964). B.R. 155C. Undersurface Warfare Division, Admiralty, London.

U.S. Navy Diving Manual (1959). Navy Dept., Washington.

British Sub Aqua Club Diving Manual (1968). B.S.A.C. Bedford Sq., London.

CHAPTER XVII

Selection and Training of Divers and Underwater Swimmers

IT MOST certainly does not need a 'superman' to make a good underwater swimmer or diver but nevertheless some rather ill-defined characteristics are desirable. It would be a great help if these could be described but attempts to do so have met with little success.

Most professional diving schools find that more than half of the students who start courses fail to complete them, a wastage which is both discouraging and uneconomical. Any recommendation which would lead to a reduction in this loss would be welcome and recently a serious attempt has been made to find out just what makes a good diver. Presumably no one starts training unless he or she is keen to become an underwater swimmer and this is the first step in selection. If, of these, only half make the grade then only a small proportion of the general public are really suitable. As with most specialized occupations there is bound to be some degree of natural selection.

PHYSIOLOGICAL RESPONSES

The special requirements of adaptation to the underwater environment suggested that some clue might be found in behaviour. Consequently three hundred divers of various experience were examined with special attention to the respiratory system. Vital Capacity, Maximum Breathing Capacity, Respiratory Patterns and sensitivity to Carbon Dioxide were all studied. For assessing the general standard of physical efficiency the Harvard Pack Test was used (Johnson, Brouha and Darling, 1942).

It was possible to compare some of the results with a similar age group of 400 National Service men. The comparison of the means of the two groups was as follows:

	Divers	Non-divers
Vital Capacity (litres)	4·8	4·3
Maximum Breathing Capacity (l./min.)	132	137
Physical Efficiency Index	86	63

In both groups the distribution and range was similar. The divers on the whole had a greater vital capacity than the others but the significant difference was in the physical efficiency index where the divers gave a

18

considerably better performance. These differences however are not very helpful. The very nature of the diver's work will tend to improve his general physique and vital capacity. It may also be to some extent true that men who take up diving are generally fitter than the average to begin with.

The big surprise of this investigation was the wide difference in breathing patterns. A fifteen-minute tracing of the movements of a spirometer in a closed double box constant volume circuit was recorded and every precaution taken to avoid external influence on respiration. The subjects used mouth-pieces and nose clips with which they were familiar in their underwater practice and were given a combined visual and manual reaction test which kept them fully occupied. Considering that every man was carrying out the same task under identical conditions it was quite remarkable what a wide range of differences occurred. Minute volumes varied from 7·6 to 33·2 litres, respiratory rates from 6 to 32 per minute and tidal volumes from 442 to 3259 ml. For convenience the patterns were divided into seven groups of which Figure 53 gives an example of each. The following table shows the fairly uniform distribution of the subjects in the groups:

Group	Mean min. vol. litres	Resp. Rate per min.	Tidal Vol. ml.	% in each group
I Shallow	11·4	12–16	Under 900	13
II Slow	12·6	Under 12	900–1500	10
III Fast and shallow	13·1	Over 16	Under 900	15
IV Middle group	16·1	12–16	900–1500	25
V Slow and deep	18·8	Under 12	Over 1500	14
VI Fast	22·5	Over 16	900–1500	10
VII Deep	25·2	12–16	Over 1500	13

There was some indication that the best divers were in Group V with the slow respiratory rates and higher tidal volume. This of course is theoretically the preferable rhythm for use with a breathing apparatus and one that is encouraged during training. It is the most economical pattern of respiration provided there is no hyperventilation as may occur in the fast deep Groups VI and VII. A rapid respiratory rhythm is unsatisfactory especially if the apparatus used has any degree of dead space for with each breath the dead space volume is wasted.

Although encouragement is given to those using breathing apparatus to try and develop a habitual slow deep-breathing rhythm there is always a fear that in an emergency they might revert to their former

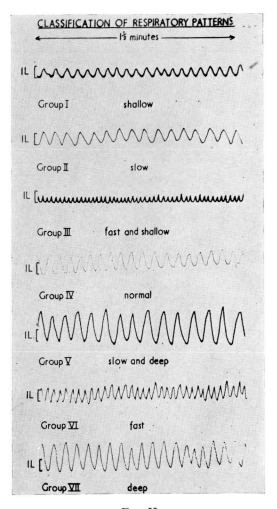

FIG. 53

pattern. More work needs to be done on the significance of breathing patterns particularly with regard to their relation with temperament. It is usual for the breathing pattern to be more regular when breathing is carried out with a mouth-piece and nose clips but even so 30% of the men showed some degree of irregularity. It is possible that an irregular breathing pattern indicates a respiratory centre more sensitive to external influence than the average whereas a steady slow deep rhythm occurs in the less sensitive individual.

There seemed to be some further correlation when the athletic histories were studied in that amongst the divers there was a high proportion of long-distance runners. Perhaps a long-distance runner makes a good underwater swimmer for the two activities demand a high degree of muscular and respiratory endurance. Whilst these investigations were being carried out consultations were held with a selection board responsible for choosing men to become air pilots. Though there were many problems in common this board expressed a dislike for long-distance runners and a preference for sprinters.

In spite of these interesting observations it is not possible to lay down any specific physical standards for would-be underwater swimmers and divers. The important factor seems to be one of temperament rather than physique and a further line of approach to the problem was tried wherein men who had started training but failed were interviewed.

PERSONAL ADAPTATION

In the majority of cases those who had failed to make the grade did so because of inadequate temperamental adaptation. This reason too was found to be the most common cause of failure in flying training. There is a tendency in such cases to label the individuals as being 'temperamentally unsuitable'. Though this may be to some extent true it is a label which tends to stick and has a somewhat discreditable ring. Undoubtedly only a minority of the community have the personality required for efficient underwater achievement and those who have not are by no means inferior and may well excel in other directions.

MOTIVATION undoubtedly plays an important part in future adaptation and this will usually be quite different in the amateur and professional. The person who takes up underwater swimming as a recreation is not influenced by financial considerations and can usually please himself when he goes under water. Both professional and amateurs are however primarily volunteers for the underwater work or recreation and must have some special reason for wishing to do so. Even with the professional money is rarely the primary motivating factor. More often it is a genuine love of water and a sense of adventure. In some cases there is a desire for individual achievement and in others a wish to belong to an exclusive group. Quite a few take up diving as a means to an end as with archeologists, photographers, cave explorers and fishermen who simply wish to extend their sphere of interest and activity.

To some extent the glamour and propaganda associated with underwater adventure, the films, books and television programmes, encourage the adventurously inclined to try their hand at the new sport. They are soon enthralled by the environment and the enthusiasm of their fellow swimmers. Both the professional demand and the popular interest are showing a world-wide increase which will continue to grow as facilities improve.

The glamour however is sometimes followed by disillusionment for those who, after a holiday or spell of duty in the Mediterranean or similar parts of the world, return to England and join a training organization. They will have seen with envy the obvious enjoyment of those who dive in the clear warm sunlit waters. Their training for such anticipated pleasure might well take place in a cold muddy harbour or bleak inland waterway under which condition they rapidly lose heart.

There seems at present no alternative to trial and error as a means of selection. During training it soon becomes apparent which members of any class will be successful and in fact the best method of selection is for a highly experienced, possibly medically qualified underwater swimmer to be in the water with the candidates observing their behaviour and reactions to various conditions. It is sometimes possible to give a fairly good assessment before the individual enters the water for generally speaking the types which are most likely to do well are those who combine a high degree of intelligence with good physique, patience and a placid, imperturbable temperament. It is however only right that, until more is known of this problem, anyone who is keen to go under water should be given a trial provided he reaches certain basic medical standards.

MEDICAL STANDARDS FOR UNDERWATER SWIMMERS AND DIVERS

The fitter a man or woman, the happier he or she will be under water. This does not mean that a high standard of medical fitness is essential and in fact the basic requirements are not particularly severe. Any person of average physique and good health is acceptable, for the underwater environment is very kind to the individual and within limits of depth and activity no undue stresses are encountered. Special attention must be paid to the respiratory system and ears which are affected by pressure changes. Some notes may be given for guidance but it is essential at all times that every case should be decided on its own merits and no hard and fast rules applied.

(i) *Age Limit.* Professional bodies do not usually accept men for training of over 35 years but many divers continue active work until very much older and a few still carry on diving in their eighties. Age is not really of great importance and provided there is a good standard of fitness it should not debar the enthusiast.

(ii) *Standard of Fitness.* Candidates should be fit enough to face the hazards of everyday life and able to carry out active work without exhaustion. They should be emotionally stable and of relatively sober habits.

(iii) *Respiratory System.* It is important that there should be no evidence of any chronic respiratory disease such as tuberculosis, catarrh, sinusitis, asthma or emphysema.

It is desirable to have a chest X-ray taken every year. Signs of active disease, or shadows in the peripheral field, should exclude. The vital capacity should not be less than 3 litres.

(iv) *Ears.* It is essential that the diver should be able to clear both Eustachian tubes. Though frequently a temporary condition, repeated failure of either tympanic membrane to give a positive Valsalva reaction is an indication for stopping diving. A perforated drum need not disqualify and each case should be taken on its merits remembering the increased risk of middle ear infection.

(v) *Cardio-Vascular System.* There must be no gross impairment of exercise tolerance or evidence of cardiovascular disease. The resting systolic blood pressure should not exceed 140 mm.Hg nor the diastolic pressure 100 mm.Hg.

(vi) *Central Nervous System.* Any history or evidence of repeated fits or attacks of unconsciousness must disqualify. So must psychological disorders especially claustrophobia.

(vii) *Teeth.* Bad teeth are usually associated with bad health. Dentures should normally be removed before diving unless they are an exceptionally good fit and normally worn continuously. If the swimmer uses a mouth-piece it is essential that, with or without dentures, he is able to make a good seal with it.

(viii) *Bones and Joints.* The possibility that repeated and prolonged exposure to high pressure has in a limited number of cases produced varying degrees of aseptic bone necrosis should not be overlooked. This is particularly important for the professional diver.

It might be advisable therefore to consider periodic radiological examination of hips, knees and shoulders say every three or five years.

TEMPORARY DISABILITIES

It has been emphasized that diving should not be carried out unless perfectly fit. Particular attention must be paid to illnesses which are liable to produce unconsciousness or vomiting, e.g. diabetes, anaemia, peptic ulcer, jaundice, etc., for this may lead to disaster in the water. Respiratory infection and ear conditions must at all times restrict diving and where apparatus and clothing is to be shared sufferers from skin diseases and venereal disease must not be allowed to take part.

What has been listed above can be no more than a guide even with regard to blood pressure limitations. Mostly the problem is one where common sense will give the answer but in cases of doubt the opinion of an expert in underwater medicine should be sought. Professional bodies and the larger amateur organizations usually have their consultants.

It must once again be emphasized that the aquatic environment leaves very little margin for ill-health. Many accidents have resulted from purely medical conditions either directly or during the period of incubation or recovery. It is essential that this is fully appreciated and medical attendants should be alert to the need for extreme care when considering illness in underwater swimmers. Chances just cannot be taken.

THE TRAINING OF THE UNDERWATER SWIMMER AND DIVER

Whatever the ultimate purpose of the training the earlier stages are very much the same and consist of a period of familiarization with environment and apparatus. Thereafter it is usual to grade the individuals according to the experience and proficiency they have achieved, limiting their activity accordingly.

Most normal persons in the early days of training experience some misgivings and even fear unless they are fortunate in being particularly familiar with the water as expert swimmers (ability to swim is in all cases a necessity). Two approaches are possible, a tough one or a gentle one.

In the 'tough' approach the instructors show little patience and force terrified candidates to keep going. When they come up and plead to leave the water they are firmly pushed under again, the instructor knowing just how far he can go with safety. The rationale of this treatment is that those who survive and qualify are more likely to deal with a subsequent difficult situation without panic. If they survive the training course they will survive anything, is the claim. This may be true but there is a very high wastage of good men and a tendency for some of the less bright characters to get through. Many of high intelligence fail who, with a little help and encouragement, would succeed and later become experienced and trustworthy divers. It is a method which today is falling into disfavour.

The 'gentle' approach is one whereby the would-be underwater swimmer is introduced to the environment by degrees. He may first spend many hours out of the water simply getting used to and familiar with his apparatus. Before being allowed out of his depth he would spend much time just cruising round until he went into deep water of his own accord in his own good time. Such a start would be made in a warm indoor pool or tank whereas the shock treatment would begin in natural water. Such a process is time consuming and though possible for the recreational swimmer is on the whole impracticable. Using such a technique a larger number of men complete training but how reliable some of them would be in an emergency is doubtful. Furthermore as men are usually trained in groups there is a need for planned programmes which must strike a satisfactory mean between the needs of the best and worst trainees.

Something between the 'tough' and 'gentle' technique is needed. The success of any training depends largely upon the instructor's ability to instil confidence into his pupils and the more time he spends in the water with his class the more likely is he to achieve this.

It is claimed by some instructors that the first two days are the most difficult and critical and if these can be overcome without fear the rest is easy. On one or two occasions tranquillizers or even barbiturates have been given with apparent success on the first two days of training. Provided there is adequate supervision and no possibility of the drug being used on any other occasion the action may well be justified, though as yet there is not sufficient evidence one way or the other. Such drugs must only be given with the knowledge and approval of the medical officer associated with the unit.

Not only must the potential diver gain confidence in his environment but he must become absolutely familiar with his breathing apparatus to such an extent that he has implicit trust in its efficiency and knows it will not fail. To achieve this he must understand its workings and be responsible for its maintenance. It is desirable, though not always possible, that each man should use only one set and be responsible for its servicing. In any case the user must make a final check and assure himself before entering the water that it is fully charged and in good working order.

It is during the early stages of training that mistakes are most frequently made and naturally these are anticipated by instructors and adequate safety organizations are prepared. In the early stages the diver, unless readily accessible, should be on a life-line and when this is discarded will depend on the confidence he has gained and the local conditions. From the beginning and throughout the underwater swimmer's career he must always take the maximum safety precautions compatible with the efficient performance of his task.

For all types of diving, confidence in the water, knowledge of and trust in the apparatus and an appreciation of the importance of safety regulations are the fundamental requirement. Thereafter special training develops to meet the needs of the particular vocation. Some confusion frequently arises with regard to names given to the different types of diver and swimmer. This depends largely on the type of apparatus, if any, which is used. A convenient terminology is as follows:

(i) *Skin-Diver*. The diver or underwater swimmer who has no breathing apparatus and must hold the breath whilst submerged. Such divers may or may not use a 'Schnorkel tube'. (The term is sometimes wrongly applied to divers using apparatus with only swimming trunks or costume.)

(ii) *Self-contained Diver*. As the name suggests the diver carries his breathing apparatus with him under water. In the Royal Navy this may be the SABA (Swimmers' Air Breathing Apparatus) diver, in the U.S. Navy the SCUBA (Self-Contained Underwater Breathing Apparatus) diver and in civilian practice the 'aqua lung' diver. In addition various types of circuit may be used by the self-contained diver, e.g. open circuit, closed circuit or semi-closed circuit.

Self-contained divers may be 'BOOTED' or 'FINNED' according to whether the needs of the occasion demand walking on the bottom or swimming.

(iii) *Free Swimming Diver*. When a self-contained diver is in no way connected with any surface group and wholly independent he is a 'free diver'.

(iv) *Frogman*. This is the specially trained 'assault swimmer' whose apparatus is designed for long endurance, relatively shallow depth and absolute concealment. He is a 'free swimming diver' used primarily for underwater sabotage and similar warlike activities. This is essentially a naval type of diver as are others such as (*a*) the 'Shallow Water Diver' who is trained for simple searches and tasks in shallow water, (*b*) the 'Clearance Diver' trained in bomb and mine disposal and (*c*) the 'Artificer Diver' who is experienced in underwater repair work.

(v) *Standard Diver*. Until recent years the Standard Diver with his heavy boots, watertight suit and metal helmet was the common practising diver. He is still used in commercial diving especially for salvage and engineering work and is dependent upon an air supply pumped down from a surface team with whom he maintains continuous contact with a life-line and frequently telephone.

(vi) *Deep Diver*. The equipment of the standard diver can be modified, by introducing a carbon dioxide absorbing canister and a semi-closed circuit, for use with a helium oxygen mixture which enables work to be carried out at depths greater than 300 ft.

(vii) *Surface Demand Diver*. More recently surface demand diving equipment has been developed which gives the diver a great deal of safety, comfort and mobility. He may be dressed as a self-contained diver with boots or fins. His air supply is normally supplied from surface cylinders to a demand valve in the face-piece through a light-weight, strong and flexible pipe. In addition an emergency self-contained air breathing apparatus is carried which automatically cuts in if the surface supply fails.

(viii) *Gas-mask Diving*. A service anti-gas respirator can be simply adapted for diving by blanking off the outlet valve. Air is supplied to the face-piece from a standard diver's air pump. A good head harness is essential.

(ix) *Saturation Diving*. This new technique involves diving excursions into the sea from a pressurized compartment in which divers remain for relatively long periods (i.e. several weeks) subject only to final and prolonged decompression routines at the conclusion of their expedition. (See Chapter XII).

The various forms of diving apparatus will be described in greater detail in the next chapter. Details of training courses are to be found in the various handbooks and manuals issued by the organizations responsible for instruction.

REFERENCE

Johnson, R. E., L. Brouha, and R. C. Darling (1942). 'A test of Physical Fitness for Strenuous Exertion.' *Rev. Canad. de Biol. 1*, 491.

CHAPTER XVIII

Underwater Equipment

EXCEPT for the short breath-holding dive which cannot exceed a few minutes, breathing apparatus is essential for diving and underwater swimming. This may vary from the highly complicated and organized equipment of deep diving to the simple single-cylinder apparatus of the underwater swimmer. All however must be constructed to supply air or appropriate mixture at the correct pressure for the diver. It must be simple, reliable and economical.

The development of underwater breathing apparatus goes back to Aristotle in 360 B.C. who described air containers for use by divers. The development from these early days makes interesting and colourful reading and a well-illustrated summary of this progress is given in Sir Robert Davis's book *Deep Diving* (1955).

Today breathing apparatus used for diving is, broadly speaking, of two types, (i) in which the breathing mixture is supplied by pipe from a surface source and (ii) where the mixture is carried in bottles by the diver. The former is used almost exclusively in naval and commercial diving, the latter is used also in recreational diving.

DIVING WITH A SURFACE SUPPLY

The supply of air from the surface to the diver can be achieved by a hand pump, compressor or a battery of cylinders containing the breathing mixture under pressure. It involves a major organization and is unsuitable therefore for recreational purposes. It is particularly applicable to static diving in salvage work and underwater construction. The heavy equipment greatly limits mobility and, though having many advantages, it denies the user the freedom which appeals to the underwater swimmer whose interest is exploration and adventure.

THE STANDARD DIVER

The best known technique of diving is that of the standard diver. This method is usually limited to depths of 200 ft. but 300 ft. can be reached by an experienced diver in an emergency.

Air Supply. In many cases this is still obtained by means of a Manual

Air Pump which does however limit the diving depth to 165 ft. (Fig. 54).

(i) *The Manual Air Pump* is a two-cylinder double-action pump. The pistons are driven by continuous rotation of two wheels on either side of the pump casing which are fitted with handles enabling two men to be employed on each wheel. Where necessary two pumps can be coupled together. In construction the pump is simple and robust but needs

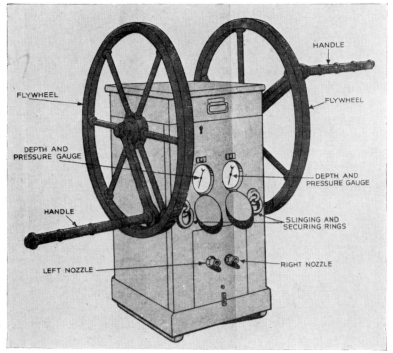

FIG. 54. The manual air pump

careful maintenance to minimize leaks. Water jackets round the cylinders prevent over-heating due to increased air pressure. These pumps need frequent testing for efficiency and may need a correction factor during use.

A diver may be breathing the same volume of air at different depths but as he gets deeper an increasing quantity of air must be pumped down to him, to make up for the increased pressure. Thus the deeper the diver the harder must the pump be worked and a second pump may be needed as the following table shows:

Depth	Air required from Surface per minute		Number of Cylinders	Revolution of pump
Feet	Cu. ft.	litres	needed	per min.
0	1·5	42·5	1	15
16	2·2	62·5	1	22
33	3·0	85·0	1	30
66	4·5	127·5	2	22
99	6·0	170·0	2	30
132	7·5	212·5	4	21
165	9·0	255·0	4	27

The depth gauges on the pump must also be frequently tested, for upon their accuracy depends the completion of any decompression schedule during ascent.

(ii) *Air Compressors* are the most satisfactory and economical means of supplying the diver with air. This method is essential for depths greater than 165 ft. A high-pressure storage system is also essential which should be of sufficient capacity to bring the diver safely to the surface if the compressor breaks down. It should also be able to supply at least two divers so that a second may be sent down if the first is in difficulties. It is essential too that the air supplied to the diver is pure. The importance of this and the need for filtration and avoidance of pollution with exhaust fumes has already been stressed.

(iii) *Compressed Air Cylinders*. Batteries of previously charged high-pressure cylinders may under some circumstances be more convenient than a compressor. Great care is needed to be sure that an adequate capacity for the proposed dive and possible emergency is available, including of course the need for decompression stops and an allowance for the increased expenditure at depth. It is advisable in addition to have low-pressure storage cylinders between the high-pressure bank and the diver.

(iv) *Air Hoses* must be so designed that they are not too heavy for the diver nor so buoyant that the floating slack may foul obstacles near the surface. The air pipe is normally supplied in two lengths 30 ft. and 45 ft. and the metal couplings of each are such that when the length of pipe is full of air the shorter one just sinks and the longer one just floats. In practice the longer length is used next to the diver and shorter ones above.

Other requirements of the air pipe are that it should be tough, flexible, non-corrosible, waterproof, smooth bored to lessen resistance and non-collapsible. An internal diameter of $\frac{5}{8}$ inch is adequate and the pipe must stand a pressure of 600 lb./sq. inch.

The pipe, which must not kink under any circumstances, is made up of four layers of indiarubber and five layers of canvas with steel wire in the centre between layers of rubber. The inner and outer layers are rubber.

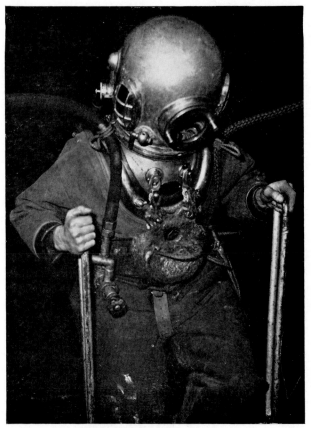

FIG. 55. The Standard diver

THE DIVER'S EQUIPMENT (Fig. 55)

(i) *The Diving Dress*. This is made of vulcanized proofed twill in one piece enclosing the feet. It has a double collar of which the outer is of thick vulcanized rubber to take the corselet. Vulcanized rubber cuffs fit tightly round the wrists and additional rubber bands are needed to make them watertight. Three sizes of dress are manufactured.

(ii) *The Corselet*. A padded oval collar is worn to protect the shoulders from the corselet or breast-plate which, like the helmet, is made of tinned copper. This is clamped on to the outer collar of the dress by brass strips which are firmly bolted down. The life-line and air hose are secured with a lanyard to the neck of the corselet.

(iii) *The Helmet* has an interrupted thread, with which it can be screwed on to a similar thread in the neck of the corselet by one-eighth of a turn. (Rather like the lid of a domestic pressure cooker.) A small catch at the back is turned down into a recess to secure it.

The helmet has three windows of $\frac{1}{2}$ inch thick glass, fixed oval ones either side protected by guards and a circular central one in front which can be unscrewed. This is left out until immediately before the diver enters the water to enable him to talk and breathe fresh air whilst on the surface.

The air pipe is attached to an INLET VALVE on the back of the helmet. This is a non-return valve which ensures air pressure being maintained in the suit if the supply fails.

Just behind the right-hand window is the OUTLET VALVE, so sited that bubbles do not interfere with vision. This too is a one-way valve allowing air to leave the helmet and no water to enter. It is set so that a pressure of $\frac{1}{2}$ lb./sq. inch greater than that of the outside water pressure is needed to lift it. It has a screw however by means of which the diver can adjust the release pressure, within limits. By tightening it he can increase the air volume in the suit, by releasing it he can get rid of surplus air more easily.

In front of the helmet is a small 'spit cock' which enables the diver to suck in water and blow it over a misted face glass. It may also be used as a supplement to the outlet valve in getting rid of air if there is too much buoyancy. A telephone can also be fitted inside the helmet.

(iv) *Other Equipment* includes two lead weights of 40 lb. each, slung in front of and behind the corselet—with facilities for quick release in emergencies. A leather adjustable 'jock strap' passing between the legs from front to back of the corselet prevents the helmet rising too far off the diver's shoulders. A sheath knife and waist belt are always worn. The boots are of tough leather with brass toe caps and wooden weighted soles each weighing about 18 lb.

A breast rope of plaited hemp, with or without telephone wires links the diver with the surface. It is usually marked every 10 ft. with a symbol indicating the depth.

The weight of a diver fully dressed is in the region of 380 lb. in air and therefore it is essential to provide him with means of getting in and out of the water. A ladder extending well below the surface and 3 ft. above the gunwale of the boat to give support is generally used.

THE DEEP DIVER

In deep diving special precautions must be taken to avoid oxygen poisoning, nitrogen narcosis and the effects of even traces of carbon dioxide in the helmet. Helium is used to replace nitrogen, the oxygen content of the mixture is reduced and a carbon dioxide absorbing canister is introduced into the circuit. Because the volume of gas to be pumped is so great and helium, a costly gas, must be preserved as much as possible, a partial recirculation is employed. The main differences are therefore to be found in the design of the helmet and the introduction of the canister.

(i) *The Helmet* is slightly larger and has two air connections, one for incoming air and the other to take expired air to the canister. The diver is provided with a mouth-piece which has valves so arranged that inhalation draws in air which is circulating in the helmet and exhalation drives expired air through the canister.

(ii) *The Canister* (Fig. 56) is worn like a knapsack on the diver's back. In size it is 13 by 11 by 5 inches and contains a compartment full of soda-lime to remove carbon dioxide from the expired gas. The oxy-helium mixture from the surface enters the container at one side and passes through a nozzle of 0·025 in. diameter. A pressure of 50 lb./sq. in. above the diver's equivalent depth pressure is needed to drive the mixture through this injector. The resulting jet is directed into the wider pipe leading to the helmet and in doing so draws gas from the canister through holes in the surrounding collar. This has already passed through the soda-lime and being free from carbon dioxide dilutes the gas from the surface, i.e. there is a partial recirculation. Surplus gas however does escape through the exhaust valve in the helmet in the normal way.

Special decompression tables are needed for deep diving and because of the long times involved it is customary to use a submersible decompression chamber (Fig. 16) in the longer dives.

SURFACE DEMAND DIVING EQUIPMENT

A recent advance which enables a diver to maintain neutral buoyancy and an increased mobility by being able to use swim fins as an alternative to boots is the surface demand system. Equipment similar to that of a self-contained diver is worn, the air being supplied by a pressure hose thinner than the standard and neutrally buoyant, to a demand valve on the diver's equipment, from which he breathes through a mouth-piece in a face mask. This type of apparatus was first developed as the 'Hookah'

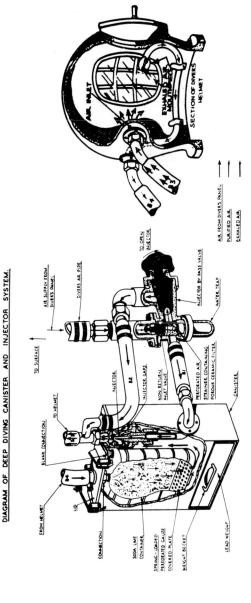

DIAGRAM OF DEEP DIVING CANISTER AND INJECTOR SYSTEM.

TO SURFACE

AIR SUPPLY FROM DIVERS PANEL

DIVERS AIR PIPE

TO OPEN INJECTOR

INJECTOR BY PASS VALVE

WATER TRAP

TO HELMET

BLANK CONNECTION

INJECTOR

INJECTOR CAPS

NON RETURN INLET VALVE

PERFORATED AIR STRAINER CONTAINING POROUS CERAMIC FILTER

CANISTER

FROM HELMET

LID

CONNECTION

SODA LIME CONTAINER

SPRING - LOADED PERFORATED GAUZE COVERED PLATE

WEIGHT BECKET

LEAD WEIGHT

THE INJECTOR IS SHOWN IN CLOSED POSITION WITH
AIR FROM SURFACE ENTERING HELMET VIA PIPES 81 & 85

AIR INLET

EXHAUST MOUTHPIECE

SECTION OF DIVERS HELMET

AIR FROM DIVER'S PANEL

PURIFIED AIR

EXHALED AIR

FIG. 56

19

breathing equipment in which the demand valve was built into the diver's face mask. The 'Hookah', widely and successfully used in Australia, is simplicity itself but has the disadvantage that no provision is made for failure of air supply as may result from kinking or fracture of the air pipe or a surface mishap. Kinking is rather more likely than with the standard equipment and air failure can be rapidly disastrous.

As at present used in naval diving the method is combined with a small self-contained breathing apparatus, which is about half the weight of that generally used independently. It consists of two air cylinders each charged to 3,000 lb./sq. inch, one of which leads directly to the same reducing valve as does the surface air supply pipe. The surface air however arrives at a higher pressure and only when this fails and its inlet valve closes does air from the first cylinder enter the breathing system. The diver does not, in fact, know whether he is breathing from the surface or his first cylinder. If however the surface supply failure is prolonged and the first cylinder empties difficulty in breathing is experienced. In such a case by pressing a sprung lever between the two cylinders the pressure in each can be equalized giving a further period of breathing. This process may be repeated but once it has become necessary it should be taken as a warning that surface supply has failed and the diver should ascend without delay.

This is a very versatile form of diving apparatus which is safe and reliable and the lightness of the self-contained breathing apparatus makes climbing in and out of boats, etc. relatively easy. It is quite likely that for most professional diving this will become the apparatus of choice and be adapted for deeper diving.

SELF-CONTAINED

OPEN CIRCUIT AIR BREATHING APPARATUS

This form of apparatus is the most popular in recreational diving and is being increasingly used in naval and commercial practice. It consists essentially of one or more cylinders of compressed air with a specially designed regulator or demand valve which supplies air as required when the diver inhales. The expired air is exhausted into the water and there is no mixing or rebreathing. Even though air only flows to meet the inspiratory requirement there is still a considerable wastage of available oxygen in the expired air and the consequent limited duration of use at depth is the main disadvantage. On the other hand this restriction does tend to limit its use to dives which require no decompression schedule for surfacing.

The design of the demand valve is an important factor for it must give the required volumes on demand with minimal resistance at varying depths.

(i) *The Demand Valve* (Fig. 57) consists essentially of two chambers separated by a flexible diaphragm. One chamber remains constantly open to the surrounding water so that the diaphragm is always subjected

THE PRINCIPLE OF THE DEMAND VALVE

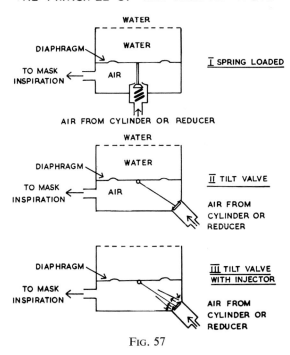

FIG. 57

to the environmental pressure on one side. The other chamber contains air and is in direct contact with the diver's respiratory system through a valve at the mouth-piece which allows inhalation only from this chamber. Also leading into this chamber but controlled by a balanced valve is the air supply from the storage cylinder which may or may not be reduced in pressure to about 100 lb./sq. inch by a regulator. Descent through the water and inspiration will both reduce the volume in the air chamber causing the diaphragm to bulge into it. The diaphragm is connected by a lever to the valve controlling the entry of air from the cylinder so that the bulging opens it, letting in air until the pressure is equalized. By this means the pressure in the respiratory system is always the same as that of the surrounding water and the requirements of inspiration met.

Three types of demand valve are available (i) a spring-loaded valve, which is less satisfactory because it introduces a part subject to wear; (ii) a tilt valve to which movement of the diaphragm is transmitted through a rigid arm causing the valve to open and (iii) a similar 'tilt' valve enclosed in a nozzle which when the valve opens introduces air in a jet. This, acting as a venturi, causes a positive pressure on the inspiratory side by keeping the valve open a little longer and so assists inspiration.

The demand valve is usually mounted with the regulator on the body of the set with the cylinder or cylinders and expired air is led from the mouth-piece into the water compartment.

Positioning of the demand valve is quite important with regard to breathing comfort. The 'Eupnoeic pressure' is that pressure of air underwater which gives the most comfortable breathing. In the prone position this is equivalent to the water pressure in the plane of anterior axillary fold and in the upright position the plane of the sternal notch. If the demand valve is mounted on the top of the set so that it is near the nape of the neck it will be above the Eupnoeic pressure level when swimming face downwards. In this position therefore an extra inspiratory effort will be needed and the mask will be slightly squeezed on to the face. Conversely swimming on the back too much air is available and there is a tendency for the mask to blow off the face. In the standing position breathing is good so long as the set is securely held in its position on the back.

In some designs the demand valve may actually be incorporated in the face mask. This has the advantage of needing less of the flexible respiratory tubing and does keep the pressure in the face mask comfortable with no tendency to squeeze or inflate and the mouth-piece can therefore be dispensed with. It is not however easy to produce a low resistance expiratory valve on the face-piece.

(ii) *Face Mask and Mouth-piece*, are less uniform in design and many types are used. An earlier variety consists of a mouth-piece, nose clip and goggles. The importance of vision has already been discussed in Chapter X. Goggles if used should be rigid and, whether these or a face glass are used, it is important to ensure that, over the range of refracted monocular vision, the front surface is flat and parallel to the plane of the eyes. Where awareness vision only is required curved surfaces can be used, and any distortion accepted provided there is no angle sharp enough to cause a blind spot. At the other extreme is the hood which encloses the head and neck and incorporates the face glass and breathing mouth-piece. Between these two are many variations some with and some without the mouth-piece.

Great care is needed in design to make sure that dead space volume is kept to a minimum. To and fro movement of air must be avoided and especially where no mouth-piece is used siting of valves should aim to eliminate this. Careful moulding of the inside of the face mask with a light rubber flap over the bridge of the nose may isolate the area enclosed by the glass from the breathing circuit.

Sealing is very important. The hood type is probably the most effective but here great care is needed to make sure that air is not trapped in the external auditory meatus. It is impossible to construct individual face masks and the air-filled seal common in land types of breathing apparatus is unacceptable for diving where increased pressure would diminish its size. Water-filled seals however have proved very satisfactory.

Although tailor-made face masks are out of the question individually fitted mouth-pieces can be produced without difficulty from a wax impression. This technique has been developed by the Royal Naval Dental Service and is proving generally popular.

Ideally it would be preferable to do away with the mouth-piece and nose clip altogether and develop a safe mask. This would increase the comfort of breathing, lessen the resistance and produce a more natural respiratory pattern. However the nose clip may have to be kept in some cases to facilitate ear clearing and the mouth-piece which many divers prefer does offer a much smaller additional dead space.

Either a full face or oro-nasal mask may be used, the former being preferable provided the 'dead space' problem can be overcome. With the oro-nasal mask, specially constructed goggles must be worn. Well-fitting goggles which are essential to keep out water, have the disadvantage that under pressure the contained air must either contract in which case the goggles press against the face or, if the goggles are rigid, the contained air remains at a lower relative pressure than adjacent tissues, e.g. the conjunctiva, which may develop oedema and haemorrhages. This problem is overcome by having on the outer side of each eye-piece a rubber air container communicating with the air inside the goggles. Contraction of these air containers enables the air inside the goggles to maintain the same pressure as the surrounding water. The construction of these air sacs can be so arranged that the goggles themselves are conveniently buoyant.

(iii) *Breathing Tubes and Valves* must meet certain requirements. In breathing apparatus at present available there is room for considerable improvement. The type of breathing tube used almost exclusively is a corrugated rubber hose of external diameter $1\frac{3}{4}$ in. and internal $\frac{3}{4}$ in. This is flexible, will stretch and being reinforced with wire is difficult to kink. It does not however have a completely smooth internal bore and any air flow through it is bound to be turbulent. An ideal tubing is one which has an internal diameter of at least $1\frac{1}{4}$ in. and a smooth bore. The requirement of flexibility, extensibility and non-kinking must also be met. Such tubing is available commercially though expensive and as yet not as pliable as would be desired.

It is theoretically impossible to construct a valve which has no resistance and frequently a compromise must be made with robustness. Simple rubber tongue valves are popular and reliable. It must be remembered too that the valves are likely to become moistened with condensation from the breath. Some sacrifice must be made and resistance accepted to avoid risk of water leaking back past valves. In many ways the mushroom valve is the most efficient and in addition may be used with the smallest dead space loss.

(iv) *The Gas Cylinders.* One, two or even three high-pressure cylinders may be used in underwater air breathing apparatus each holding from 1200 to 1500 litres. A choice lies between steel and light alloys. The relative merits involve a number of technical considerations which are hardly relevant since the law in this country at present restricts commercial sets to steel cylinders. In naval usage light alloys are preferred because of the better buoyancy for volume ratio.

The importance of ensuring the purity of air with which the cylinders are charged has been repeatedly emphasized. Air only should be used with the open circuit breathing apparatus. Oxygen may be available but has no advantage and is dangerous in that slight amounts of oil or grease present may result in an explosion during charging. So great is the volume of gas used at depth that to replace air by oxyhelium mixtures for deep diving would be prohibitively uneconomical. For example the endurance of a breathing set on the surface is reduced to $\frac{1}{4}$ at 100 ft. and $\frac{1}{7}$ at 200 ft. Work also further reduces the endurance.

Tables can be worked out for the various capacities of cylinder to relate endurance with depth and work being done. A diver working so that he breathes 30 litres per minute would get 40 minutes' use from a 1200-litre cylinder at the surface, 20 minutes at 33 ft., and 10 minutes only at 100 ft.

Only one-fourth of the available oxygen in the cylinders is used and expired air is discharged into the water. There is thus a continuous evolution of bubbles which expand as they rise to the surface thus making the presence of the underwater swimmer very obvious. For this reason, and also because of the noise the apparatus produces it is unsuitable for military operations which demand concealment.

WARNING OF EMPTYING CYLINDERS

It is most important that some warning device should be fitted to each breathing set to indicate to the user when the gas supply is running out. A pressure gauge fitted to each cylinder, though useful to show they are full before the dive may be difficult to read underwater. In any case to be readable a long air tube to the gauge is necessary and this adds an appendage to the set which may become entangled or knocked off. Where pressure gauges are fixed to the apparatus the orifice leading into them should be so small that if they are displaced no great loss of air occurs.

Many methods of warning are in use, the simplest being in a multi-cylinder set to have one bottle solely as a reserve. This may even be of smaller capacity. Another method is to have a valve on the supply line which makes breathing difficult when pressure drops to a set value, say $\frac{1}{4}$ of the full pressure. When this occurs the valve may be released by hand to allow the full capacity of the cylinder to become freely available. It does however give only one warning.

An attractive method which can be applied to sets with two or more cylinders is one used in the Royal Naval Diving organization. In a twin-cylinder apparatus, for example, only one cylinder is used to begin with. When this empties the diver, feeling the restriction on his breathing, can immediately by pressing a spring-loaded lever, or turning a cock, connect the second cylinder to the first so that pressure is equalized and both become half full. It is then the practice to turn the cock to close the valve. In the spring-loaded type this is done automatically. The diver is thus warned that he has used one cylinder. He may continue until his first cylinder is again exhausted when the process of equalization can be repeated. When this is done the second time each cylinder is a quarter full and he should consider terminating the dive. If the third equalization becomes necessary he must surface without delay for then he will have used $\frac{7}{8}$ of his available supply.

Simplicity of charging cylinders is important and whatever method is used it is important to ensure that all are fully charged and that emptying warning devices are re-set and not allowed to interfere with filling. Connecting points must be airtight at very high pressures and joints must therefore be well sealed. Metal to metal contacts are susceptible to leaks if not absolutely clean and fibre washers need tight screwing home. The best perhaps is the coupling which contains a hollow rubber ring so placed that the increased pressure within the tube forces it against the connecting rims to give a complete seal. Such a method is satisfactory and connection can be made and broken by hand-turned nuts.

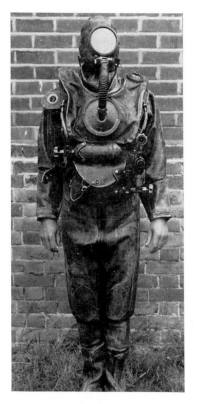

FIG. 58. Closed circuit breathing apparatus

CLOSED CIRCUIT BREATHING APPARATUS

The principle of such a circuit is the enclosure of a given volume of breathing gas from and into which the diver breathes (Fig. 58). The carbon dioxide exhaled is absorbed and replaced by an equivalent volume of oxygen. The essential features are the face-piece, the CO_2 absorbing canister, the breathing bag and the oxygen supply cylinder.

With such a system no oxygen is wasted, no bubbles need escape and the apparatus is relatively silent. Care must be taken that the oxygen in the rebreathing bag does not become diluted with nitrogen from the atmospheric air or the body tissues. To lessen this possibility the lungs are flushed out with oxygen which is then breathed for two minutes followed by a further flushing out before entering the water. Great care must also be taken that no water enters the absorbing canister as this would greatly reduce its efficiency and might lead to caustic burns of the mouth.

The simplest form of closed circuit breathing apparatus utilizes pendulum breathing whereby the user breathes to and fro in a single

CLOSED CIRCUIT BREATHING APPARATUS

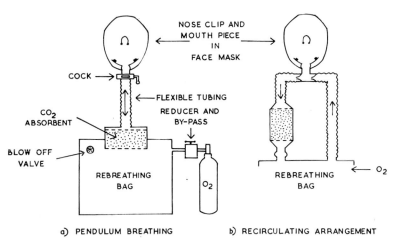

FIG. 59

tube, through the canister and in and out of the breathing bag which must be refilled from the supply cylinders as it empties (Fig. 59a).

(i) Whether a FACE MASK or GOGGLES are worn depends on circumstances but in all cases at present both a MOUTH-PIECE and NOSE CLIP are used. Immediately adjacent to the mouth-piece, outside the face mask if used, is a cock with which the diver can cut off his connection with the apparatus and breathe directly the atmospheric air. This is an advantage when he is on the surface but its main function is to enable him to take oxygen from the set into the lungs and then exhale it to the atmosphere to wash out any residual nitrogen from his lungs. This action is essential before using the set and also on every occasion when air has been breathed during use. In pendulum breathing the mouth-piece leads directly to the canister and there are no valves. With the recirculating system the mouth-piece connects to a 'T' junction which contains two valves and is connected by one arm to the canister and the other to the breathing bag (Fig. 59b). The valves are so arranged that on inspiration gas is drawn directly from the bag and not the canister and on expiration it passes through the canister only. With pendulum breathing both inspired and expired air pass through the canister.

(ii) *The Canister* is a vital unit in the apparatus and must function efficiently for as depth increases even small amounts of carbon dioxide may be dangerous. It should as far as possible have a capacity to give it an effective life equal to that of the oxygen carried.

In designing the canister many factors must be considered. The gas stream must be distributed through the absorbent to ensure its complete use. Excessive baffling however must be avoided for it will increase resistance. Packing of the absorbent must be tight or channelling will occur and care must be taken that water cannot enter. The absorbent itself is of great importance. Soda-lime has been found most satisfactory, with a granule size of 2–4 mm. and a freedom from dust. A convenient size of canister for pendulum breathing is $5\frac{1}{2}$ in. diameter by 3 in. deep which holds 2 lb. of soda-lime granules. When filling, gentle tapping on the side will ensure efficient packing and diminish the risk of channelling. Mechanical packing will achieve an even greater compactness. It is customary for each swimmer to accept the responsibility for packing his own canister. When the soda-lime is well settled down a metal gauze filter and gas spreading diaphragm secured with a sprung locking ring, tightly hold the absorbent. The soda-lime must be inspected before use and discarded if wet or pasty. Excess dust can be removed by sieving. The absorbing power of such a canister is about 180 litres of carbon dioxide which is about $1\frac{1}{2}$ hours' usage with fairly heavy work.

(iii) *The Breathing Bag*, or 'counter lung' is a collapsible bag made of reinforced rubber and holding about 7 litres of gas. It can be filled up as necessary from a high-pressure oxygen cylinder but in order to maintain a constant flow of oxygen into the bag it is usual to fit a 'reducing' valve. This can be set to give a constant flow of oxygen into the bag of $\frac{3}{4}$ litre to $1\frac{1}{2}$ litres per minute. The facility to fill the bag directly from the cylinder must also be retained as this reducer flow is not sufficient to meet the demands of hard work and compression due to going down. Were it so the bag would over-inflate during periods of rest or light work. Where a reducing valve is used therefore a hand-operated by-pass valve is also included. The breathing bag is fitted with a relief valve to avoid over-inflation with excess pressure which might otherwise cause the mouth-piece to be blown out of position. This valve, which is spring-loaded, can be controlled by the diver to blow off with an excess of pressure within the range of 4 to 12 in. water above that of the surrounding water. The surface of the bag away from the diver can be adapted to receive the base of the canister so that gas passing in and out of the bag is widely distributed through the absorbent. In order to keep the distance from the bag to the mouth as low as possible and to give comfort in breathing the bag is worn on the upper part of the chest with extensions over each shoulder, the blow-off valve being in one of these. From the canister, clamped into the front of the bag, a relatively short tube connects it with the mouth-piece. Where a recirculating system is used the position of the canister and length of breathing tubes is less important.

(iv) *The Oxygen Cylinders* are much smaller than the air cylinders of the open circuit apparatus holding about 400 litres of oxygen. Two cylinders are used one above the other as the main source of supply and are supported below the breathing bag with the by-pass valve or bag inflating valve easily accessible to the diver's left hand. These cylinders have a life of up to 2 hours according to activity.

In addition a third similar cylinder is attached in front also connected to the bag and controlled by a valve reached by the diver's right hand. This is for use in emergency only and allows the diver to surface when his main cylinders are empty. Once on the surface, by inflating the bag and turning the mouth cock to atmosphere, he will be kept afloat and be able to breathe air. Weights also can be discarded.

(v) *Weights*, usually in the form of lead balls of 12 oz. each, may be carried in a pocket on the back from which they can be released quickly in an emergency by pulling a ringed wire which is attached to a securing pin.

COMPARISON OF PENDULUM AND RECIRCULATING BREATHING

Pendulum breathing needing no valves has the advantage of simplicity. The fact that the gas is drawn through the canister on both inspiration and expiration improves greatly the efficiency of carbon dioxide absorption. It does however have the big disadvantage of added dead space which may be as much as 180 c.c.

In the recirculating system the dead space is insignificant but valves and more tubing are used. The canister is fitted to the expiratory side of the system and only expired air passes through it. It is usually designed with its length greater than its diameter which is the reverse of that used with pendulum breathing. Ideally the canister should be on the inspiratory side as it is undesirable to have expiratory resistance greater than inspiratory. In practice however the canister does not function efficiently on the inspiratory side being more effective with the warm moist air of expiration.

The proof of the pudding is in the eating and the pendulum system has been widely and successfully used with no evidence of ill-effects due to the increased dead space and therefore, being the simpler it would appear to be the one of choice.

Commercially and recreationally this type of apparatus is not widely used. Its limitation of depth to 30 ft. makes it unpopular though for the frogman this is enough. It has been used successfully by 'cave divers' where great depths are not encountered and the long endurance and compact size is welcome. A set of this type manufactured by Pirelli is available and this firm also produce a smaller model which is designed for use by spear-fishermen allowing intermittent use for pursuit. At other times the diver breathes surface air through a Schnorkel tube.

SEMI-CLOSED CIRCUIT BREATHING APPARATUS

In an attempt at compromise to avoid the limitation of depth of closed circuit oxygen and to improve on the restricted duration of the open circuit air set the semi-closed circuit apparatus has been developed. This makes use of various mixtures of oxygen and nitrogen according to working depth.

The design of the apparatus is in every way similar to the closed circuit apparatus except that a chosen gas mixture is supplied at a rate according to depth. Excess gas escapes from the bag through the exhaust valve. A mixture richer in oxygen than air is used, the object being to keep an adequate oxygen partial pressure within the bag, absorb carbon dioxide and get rid of nitrogen with as little oxygen wastage as possible. Essentially oxygen must be supplied at a greater rate than the possible maximum consumption rate. In considering the mixture requirement, allowance must be made for the fact that the diver may need to come to the surface without delay and therefore, in spite of any increase in oxygen partial pressure with depth, the percentage of oxygen in the bag must never be allowed to fall below 20%. In practice it is assumed that the maximum rate of consumption of oxygen will be 2 litres per minute. Higher rates can be achieved under water but not maintained and the occasional excess will be allowed for by the bag volume.

(i) *Mixture Flow Rate*

Knowing this requirement and the need to maintain 20% oxygen in the breathing bag the correct flow rate has been calculated and is as follows:

% Oxygen	Flow Rate (litres/min.)
40	8·00
50	5·33
60	4·00
70	3·20

(ii) *Maximum Safe Depth*

A further consideration is the maximum depth to which a mixture may be used without any risk of oxygen poisoning. When work is being done the oxygen content in the bag will tend to be kept down to the 20% level but when no work is being done it will approach the level in the supply mixture. At rest the safe depth for pure oxygen is 33 ft. (2 atmospheres absolute pressure).

A convenient figure to take for resting oxygen consumption is 250 ml. or 0·25 litres per minute.

The total flow rate can be determined and the oxygen flow rate calculated from its percentage in the mixture.

For example a 40% oxygen mixture would be used with a flow rate of 8 litres per minute and therefore an oxygen flow rate 3·2 litres per minute. For this a safe depth will be found to be 140 ft.

For other mixtures the safe depth is calculated to be:

% Oxygen	Safe Depth in feet
40	140
50	106
60	82
70	65

(iii) *Equivalent Air Depth*

It is quite possible that one of these mixtures may be used at a given depth and for a period of time such that subsequent decompression may be necessary as a result of absorbed nitrogen.

The diver will be subjected to a higher percentage of nitrogen when he is working than when he is resting and as he will be doing both during the dive it is usual to take an intermediate figure for oxygen consumption. In practice an oxygen consumption of 1·3 litres per minute is used.

In actual practice at present only three oxy-nitrogen mixtures are used and these may be tabulated as follows showing flow range and maximum depth.

Mixture		Flow	Max. Depth
% Oxygen	% Nitrogen	l./min.	Feet
60	40	4	82
40	60	8	140
32½	67½	13	180

EQUIVALENT AIR DEPTHS

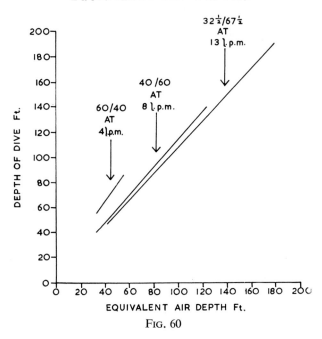

FIG. 60

Where there is a likelihood of going beyond the depth and time which need no decompression the schedule for ascent must be worked out as for the equivalent dive to the same depth using air. These equivalents are shown in Figure 60.

DRESS FOR THE UNDERWATER SWIMMER

For short recreational dives in warm waters and temperate waters many prefer simply bathing trunks or costume. This can be very pleasant but it is believed that the diver wearing a dark coloured suit has a greater immunity to shark attack. The suit furthermore does give some protection from sharp coral, sea eggs, the playful buffeting of friendly sharks and sharp edges on wrecks. Even in tropical water prolonged immersion may produce some chilling if no suit is worn. The comfort of the diver between dips must also be considered.

The most important requirement of the swimmer's suit is that it should maintain a heat balance in relatively cold water. It may also be designed to keep him dry though this is by no means essential.

The suit should be well fitting, flexible, smooth, easy to take on and off and provide adequate insulation. In most other fields air is used as the important insulating medium—cellular garments, e.g. string underclothes, etc., being particularly effective. Unfortunately the compressibility of air causes the cells in insulating garments to contract and lose their effectiveness. Contraction of trapped air within a suit may also, when external pressure increases, cause severe bruising and pinching and thus involve the need for suit inflation from a pressure cylinder. Consequently 'wet suits' have been developed and offer many advantages. There is still some doubt as to which is to be preferred and each must be considered.

Any suit which keeps water out will also prevent the evaporation of sweat with the result that when the suit is worn out of the water in moderately warm weather it becomes unpleasant.

The ideal suit has not yet been produced but improvements are continually appearing. The environments in and out of water are so removed from one another as to demand in most cases quite different requirements in the way of protective clothing. The compromise is difficult and not always satisfactory. There is still a long way to go before a satisfactory recommendation can be made.

(i) *The Dry Suit*

Many materials are today available, mostly of the rubberized fabric type. Ideally, and this applies to all varieties of suit, the swimmer would be individually fitted but expense invariably prohibits this. Where large numbers of divers are concerned suits may be ready made in a range of sizes which necessitates some elasticity in material if a good fit is to be achieved.

Rubberized nylon is at present widely used with reinforced feet and a lighter rubber for the cuffs to seal them on the wrists. To allow entry the neck and surrounds are made of stretchable rubber, and so designed that a watertight joint may be made between this and a rubber hood which fits lightly over the face. For this a metal neck ring is used. Dressing may need the help of an attendant. Because of the difficulty of dressing and undressing it is usual to fit the suit with a screw-out urinal port for use out of water only. The suit may be worn with swim fins or boots as necessary.

The hood, made of rubber, fits closely over the head with the face only exposed so that no water can enter it. The exposed face is covered by the face mask of the breathing apparatus. Foam rubber pads over the ears allow for pressure equalization but if depths deeper than 30 ft. are intended facilities must be available to ensure sufficient air in the suit to prevent a relative fall in pressure in the external ear.

Entry into the suit is always a problem because of the need for watertightness. Other forms are available with (a) entry through a rubber sleeve in front which can then be folded and clamped or (b) a watertight zip-fastener. Two-piece suits with a mid-line seal are also made.

Whatever form of dry suit is used it is almost certain that air will be trapped within it. For this reason a tongue valve is fixed to the back of the hood so that when the diver enters the water excess air can escape. Where the diver goes deep however what little air remains in the suit will be compressed and contract so that, as well as losing insulation, bruising may occur and marks of underwear be imprinted on the skin. This may be prevented by including with the suit an additional small gas cylinder with which the suit may be inflated. This too will give additional buoyancy in an emergency. The blow-off valve in the hood may be supplemented by additional ones in the sleeves.

The dry suit, with suitable underwear such as woollen 'combinations' with long sleeves and legs and a stockinette, or equivalent, streamlined well-fitting undersuit with a zip-fastener entry, will give adequate comfort in most sea conditions.

(ii) *The Wet Suit*

With the wet suit no attempt is made to maintain watertightness though some areas where the suit fits closely may remain dry for some time. The suit may be made in several pieces or enclose only the arms and trunk. The type will depend largely upon the conditions under which it is proposed to operate. Any clothing worn underneath the suit will become wet. However since the suit itself is usually made of unicellular foamed neoprin there is little movement of the trapped water which becomes warmed by the body and acts to some degree as additional insulation. The wet suit may be cold at first but warms up later even in colder waters particularly when exercising.

The wet suit has the advantage of comfort and though there is no problem of squeeze from trapped air there is some loss of buoyancy. If worn out of the water for any length of time the swimmer may become extremely uncomfortable. Even if lined the material tears easily which demands careful dressing though repair is usually easy.

OTHER UNDERWATER EQUIPMENT

(i) *Compasses, Watches and Depth Gauges*

The difficulties of maintaining a desired course under water and of knowing accurately one's personal orientation are well known. The swimmer in many cases therefore will need the assistance of instruments. These are specially constructed to withstand changes in pressure and to remain watertight. Luminous dials assist in their underwater reading. For convenience watches, compasses and depth gauges may be worn on the wrists. The watch is an important safety check on cylinder endurance and necessary for keeping within non-decompression limits or timing decompression stops where necessary. The use of the compass is obvious and the depth gauge is an important safety measure particularly when high oxygen mixtures are being used. The principle of the depth gauge generally depends on the changing volume of an enclosed bubble of air subjected to the ambient pressure changes.

(ii) *Communications*

Modern methods of communication including radio and telephone are being applied under water as well as the simpler rope signals and message slates. Improved and smaller earphones and microphones and transistorized amplifiers enable more equipment to be incorporated in the breathing apparatus or suit.

Some form of communication is essential and whenever a diver or swimmer is in the water someone must know he is there, where he is and have a reasonable means of contact. Explosive signals and tapping on ladders are also used.

(iii) *Tools*

The development of underwater tools is a specialized subject outside the scope of this book. There is little the artificer can do on land which he cannot now do under water. Power tools, burners and explosives are all in common use. Underwater cameras and supersonic or electronic detecting apparatus has been used in the examination and location of lost underwater objects such as wrecked ships or aircraft.

20

(iv) *Lighting and Welding*

Electric appliances are safe under water, any faulty wiring being immediately 'earthed'. Lights and electric welding apparatus are widely used. The diver who leaves the water dripping wet and often so soaked that rubber gloves or clothing are useless as insulators is very vulnerable to any live electric source which may be about. Great care must always be taken to eliminate this risk.

(v) *Propulsion*

The progress of the unaided underwater swimmer is slow and his range is limited. Artificial means therefore are used to move him

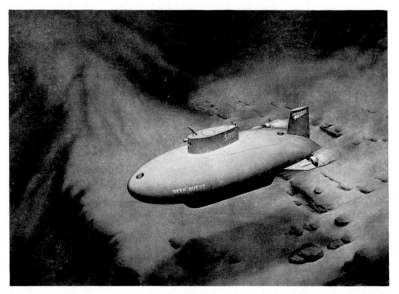

Fig. 61. Deep Quest research submarine (courtesy of Lockheed Missiles and Space Company)

quickly of which the commonest practice is to tow him by a surface boat. He is usually towed, not directly which would pull him to the surface, but by some form of underwater sledge or hydroplane so constructed as to remain submerged when towed or have its depth controlled by the diver. Self-contained, neutrally buoyant controllable towing devices have been used which range from simple battery-driven motors, which the swimmer holds on to and controls, to the complicated torpedo-like 'chariots' used by frogmen in wartime.

Many ambitious underwater swimmers have also been towed by marine animals such as Dolphins, Manta Rays and Seals. The Dolphins and Seals are very responsive to training and there is a great unexploited potential in this field.

Recent years have seen a remarkable advance in the development of underwater equipment of all forms. Of particular interest are underwater vehicles which may submerge with atmospheric or increased internal pressures according to design and requirement. These give increased range of activity to the diver and are of particular value in search and rescue. Indeed they are bridging the gap between the diver and the submariner and although most at the moment are propelled by jets or screws it is not inconceivable that the future may produce tractor like vehicles which can travel along the sea-bed. As on land the range of possibilities is unlimited. (Fig. 61.)

READING AND REFERENCES

Davis, R. H. (1955). *Deep Diving and Submarine Operations.* Siebe Gorman & Co. Ltd., London.

The manuals and handbooks listed at the end of Chapter XVI.

CHAPTER XIX

The Submarine

THE diver goes into the underwater environment and adapts himself to it as completely as possible. The submariner encased in a rigid waterproof cylinder keeps the environment at arm's length. Provided his vessel is robust enough to withstand the external pressures of its operational depth he is concerned only with the problem of keeping his own environment, which he has borrowed from the atmosphere, in a state of purity which will enable him to carry out his duties without loss of efficiency.

The problems of submarine medicine would therefore seem, at the outset, to be vastly different from those of diving medicine. In many ways they are but, as the story unfolds, it will be seen that the two disciplines have much in common.

HISTORICAL

Various attempts to construct a boat which could move under water and re-surface have been on record since 1578 when William Bourne described how to construct a 'ship that may go under water' with wood and watertight decks. Entrance was made through leather sleeves which could be clamped to seal and a hollow mast provided air for the crew. Ballast was used to keep the ship upright and slightly buoyant and care was recommended that it was not used in water so deep that the top of the mast would submerge. Either side were huge concertina-like bellows with screws like a cider press so that they could draw in water to make the boat submerge or squeeze it out to make it rise.

Many attempts followed this but with equally little success. The first to be used in war was a 'one-man' egg-shaped submersible with hand-driven screws pointing vertically and forwards. The former took the 'egg' up or down, the latter backwards or forwards. This craft called the *Turtle* was built in Bushnell in 1776 and used against the British in the American War of Independence but without success. In 1801 Fulton, another American, built the first *Nautilus*. She was only 21 ft. long by 7 ft. diameter and made of copper with iron framework. Under water she was moved by a hand-turned propeller, on the surface she had a sail and in both cases was tolerably successful.

The first submarine 'kill' occurred in the American Civil War in 1864 when a small hand-propelled submarine blew up and sank an enemy frigate—and herself. About the same time the first power-driven boat *Plongeur* was built in France. From here on steady progress was made, stimulated by two world wars. One hundred and fifty-eight years after Fulton's tiny *Nautilus* made her limited and erratic dive her namesake created history with an epic voyage beneath the north polar ice cap.

THE SUBMARINE TODAY

The submarine has developed essentially as an instrument of war and has shown so much promise that in 1958 the Financial Secretary to the Admiralty stated:

'It is my belief that the fleet of the far distant future may be largely submersible.'

The advantages of the submarine in this respect are obvious but the exploits in recent years of nuclear-powered submarines have underlined the possibility of their being used for commercial purposes particularly as carriers of cargoes. Already research into the construction of such a vessel is well advanced with the suggestion that this first nuclear-powered underwater freighter, capable of carrying 28,000 tons of cargo at 25 knots, should be called *Moby Dick*. Such a vessel would avoid surface winds and storms and might open up new trade routes beneath the polar ice. Whether the submarine will become popular as a passenger carrier is doubtful. Little can be expected in time saving and the only true virtue is the smoothness of the passage.

Three major steps have occurred in development since the introduction of power. The first problem in the power unit was that during submergence the internal combustion engine, because of its need for air inlet and exhaust systems, was unacceptable. Underwater battery-driven motors were therefore developed and used. With such however, the activity was limited to the life of the batteries and periodic surfacing was necessary to recharge them. Thus there was a need for two engine systems, electric whilst submarged and piston engines for surface propulsion and battery recharging. The time the submarine could remain submerged depended upon its activity and battery capacity but under the best conditions rarely exceeded 48 hours. Surfacing as well as charging the batteries gave an opportunity of replacing stale air in the boat with fresh. The need to surface however at such frequent intervals greatly interfered with the strategic value of submergence.

The second step was the introduction of the Schnorkel mast which allowed both charging and air replenishment without complete surfacing, in fact from periscope depth. The Schnorkel mast however still had disadvantages apart from bringing the vessel very near the surface. For structural reasons its diameter was limited to about 8 inches which meant that the exhaust requirements of the engines could only be met at the expense of a drop of pressure within the submarine. If, as a result of prolonged submersion, the internal oxygen pressure was dangerously low, this could result in a further lowering of oxygen tension which might be dangerous. Furthermore in a rough sea each time the mast dipped below the water it would automatically close giving a brief but unpleasant drop of pressure within which at times could be especially painful to the ears of the crew. A third though less common hazard was that under certain weather conditions exhaust fumes from the diesel engines might be taken in again by the Schnorkel tube.

In spite of this disadvantage the Schnorkel tube made the submarine a much more formidable weapon. It was not however until the third major step, the introduction of nuclear power, that the 'true' submarine was evolved. The 'true' submarine requires no intermittent contact with the surface atmosphere throughout its operational cruise. No air inlet or exhaust is required by the engines which serve equally well on the surface and submerged. In brief, the nuclear reactor produces heat which evaporates water the steam from which is used to drive a turbine engine.

SUBMARINE HABITABILITY

The medical problems of the submarine are those of habitability which in its simplest form means that a group of men, possibly one hundred, are to be placed in a sealed tube containing about 25,000 cu. ft. of air, completely isolated from the rest of the world and surrounded by sea. In this they must carry out their daily work, eat, sleep and play for a period of months, indeed for as long as the habitable environment can be maintained. They must be kept in good health physically and mentally and maintain a high morale.

In the earlier submarines, in spite of the periodic contact with the surface it was not always easy to maintain comfortable conditions especially where a wartime engagement forced a prolonged dive. The problems however may be studied as they occur in the true, nuclear-powered, submersible for these are after all no more than an extension of the problems of the conventional submarine.

The fundamental difference is that in the conventional submarine the endurance of complete submersion is limited by the life of the batteries whereas in the 'true' submarine the limiting factors are the facility to maintain tolerable environment and the ability of the men to endure it. The 'true' submarine thus introduces an entirely new environmental concept. The enclosed volume of air must be so treated as to remain adequate for the welfare of the personnel for an indefinite period with no facility for replacement in part or whole from the atmosphere. This is quite different from what has hitherto been the basis of atmospheric control. In the factory, for example, even if the environment is below the desired standard, the men, working in shifts, may escape to clean air for long intervals.

In the modern world the submarine is not alone in presenting this

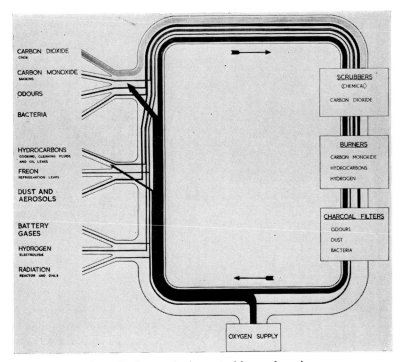

FIG. 62. Atmospheric control in a submarine

problem. The space ship is likely to spend even longer periods in complete isolation and if nuclear war should come the need will arise for key personnel to live and work for prolonged periods in sealed underground shelters. It is necessary therefore to consider this new situation and revise the present accepted industrial limits for impurities in the atmosphere.

As well as the atmospheric purity of the environment attention must be paid to the supply of food and drink when storage space is at a premium. Physical and mental exercise must be seriously planned and the psychological aspect of prolonged existence in a confined space studied.

(i) *The Submarine Atmosphere* (Fig. 62)

Every attempt must be made, in view of the possibility of lengthy exposure, to provide in a submarine an atmosphere which is of the highest standard of purity. One in fact which might be defined as 'country air'.

In a closed environment any toxic agent produced will be cumulative. Any leak of such an agent, however small or slow the evolution, will in time give rise to a toxic level. This can be very well illustrated by studying the effects of cigarette smoking. One cigarette will produce about 0·001 cu. ft. of carbon monoxide and if in a submarine there are 100 men smoking on an average 5 cigarettes each per day the daily production of this toxic substance will be 0·5 cu. ft. In four weeks of such smoking in the confined environment a concentration of 600 parts per million would arise. Since absorption would have been going on during the period of exposure it is unlikely that any of the occupants would have lived this long. The important fact is that, with adequate oxygen replacement and carbon dioxide removal, the everyday habit of smoking could become lethal to smokers and non-smokers alike. A similar danger could be present with any other potentially toxic substance.

This example may serve to show the necessity for a new approach and in considering the problem as a whole three sources of information are available. These are:

(i) Past experience in industrial and academic toxicology with an intelligent anticipation of likely hazards.

(ii) Continuous monitoring of the atmosphere during the period of exposure.

(iii) Clinical observation of the men during and after the exposure.

Such commonplace impurities as carbon dioxide, cooking and body odours, bacteria, battery gases and oil fumes can be anticipated and an accurate assessment of the levels or presence of respiratory gases, carbon monoxide, radiation and rarer gases can be obtained from monitoring instruments. In spite of anything which may be expected it is still possible that unsuspected impurities may accumulate. These may be quite unrecognized until untoward symptoms appear in the men during or after the exposure. It is therefore of the utmost importance to be on the alert for such conditions and to follow the medical records of submarine personnel throughout their careers.

So much for the general problem. There are many well-known constituents, normal and abnormal, of the submarine atmosphere which merit special attention:

(*i*) *Oxygen* must be replaced as it is used by the personnel. Ideally the percentage breathed should never be allowed to fall below 20%. This is achieved in the nuclear submarines but in conventional submarines in order to obtain increased submersion time a limit of 18% is accepted. Although lower percentage will support life this is undesirable. At 17% there is impairment of night vision and 15% may result in some diminution of mental skill. As low a concentration as 10% will support life for a little while but the danger lies in the false sense of well being which accompanies this and the complete unawareness of the danger until consciousness is lost.

Oxygen is supplied either from high-pressure cylinders or by the ignition of a compress of potassium chlorate and iron filings stored in metal cylinders. There is little to choose between these two methods. Both have the disadvantage of occupying a considerable amount of space if a supply for many weeks is required and this must ultimately put a limit on the length of the voyage. The atmosphere can be replenished with oxygen according to a pre-determined schedule calculated from the number and activity of the crew or it can be added as indicated by oxygen meters. There is a need for an alternative method of oxygen production and the most obvious one is to obtain it from sea water by hydrolysis. There is plenty of power available in the nuclear submarine and unlimited water. Snags in technique have still to be mastered and the satisfactory elimination of hydrogen is no easy matter. Space scientists, to whom oxygen production is even more vital, are investigating biological methods such as the culture of certain algae which in the presence of light waves will absorb carbon dioxide and give off oxygen. In addition the culture may grow and be available as extra food. The reluctance of submariners to carry oxygen in liquid form has always been puzzling.

Oxygen supply is thus of the greatest importance and, if it runs short, some extension of its availability may be obtained by increasing pressure within the submarine which increases the oxygen partial pressure. This is satisfactory up to a point but the drop in pressure on return to the surface must not reduce the partial pressure of oxygen to a dangerous level and atmospheric replenishment must take place as quickly as possible. A more realistic approach to the conservation of oxygen which is always a desirable practice is to avoid all superfluous activity. As far as is compatible with a healthy existence personnel not doing essential work should rest.

(*ii*) *Carbon Dioxide* must be removed from the atmosphere in just about the same volumes as oxygen is added. The atmosphere in a submarine is kept circulating and arrangements are made at certain points for it to be drawn through large canisters which contain an absorbing chemical. Carbon dioxide gauges are placed at convenient sites in the boat and according to their reading so are the canisters introduced into the atmospheric circulation. When exhausted, usually indicated by timing their period of use, they may be replaced. Conventional submarines may use in these canisters soda-lime or lithium hydroxide. Where many weeks of use are required the problem of storage of an adequate supply again appears. A technique however is available which employs a solution of monoethanolamine as a spray which removes carbon dioxide from air passing through it. The spray is collected and heated to liberate carbon dioxide which can be pumped overboard and the solution used again (Rigshee, 1959). Great care must be taken to prevent contamination of the atmosphere with the amine which is volatile and toxic.

Under ideal conditions all the carbon dioxide would be removed from the atmosphere. In practice however, and this applies to the removal of other impurities, it is usually very much more difficult to remove carbon dioxide completely than to maintain a low concentration. Consequently to achieve an economical compromise it is necessary to know how high a percentage of carbon dioxide can be accepted in the atmosphere without discomfort or detriment. In conventional submarines 3% is usually regarded as the upper limit for safety. Ebersole (1960) describes an experiment where 23 men were exposed to an atmosphere containing $1\frac{1}{2}\%$ for 42 days. There was no change in basic physiological function but some evidence of stress. As a result of this well-conducted trial $1\frac{1}{2}\%$ CO_2 has been accepted as the upper limit for long exposures and in practice the concentration is kept below 1%. With improved techniques and apparatus the American nuclear submarines have, as their submergence time has increased, continued to improve on this figure.

(iii) *Carbon Monoxide* has already been mentioned as a by-product from smoking and in Schnorkel-fitted submarines as an occasional hazard from indrawn exhaust fumes. An obvious way to reduce the risk would be to stop smoking in submarines. This has been from time to time considered but if the boast of the ventilating engineers that they will provide 'country air' is to be fulfilled smoking must be accepted for 'country air' can be smoked in without harm. Moreover the life in a submarine is such that smoking can be a very helpful contribution to the emotional comfort to many of the crew. In conventional submarines smoking is automatically restricted because cigarettes will not burn when the oxygen content drops below 19%. In nuclear submarines smoking has been accepted as a necessity and repeated estimations of carbon monoxide content of the atmosphere are carried out. As a means of removal combustion is used, the atmosphere being circulated through 'burners' which consist basically of red hot marble chips. These burners, as will be seen, are useful in removing other impurities. By this means it is possible to keep the carbon monoxide concentration below 50 parts per million which is generally accepted as a harmless level. Ebersole (1960) however, from his experience in nuclear submarines, considers that when this concentration is encountered continuously for many weeks it may well be unacceptable and is possibly the cause of frequent headaches. This may be especially so if traces of other impurities such as carbon dioxide are also present.

There is some evidence that if an atmosphere contains a number of toxic impurities each in a concentration below the symptom-producing level, there will be an additive effect with possible adverse results. This is a subject on which more work must be done.

(iv) *Bacteria* in the atmosphere have on the whole produced less of a problem than might be expected. Wherever possible 'carriers' are eliminated from personnel embarking in submarines. Frequently there is an outbreak of upper respiratory tract infection at the outset of a cruise and thereafter, little else. Suspended bacteria appear to settle in ventilating trunking, are destroyed in the burners and removed by filters. Ebersole (1960) gives a sickness table for U.S.S. *Seawolf* in which 116 men were completely submerged for two months. Only 18 cases of upper respiratory tract infection occurred, one only being febrile with a loss of 5 days' duty. The only other possibly infectious cases were 3 of mild diarrhoea. Throughout the whole voyage there was no other loss of working time through sickness.

(v) *Odours* must be eliminated from the atmosphere and this is not usually difficult with careful placing of exhaust fans and charcoal filters which are essential in such places as galleys and toilets. Body odour was somewhat of a nuisance in the older submarines, not so much to the men, who got used to it, but to their first contacts on return to shore. The wife always knew when her husband had been to sea in his submarine and a saying popular in the service was that 'Submariners never die, they only smell that way'.

In actual fact you could not wish to meet a cleaner lot of men than those in the submarine service but in the earlier boats on many occasions there was no opportunity for changing clothes, even for sleeping, and the body seemed to absorb suspended matter from the closed atmosphere. In the modern—luxurious by comparison—accommodation of the nuclear submarine, where ample space, bunks, an abundance of water and air conditioning, make life so much pleasanter, even the lowliest crew member can maintain throughout his long confinement the freshness of a well-scrubbed schoolboy.

Carbon dioxide, carbon monoxide, bacteria and the odours are primarily the man-made contaminants, the next group to be considered may be regarded as domestic.

(vi) *Hydrocarbons* are always liable to be present in the atmosphere where oils, fats, wax polishes, cleaning materials and various solvents are used. Even newly applied paint may give off aromatic hydrocarbons for a week or more. This condemnation of household practice must come hard to those who as recruits to the service were indoctrinated with the traditional belief that 'if it moves salute it, if it's stationary paint or polish it'. A complete revision of painting and cleaning routines must therefore be adopted. Even this will not eliminate the odd oil leak or the fumes from cooking fats. Fortunately the burners which are destroying carbon monoxide will also destroy some of these hydrocarbons. The total elimination of hydrocarbons is not always easy as the range of common substances which can produce such contamination is very wide. Even such simple things as mimeograph ink, lighter fuel and adhesives must all be considered.

(vii) *Freon* or dichlorodifluoromethane has for many years been used in refrigerating equipment. In a submarine where the system may need dismantling for repair and inspection it is very difficult to make the freon system absolutely free from leaks especially if subject to vibration or other shock. Freon from time to time may therefore leak into the atmosphere. In itself it is not particularly toxic but when it passes over the burners or is inhaled through a lighted cigarette it decomposes into hydrochloric acid, chlorine, hydrofluoric acid and fluorine which are both corrosive and irritating.

There is at present no solution to this problem other than making sure that the refrigerator plumbing is sound and absolutely leak proof. Where freon is present in the atmosphere there is little alternative but to come to the surface, and having ensured that the leak is repaired replenish the submarine with atmospheric air.

(viii) *Dust and Aerosols* are always a problem and anyone who has lived or worked in an air-conditioned space will know how quickly dust accumulates in ventilation trunking and filters. The ventilating system of a submarine is no exception and filters rapidly become thick with dust. Much of this is from clothing, blankets and bedding and it is at once apparent where a hole in a pair of socks gets to. Over a long period of time dust and fluff will lower the efficiency of the ventilating system. This may be considerably lessened by the use of synthetic non-fluff materials.

The chief sources of aerosols are tobacco smoke, cooking and cleaning. They may irritate and carry other contaminants into the respiratory system. Aerosols cannot always be removed by the method described and may justify the use of electrostatic precipitators. These though very effective have the disadvantage of producing ozone, an additional irritant.

As well as contaminations from man and his domestic arrangements there are other impurities produced by the machinery and equipment of the submarine. These include gases evolved in the use and charging of any batteries which may be used for purposes other than propulsion. Their nature will depend on the type of battery and in some cases difficulty in removal may occur. Design of batteries for use in submarines is an important consideration and freedom from the production of impurities is essential. Some hydrogen will however result from charging and this is quite simply removed in the burners.

Finally in the nuclear-powered submarine there remains the problem of radiation.

(ix) *Radiation* must be considered as a potential hazard especially as the men are living in close proximity to the reactor day in day out for maybe many weeks. For information on this problem it is necessary to turn to the experiences of American nuclear submariners and further reports by Ebersole (1958) of his experiences in *Nautilus* and *Seawolf*. In the early stages radiation from luminous dials and wrist-watches gave a misleading picture of the radiation hazard but since these articles are no longer permitted on board there has been remarkably little evidence of any radiation hazard. If a permissible exposure limit of 100 m.rem. per week is accepted the exposure levels recorded so far have been less than 5% of this figure. In construction the screening of the reactor is very efficient and once submerged there is natural protection from the basic radiation to which man is exposed on land.

The apparent radiological safety must not however be allowed to blind those concerned with the importance of maintaining a continuous atmospheric monitoring service and also a personnel exposure measurement organization. Clinical laboratory examinations are not sensitive enough for this purpose and every man must carry his film badge and pocket dosimeter. Facilities are available for developing the films and recording dosage on board.

Medical personnel in a modern submarine spend little time treating routine sickness but have a grave responsibility in assessing habitability and giving advice on toxicological matters. They may also make a valuable contribution to general morale.

It is inevitable at the present time that American experience is the main source of practical knowledge. Great credit is due to Commander John Ebersole of the U.S. Navy Medical Corps who as the first medical officer of a nuclear submarine has spared no effort to make his experiences widely available. His many papers and lectures show a profound practical approach to this new and interesting branch of naval medicine.

Atmospheric purification and maintenance are without doubt the tasks which will continue to assume major importance in submarine medicine. Nevertheless other problems which need attention are food, drink, recreation, exercise and above all morale.

FOOD AND DRINK

American nuclear submariners have laid great stress on the importance of diet. A varied menu is a strong weapon in the fight against boredom. Cooks need special training not only in presentation and variety but in adapting their technique to a situation which introduces certain restrictions, the main one of which is shortage of storage space. Desiccated foods and deep freeze equipment are fully used and clean fumeless cooking encouraged, e.g. the infra-red grill or oven. Canned foods today inevitably occupy a large share of the menu but for convenience of manufacture cases are usually cylindrical. A very great saving in space could be achieved by the use of square tins. If the tins could be filled with square peas for example, the saving would be still greater!

Just as a 'new look' is essential in the atmospheric control so must the catering organization be completely re-fashioned to the new condition. Fortunately there is no shortage of water which, with unlimited heat available, can be freely distilled from the sea. In this respect the submariner scores over the space traveller being spared the sordid processes of redistillation of urine and cyclical feeding.

RECREATION AND EXERCISE

It is difficult to be dogmatic about the need for exercise which must be weighed against the need to conserve oxygen. Experience will no doubt produce the answer and it would seem desirable to have at least some organized games. Physical training instructors of today can devise efficient routines of a modified circuit training which can be conducted in a confined space. Some indoor party games, e.g. table tennis, can be quite exhilarating and the steadiness of the craft underwater makes many more of them possible. Whatever is done it is difficult to find replacements for the outdoor activities available ashore or even in surface ships and unless care is taken constipation may become a nuisance.

Recreation is again not difficult to produce. Cinema shows, recorded music, libraries and card games are all freely available and popular but as the days pass interesting changes in mood occur. In the early days the demand is for 'pop' records and popular fiction. This changes eventually to an interest in more serious music and a demand for classical literature. There is no doubt that a prolonged voyage in a submarine gives a leisure and freedom from the rush and bustle of civil life which is rarely available and with it an opportunity to enrich the mind which is unlikely to occur otherwise.

MORALE

Thought must be given to the mental and emotional welfare of personnel embarking for long submarine voyages. Few will be adapted to such conditions and some may not be able to adjust themselves to it.

In the earlier cruises of the American nuclear submarines there was always for the crew the strong motivation of adventure and novelty and the element of challenge. Few men would not gladly accept even months of confinement to be members of a group which made history in record dives and sub-polar voyages. What is more important is to ensure that, when underwater voyages of weeks or months become routine affairs, the men are conditioned to accept it without distress.

Submariners are largely volunteers and may be hand picked for special missions. Already experience is pointing out ways and means to make the life more acceptable. There is a tendency for older men to replace the younger restless types whose immaturity is emphasized by the restricted sphere of activity and who, when the juke-box palls, lack the depth of character to profit from the opportunities of enforced idleness.

One of the most valuable approaches to the problem is in the organization of planned courses of study, not only the development of manual and constructive hobbies, but more academic training such as courses in mathematics, science, a language or one of the arts. Where such a method succeeds is that on completion of the cruise the men may go ashore having accomplished something positive which in other circumstances they would never have achieved.

The psychologists naturally have had a 'hey-day' with this problem and much investigation has been carried out under artificial conditions. In spite of this the need for a realistic and practical approach is essential and the experience of the submarine personnel themselves is invaluable. Ebersole (1960) is very firm about this and discourages any attempt to suggest an emotional stress by too much psychological testing. In fact he goes so far as to state a belief that 'if there had been a psychologist on the *Santa Maria* they wouldn't have made it'.

READING AND REFERENCES

Bourne, Wm. (1578). *Inventions and Devices*. Thomas Woodcock, London.

Ebersole, J. H. (1958). 'Submarine Medicine on U.S.S. *Nautilus* and U.S.S. *Seawolf.*' *Proc. Roy. Soc. Med. 51, 63.*

— (1960). 'The New Dimensions of Submarine Medicine.' *New England Med. Jour. 262,* 599.

Rigshee, J. T. (1959). 'Man made air.' *U.S. Nav. Inst. Proc. 85,* 30.

CHAPTER XX

Submarine Escape and Free Ascent

MAN's deep-rooted distrust for anything mechanical and a healthy respect for the violent moods of the elements, has, wherever possible, led him to make every effort to ensure that, should his machines fail or the elements overcome them, every means is provided to prevent loss of life. It is consequently an accepted practice to make provision for personnel to leave a submarine should the rare event occur of its being unable to surface of its own accord. Similarly if the breathing apparatus of an underwater swimmer breaks down he should at least be given a chance to surface without it.

In working out ways and means by which personnel may safely abandon a disabled submarine it must be remembered that, as long as the hull is intact, the pressure of the air within will be more or less that of the atmosphere. Under certain circumstances it may be possible, either by raising the submarine or with specially constructed diving chambers, to rescue the occupants without subjecting them to pressure changes. More often, however, to reach the surface the submariner must first be compressed to the pressure of the water surrounding the submarine and then be decompressed again as he rises through the water. Furthermore it is quite impossible for any hatch in a submarine to be opened from within until the pressure inside has been raised to that outside. Even at a shallow depth of 33 ft. the hatches are kept shut by a pressure of about seven tons on each one.

Getting a man out of the submarine is one problem, getting him safely to the surface another and once on the surface it is still necessary to provide every chance of survival until he can be picked up. These problems are largely physiological and an application of the principles outlined in earlier chapters will be necessary. Before the details of possible methods are studied a review of the history of submarine escape would seem to be appropriate.

THE HISTORY OF SUBMARINE ESCAPE

A great deal has been written by various authors on the history of submarine escape. Much of this makes exciting reading, emphasizing the bravery of many individuals and the gradual application of scientific knowledge to produce the improved methods in use today. For these accounts reference should be made to the publications of Davis (1955),

21

Schilling and Kohl (1947), Taylor (1953) and the Royal Naval Submarine Base (1959). Meanwhile a brief summary is presented.

Submarine disasters fortunately are not common and are becoming less frequent. In wartime operational losses are accepted but in the anticipation of prolonged intervals of peace the submarine must be made as safe as possible and given maximum escape facilities. The commonest cause of disaster is collision with a surface vessel which is most likely to occur in the relatively shallow waters at the approaches to harbours. Alternative causes are navigational, structural or mechanical failure. In the earlier accidents where facilities for escape were limited survivors were few and those who escaped were blessed with an element of luck as well as courage.

The first recorded escape took place from a German submarine which sank in 1851 in Kiel Harbour in 60 ft. of water. An intelligent Army corporal, Wilhelm Bauer, realized that the only hope of opening hatches was to raise the internal pressure by flooding. This caused the flimsy hatches to burst open and a number of men shot to the surface.

The first British submarine to be lost was strangely enough the A-1 which was rammed by a liner and sank with the loss of all hands. Between this accident and the beginning of the First World War in 1914, a further five were lost, three from collision. The only survivors were those who, where the collision occurred on the surface, floated off before the sinking.

Compared with modern submarines these vessels were small and four out of the six were salvaged within a few weeks of sinking. These submarines were not divided by watertight bulk-heads and any break in the hull meant complete flooding. The introduction of such bulk-heads and the fitting of a hatch at the bottom of the conning tower greatly increased the chances of escape from later submarines.

Although everything possible is done to improve chances of survival, and the Admiralty has a Standing Committee on Submarine Escape, there has, from the very beginning of the Submarine Service, been the overall realization that the only satisfactory technique of submarine escape is to ensure that accidents never happen.

When bulk-heads were fitted and flooding limited, survival within the submarine became possible. In 1916 when two submarines collided and sank, many men had already escaped from the conning towers. One man however, a Stoker Petty Officer Brown, was trapped in the engine room of one of them. The story of this man's escape, the first in the Royal Navy, has been told many times and for sheer calm courage takes some equalling. Brown flooded the engine room to equalize the pressure and was able to open the hatch but each time he did so a bubble of air escaped, the pressure dropped and the hatch slammed shut. This was repeated many times following further flooding until almost all the air was lost and the hatch remained open letting Brown escape. And all this in darkness!

Less than six months later, a submarine K-13 dived in the Gareloch, with an engine induction valve open which flooded the after part, drowning the occupants. She remained on the bottom in 38 ft. and divers were able to connect an air supply line for those men still alive in the

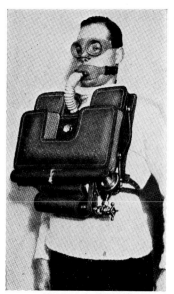

(*By courtesy of Sir Robert Davis*)

Fig. 63. The Davis submarine escape apparatus

forward end. Two days later she was raised and 46 men rescued. This success gave a great boost to salvage as a method of rescue but in the six years following the First World War there were four submarines lost with no survivors. It was quite apparent therefore that only in very limited circumstances could salvage hold out any real hope of success and other methods were needed. Thoughts turned to individual methods and the supply of some form of breathing apparatus was considered. The Germans had developed the Draeger Breathing Apparatus and the Americans the Momsen Lung. This was not an entirely new idea for in 1914 a self-contained breathing apparatus had been issued to submarines. This 'Hall Rees' apparatus had a helmet like a diving suit and because of its bulk and doubtful safety it was abandoned. In 1929 the Davis Submarine Escape Apparatus (Fig. 63) was tested and the following year issued, one for every man in submarines.

In order to avoid the experience of Petty Officer Brown in losing air with flooding every time the hatch opened, those hatches which were chosen as convenient for escape were fitted with twill trunks, which could be lowered below the water level after flooding. Outside this trunk air is trapped above the water and the hatch can be opened without losing it. Men waiting to escape have their heads above water and simply dip under the lower lip of the trunk to escape.

Shortly after this, in 1931, the *Poseidon* sank after a collision in the China Seas and settled at a depth of 120 ft. Twenty-seven men got away before she sank and a further six made successful escapes using the Davis Apparatus. Three of these survivors who, whilst waiting to escape, had been subject to prolonged high pressure followed by rapid decompression, developed decompression sickness on surfacing and bony changes later in life.

However the value of the Davis Escape Apparatus had been demonstrated as well as the need to limit time under pressure prior to escape. Unfortunately another surface collision about the same time in quite shallow water had no survivors and salvage failed completely.

In consequence salvage was abandoned as a rescue method and all submarines were fitted with escape hatches, trunks and enough Davis Escape Apparatus for every man plus a $33\frac{1}{3}\%$ excess. In addition equipment was supplied to give searching craft a better chance of locating the disabled submarine.

The Davis Submarine Escape Apparatus was thus fully accepted by the Royal Navy. As an alternative to the twill trunk which could be lowered into the boat's compartments consideration was given to the design of special escape chambers to hold one or two men. The object of these chambers was to limit time under pressure and in water whilst waiting to escape. They were simply small upright cylinders with a hatch at the top and bottom, the lower giving access from the submarine, the upper to the sea. To escape one or two men climbed into the compartment which was then sealed and flooded until the pressure was the same inside as in the sea above. This allowed the hatch to open and the occupants to ascend to the surface. The upper hatch could be closed from within and the chambers drained down and made ready for use again. This method though attractive physiologically had the disadvantages that a considerable time would be taken for a large number of men to pass through and any accident to a man within, such as loss of consciousness or death, might well block the hatch of the chamber and make its further use impossible.

Chamber escape was soon to have its test for in 1939 the *Thetis* sank during trials in Liverpool Bay with 103 persons on board who were all alive in the after end of the submarine. Difficulty was encountered in finding her and help did not arrive for about 17 hours during which time attempts by the crew to surface the submarine had resulted in her stern being out of the water. Unfortunately the hard work this entailed with the large number of persons on board, had resulted in the air becoming very foul.

The *Thetis* had two escape chambers each designed to hold two men, but no escape trunks. Two men using the Davis Apparatus got out safely but realizing that the air was becoming foul those remaining made the mistake of putting four men in the two-man chamber. Of these three died and subsequently only two more men escaped.

This disaster, with what at the time was considered to be adequate escape arrangements, shook the confidence of the authorities and the whole question was re-examined. The risk of carbon dioxide poisoning was studied and balanced against the risk of oxygen poisoning if the Davis Apparatus—which supplied pure oxygen—was used whilst waiting under pressure. Moreover the risk of oxygen poisoning was found to be increased in the presence of carbon dioxide.

The Second World War commenced later in the same year and attention was rightly diverted to increasing the submarine's fighting efficiency. Nevertheless the physiologists were busy investigating the problems of the effects of high pressure with particular reference to oxygen and carbon dioxide poisoning. Seventy-seven submarines were lost of which two were due to collision on the surface. Many men escaped from the conning tower before sinking and quite a few from the bottom by flooding up and using the trunks. Only about half these survivors had Davis Apparatus and a number were lost after reaching the surface. Two other craft were lost during exercise, one with all hands was never found, and in the second, although all were alive when flooding was commenced, a defective valve so delayed the equalization of pressure that the depth being 150 ft. all died from carbon dioxide poisoning before they could escape.

Following the war the Admiralty appointed a committee under the chairmanship of Rear Admiral Ruck-Keen to look into the whole question of submarine escape. Two very important findings were reported:

(i) The major hazard is within the submarine prior to ascent.

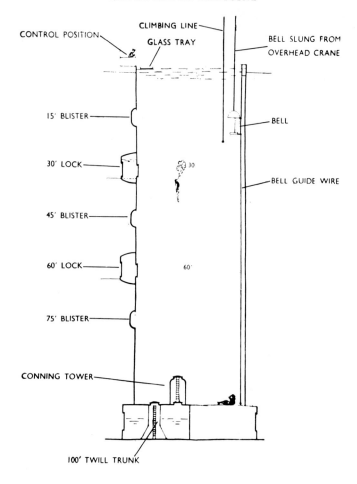

CONTROL POSITION

CLIMBING LINE

GLASS TRAY

BELL SLUNG FROM OVERHEAD CRANE

15' BLISTER

BELL

30' LOCK

30

45' BLISTER

BELL GUIDE WIRE

60' LOCK

60'

75' BLISTER

CONNING TOWER

100' TWILL TRUNK

100' ESCAPE TRAINING TANK

FIG. 64

Three-quarters of all submarine escape casualties occurred during the period of flooding.

(ii) During the war as many men made an escape ascent without breathing apparatus as did with it.

The importance of training was emphasized and a 100 ft. training tower built at the Submarine Base in Gosport (Fig. 64). This enabled every man who went to sea in a submarine to have absolute confidence in his ability to escape should the need arise. The technique of ascending without apparatus other than a life-jacket (Buoyant Ascent) was at the same time developed and taught.

As far as the period in the submarine during flooding was concerned, realizing that acceptable limits of carbon dioxide rapidly decreased with pressurization, the supply of an air breathing apparatus to every man was considered but could not be accepted because of the demand on stowage space. It was possible however to build into submarines a breathing system which consisted of a battery of high-pressure cylinders from which a mixture of 40% oxygen and 60% nitrogen was piped round the compartments designated for escape. At intervals along the pipe were connections into which could be plugged, prior to starting flooding, flexible tubes on the end of which hung mouth-pieces and demand valves. During the flooding and whilst waiting to escape men were able to breathe a mixture which was pure and independent of the atmosphere in the submarine.

Two submarine disasters have occurred since the introduction of these techniques. The *Truculent* sank after a collision in 1950 in the relatively shallow water of the Thames Estuary. Fifty men were trapped below and all escaped by the method taught. Unfortunately as the escape took place during bad visibility and a strong ebb tide, only ten of these were picked up alive.

The other accident, the loss of the *Affray* in 1951, remains a mystery and all personnel were lost. She was found by underwater television at a depth of 280 ft. but never salvaged.

The unfortunate loss of men who have actually reached the surface, as occurred with *Truculent*, hastened the development and issue of a submarine escape immersion suit designed to keep men warm, dry and afloat until picked up.

To complete the brief history of submarine escape, reference must be made to a disaster which occurred in the American Navy in 1939, that of the U.S.S. *Squalus* which due to the failure of an induction valve to close during a dive became partially flooded and stuck on the bottom in 240 ft. of water. The submarine was quickly located and the following day a rescue chamber reached the scene. This was lowered to make a water-tight seal around the submarine escape hatch. Men then entered the chamber and were brought to the surface. Four descents with this chamber brought all the men remaining alive in the unflooded compartments safely to the surface.

This is a very satisfactory method of rescue eliminating problems of pressurization in the submarine and survival on the surface. It does however demand an early location of the submarine, relative freedom from currents, a fairly calm sea and the submarine on a fairly even keel. It is costly to maintain especially if a world-wide service is desired.

SUBMARINE ESCAPE TODAY

It is very important when studying the overall problem of submarine escape to keep a balanced view. Over the years during which submarines have been in operation the loss of men from submarine disaster compared with other accidents is relatively low. When a submarine fails to surface there is an immense impact on public feeling. Unlike the crash of an air liner, the outcome of which is decided in seconds, there are hours or even days of uncertainty during which hope for trapped men rises and falls with changes in circumstances. It is very much akin to the major mine disaster where men are likewise trapped and no one quite knows how they are faring.

Furthermore it is important not to lose sight of the fact that submarines at present in use are vessels of war and although feelings of humanity demand every facility for rescue be provided, the very nature of their purpose equally demands that nothing shall be done which would in any way lessen their striking power. It would be quite unacceptable to sacrifice stowage space for torpedoes to make room for inflatable life rafts. This requirement sets a stiff task for those responsible for escape arrangements and an intelligent compromise must be achieved. The submariners themselves are very modest in their demands for escape equipment especially in wartime. It must be remembered that, in spite of their selflessness, they are trained and valuable men and even if their submarine is lost it is most important to do everything possible to retain their services. There is thus a practical as well as humanitarian stimulus in the development of escape procedure.

In no other field is there a greater opportunity for imagination and a long list could be given of alternative suggestions for rescuing men from a disabled submarine, some quite reasonable many utterly fantastic. They include capsules which can be let up from the submarine, whole buoyant compartments and facilities for one submarine to couple itself to another.

In planning escape from present-day submarines and also those of the future, consideration must be given to possible improvements in design and strength of structure which will enable operation at greater depths. Increase in depth greatly adds to the difficulty at all stages but from a survey of all submarine disasters it will at once be realized that three-quarters of them occurred as a result of collision or during trials. The risk of collision is almost wholly limited to the harbour approaches where shipping lanes converge and trials, too, are usually carried out near to the bases. The greater proportion of accidents are therefore likely to occur in inshore waters of depths not likely to exceed 300 ft. or 400 ft. This fact must influence thought on the subject and justify the adoption of methods which may not be effective from the submarines' maximum operating depths. Planning however must be flexible and though the submarines are provided with the best compromise between escape facilities and working efficiency, there can be no relaxation in attempts to improve techniques.

The more recent loss of two nuclear submarines in deep water and two conventional submarines in the Mediterranean has necessitated further study of escape techniques to give increased chance of survival from greater depths. It is logical to assume that military requirements will demand operation at greater depth and longer patrols more distant from the home base.

Escape procedures must fall into two major groups, those in which the survivors remain at atmospheric pressure throughout and those where the pressure in the submarine is raised to that of the surrounding water. Both methods are in use today.

(i) *Escape with No Pressure Change*

When any ship is lost at sea it may be left to its own resources or help may be immediately to hand. In the former case lifeboats or rafts are launched and facilities for survival until picked up must be provided. In the latter another vessel may come alongside and take off survivors directly. This direct rescue is analogous with the 'non-pressurized' submarine rescue, which is dependent upon the early arrival of highly technical surface assistance. It may include salvage or the use of a rescue chamber.

The major objection to such methods is that much time may well be needed for rescue ships to reach the area. For this reason salvage as a method of rescue was abandoned. However with the introduction of nuclear-powered submarines the picture must change. A situation may well arise where such a vessel, though disabled and unable to leave the bottom, is able to maintain its domestic services and air purification facilities for weeks. This opens up possibilities of unhurried salvage and improves chances of obtaining ideal conditions for use of the rescue chamber.

The Rescue Chamber is standard equipment in the American and some other navies and demands an immense organization to maintain it. In practice the chamber is carried by rescue vessels which have on board trained and experienced divers.

Once a distressed submarine is located a guide line is attached from the rescue vessel to a convenient ring near the escape hatch on the submarine. The rescue chamber consists of two compartments. The upper one, roomy enough to accommodate six or more survivors, has a hatch above and below and remaining at atmospheric pressure is refreshed by air piped from the parent vessel. An attendant travelling in this compartment is in constant communication with the surface and can control the working of the chamber. The lower compartment is less roomy and open below. It is a cylinder whose diameter is greater than the escape hatch of the submarine and, having round its lower rim a rubber

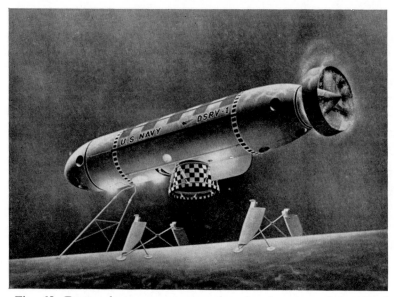

Fig. 65. Deep submergence rescue submarine (courtesy of Lockheed Missiles and Space Company and U.S. Navy)

gasket, it can be lowered until it rests snugly around the submarine's hatch where it can be further secured. The lower compartment will contain water which can be forced out with compressed air. When the chamber is securely in place the lower hatch of the upper chamber and that of the submarine can both be opened to allow men through. When the rescue chamber has received its quota of survivors both hatches are closed and it is raised to the surface. The process is repeated until all men alive in the submarine have been withdrawn.

The advantages of this technique are obvious. The men are not subjected to the hazards of increasing pressure, they remain dry, they do not ascend through water and on reaching the surface are assured of attention. On the other hand it demands a vast organization and may be rendered useless by adverse weather or the submarine lying at too great an angle.

A considerable advantage would be gained if the 'bell' could be more mobile and independent, in other words a deep rescue submarine with its own source of power (Fig. 65).

This will be achieved by enclosing the rescue chamber—possibly enlarged to take more men, in an outer streamlined shell which could flood under water except for pressure resistant compartments for the crew and survivors. It would operate only in the disaster area and thus would need to be small enough to be carried by aircraft to the nearest port and there by rescue vessel or other submarine. The development of the rescue submarine capable of operating down to the collapse depth of all operational submarines and having transfer facilities at atmospheric pressure is inevitable.

(ii) *Escape using Pressure Equalization*

This method, at present widely taught in the submarine service of most navies, depends on the man being able to leave the submarine on his own. For this it is necessary for the pressure within to be raised to that outside before any hatch can be opened. With such a procedure there are four stages all of which must be fully considered. These are:

(*a*) In the submarine before flooding and pressure equalization is commenced.

(*b*) The period of pressure equalization.

(*c*) The ascent.

(*d*) Survival on the surface.

(*a*) PRE-FLOODING PERIOD

What happens during this period will depend upon the conditions within the hull immediately after the accident. In some cases where there is structural damage and general flooding, escape of toxic fumes or other immediate danger, escape must be made at once, at the rush, the object being to abandon the submarine as quickly as possible. In such a situation all available means must be used and the risk of being lost after surfacing accepted.

On the other hand the damage may be isolated and men be alive and secure in undamaged compartments. Consideration must be given to the number of men, the state of the atmosphere and how long it may be maintained breathable. If possible escape should be delayed until help is known to have arrived at the surface but not if this results in the men being exhausted and unable to carry out the escape routine. This calls for great courage and judgment and at the same time attempts will no doubt be made to refloat the vessel, though this too must not exhaust the men so as to destroy their chances. In the *Thetis* the men were exhausted and waited too long, in the *Truculent* they did not wait long enough.

During this period which demands hard thinking and planning the men may have an opportunity to don warm clothing and survival suits. If hot drinks are available they should be consumed and possibly a tot of rum. (Research is still in progress to examine the effect of alcohol taken prior to immersion in cold water.) It is important that only essential work should be done for rest is important in conserving the oxygen supply. Correct timing and good use of this waiting period may well determine the success of the whole operation.

(b) PRESSURE EQUALIZATION

When the time comes to prepare for escape pressure within must be raised by letting water come in from valves in the lower part of the submarine. This process may be speeded up in some instances by using compressed air also if any is available.

The hazards of this period are not unlike those which beset the diver. The worst of these is the submarine atmosphere which must contain some impurities notably carbon dioxide. At atmospheric pressure they may be harmless but pressurization can produce lethal concentrations. Because of this the built-in breathing system is used and as soon as the flooding starts each man breathes from this independent and pure supply of breathing mixture.

Having eliminated the risk of carbon dioxide poisoning the effects of pressure must be considered. Flooding may take about five minutes, according to depth, and it may be another ten before the last man can get out. He will have been exposed to 10 minutes at pressure and 5 minutes being compressed and for convenience may be regarded as being under the pressure equivalent to depth for $12\frac{1}{2}$ minutes. If the submarine is deeper than 145 feet there will be a risk of decompression sickness if air is breathed. At 200 ft. the safe time for exposure if 'bends' are to be avoided is 6 minutes, at 300 ft. it is 3 minutes. If a mixture containing 40% oxygen and 60% nitrogen is used these safe times are longer as less nitrogen is absorbed. At 200 ft. the time is 13 minutes and at 300 ft. $5\frac{1}{2}$ minutes. The mixture does therefore give a better chance of escaping decompression sickness.

Oxygen poisoning however must be considered and in this respect the mixture is more dangerous, the limit of safety being 130 ft. as opposed to 300 ft. with air. Moreover cases of oxygen poisoning would occur whilst men were still in the submarine, and of decompression sickness only on reaching the surface. The former might easily impair the orderly routine of escape and endanger morale as well as producing fatal casualties. It is for this reason that air is used in the built-in breathing system instead of the mixture as first introduced.

Nitrogen narcosis is also a risk but it is considered that the urgency of the situation coupled with good discipline will enable the personnel to withstand its effects.

The times quoted for flooding and the escape of a large number of men refer to the use of a compartment. In those submarines which are fitted with escape chambers, e.g. for two or more men it is possible to save a great deal of time under pressure. These chambers are relatively small and once two men have entered and hatches are closed pressure equalization can be completed in as little time as two minutes and the occupants can be out seconds later. These chambers, and the conning tower which can also be adapted for this type of escape, are also fitted with breathing points from the built-in system. The chamber method is likely to be much safer from greater depths as the remainder of crew wait their turn at atmospheric pressure. The main drawback is that for a number of men to escape a much longer period of time is needed.

(c) THE ASCENT

Pressure being equalized the hatches can be opened and no time is lost by the men in escaping either from the compartment or the chamber. It is usual to provide some aid to buoyancy and a standard life-jacket of the 'Mae West' type is used. With this a man will ascend through the water at about 4 ft. per second. Without added buoyancy he would come up at about half this rate.

Before a man leaves a submarine he will take a last full breath from the breathing system so that at the commencement of the ascent his lungs may contain as much as 6 litres of air (vital capacity and residual volume). This as the pressure decreases must expand and if lung damage is to be avoided the excess must escape through the mouth. This 6 litres if the submarine was at 100 ft. would expand to 24 litres by the time it reached the surface though of course some of this expansion would take place after the air left the body. The expansion increases as the survivor nears the surface and to give some idea of this it is possible to calculate the rate at which air flows out of the respiratory system if the man is ascending at a known rate, e.g. 4 ft. per second.

Depth during ascent feet	Rate of flow of expanding air litres per minute
100	10·8
80	13·2
60	15·6
40	20·4
20	28·2
10	34·8
2	43·2

This outflow of air helps to prevent an accumulation of carbon dioxide which might otherwise bring breath holding to an end and at the same time there is sufficient oxygen partial pressure to maintain consciousness. The increase in rate of air escape can be seen, if a man is followed up through the water, as a gentle stream of bubbles to begin with and a massive one near the surface. If there is no obstruction to this escape of air there is no danger in coming up through the water. Experimental escapes have been made from depths over 300 ft. both in laboratories and at sea. At such a depth rapid compression in a chamber prior to escape is used.

The most convenient way to ascend is to be completely relaxed, particularly the respiratory muscles. If a gentle blow is started immediately after leaving the submarine no difficulty should be encountered in getting rid of the expanding air. It is usual to start the ascent with the lungs full especially if the depth is great. Opinions have been expressed that, if on leaving 100 ft. the escaper blows right down to his residual volume before ascending, it is quite impossible for the lung to be over-distended. This is true from a hundred feet but is certainly not so from greater depths. Starting with an empty lung often results in discomfort and a desire to breathe before the surface is reached. With a full lung the ascent is comfortable and indeed exhilarating and in training, which is given to all submarine personnel, repeated attempts are made to ensure complete confidence. This will undoubtedly be of the greatest value should escape in earnest ever be demanded. In addition American workers are successfully experimenting with a hood which is refreshed with expanding air from the life-jacket. This enables free breathing to be carried out during the ascent.

It will have been realized that circumstances may arise when the time, for which men have been subjected to excess pressure prior to the ascent, demands that decompression shall be interrupted by stops if decompression sickness is to be avoided. This is of course impossible in the buoyant or free ascent technique and could only be done if the escaper was a trained diver using a breathing apparatus. At present therefore nothing can be done during the ascent to prevent decompression sickness but it should be remembered that, at least, the victims do reach the surface alive where the possibility of treatment may exist and not every case of bends is fatal. Even if the effects are permanent they are not incompatible with a happy and useful life.

Other things being equal it should be possible for all of a submarine's complement to escape without difficulty by the compartment method from 250 ft. and by the chamber method from 300 ft. There would be a good chance of many survivors if the depths were 300 ft. and 400 ft. Bearing in mind that the majority of submarine disasters are within these limits the present situation is highly satisfactory.

If escape from deeper depths by these methods is contemplated an alternative mixture will be required for breathing during the flooding period, e.g. a 10% oxygen in helium. The problem of decompression still remains and is difficult to control with the resources at present available.

Looking a very long way ahead it might be possible that submarine personnel will be trained divers with breathing apparatus which will allow them to leave a submarine as if they were completing a routine dive.

Thought is also being given to the use of pressure suits. If suitable fabric could be found and a suit made to hold a set pressure of say 25 lb. per sq. inch, it would be possible for the man to reach the surface and, provided he was totally enclosed, remain at what would be equivalent to a decompression stop at 50 ft. He could breathe the air contained within the suit which may need a means of purification. Such a practice would, if it could be achieved, go a long way to reducing the danger of severe decompression sickness.

More immediately practicable however, in cases where controlled decompression is necessary, is to use the technique of 'surface decompression'. This needs the attendance of surface ships with pressure chambers. If a large chamber is available many men may be treated at the same time. Alternatively, though less satisfactory, a compartment of an accompanying submarine may be adapted for this purpose. Small one-man chambers, possibly of fabric or light construction, may even be flown to the scene of the accident.

It may be difficult in actual practice to persuade men who are overjoyed at being rescued to submit to recompression but if there is reason to suspect that they may develop decompression sickness, or indeed if they already show signs of it, this must be enforced and it may well be necessary to recompress the survivors in groups as they arrive on the surface.

(d) HOOD SYSTEM

The disadvantage of the free ascent or buoyant ascent methods is the risk of pulmonary barotrauma. If unrestricted breathing could be provided during ascent the risk would be greatly lessened. The possibility can be demonstrated in the escape training tank by ascending with an inverted bucket of air over the head which allows relaxed and unrestricted breathing.

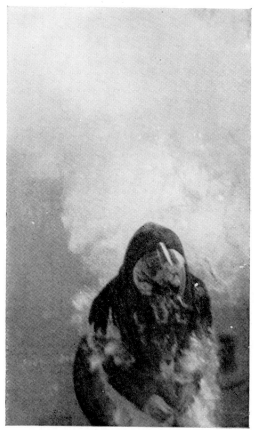

FIG. 67. Escape Hood in use

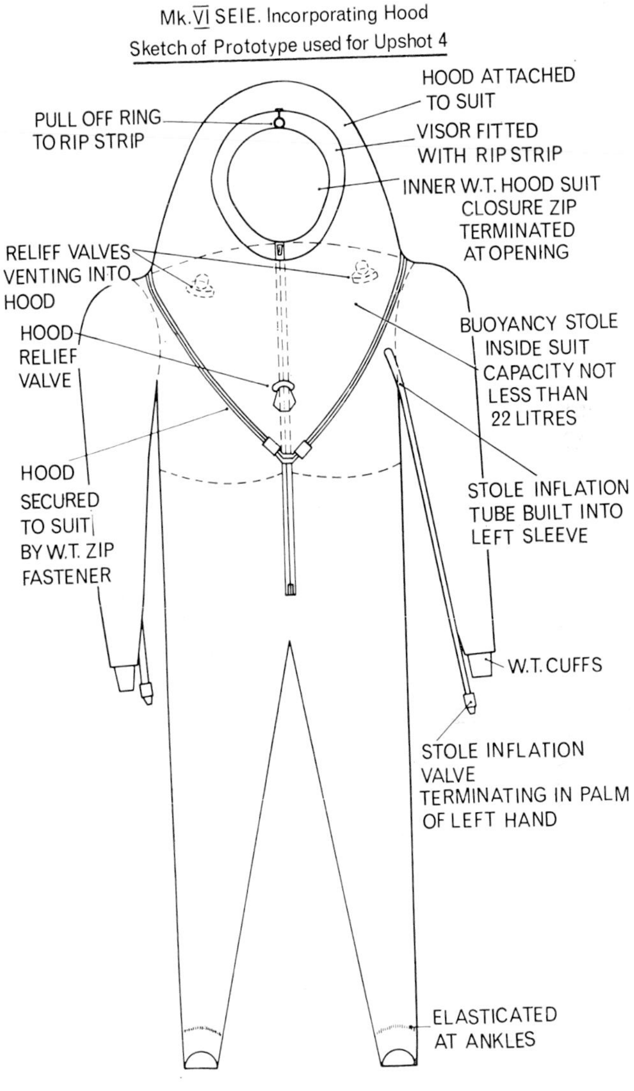

Mk.VI SEIE. Incorporating Hood
Sketch of Prototype used for Upshot 4

HOOD ATTACHED
TO SUIT

PULL OFF RING
TO RIP STRIP

VISOR FITTED
WITH RIP STRIP

INNER W.T. HOOD SUIT
CLOSURE ZIP
TERMINATED
AT OPENING

RELIEF VALVES
VENTING INTO
HOOD

HOOD
RELIEF
VALVE

BUOYANCY STOLE
INSIDE SUIT
CAPACITY NOT
LESS THAN
22 LITRES

HOOD
SECURED
TO SUIT
BY W.T. ZIP
FASTENER

STOLE INFLATION
TUBE BUILT INTO
LEFT SLEEVE

W.T. CUFFS

STOLE INFLATION
VALVE
TERMINATING IN PALM
OF LEFT HAND

ELASTICATED
AT ANKLES

FIG. 67. A sketch of the escape immersion suit used in these trials

22

The principle has been introduced as the 'Hood Inflation System' (Elliott, 1966). In brief, this is little more than a large hood with transport face piece which passes over head and shoulders to be attached to the immersion suit described under the sub-heading. The hood is used for escape from a one-man escape chamber and is filled with air which the escapee breathes during the rapid flooding and pressurization of the chamber to the outside pressure. When this is complete the hatch is opened and he surfaces breathing freely from the air in the hood. The hood is fitted with a relief valve which allows free escape of expanding air. The transparent face piece has a ring with which it can be removed to allow the occupant to breathe fresh outside air when he is afloat on the surface if the hood itself cannot be conveniently removed. (See Fig. 66 and 67.) In trials successful escapes in the open sea have been made from keel depths of 500 ft. This method thus represents a considerable advance both in increase of escape depths and the fact that during ascent which is at about 9 ft. per second natural breathing can continue.

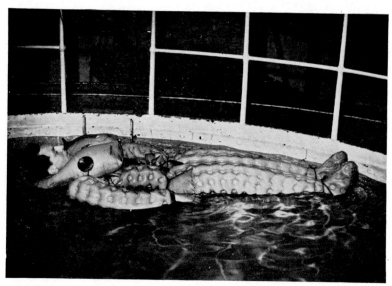

Fig. 68. The submarine escape immersion suit

(e) SURVIVAL ON THE SURFACE

There can be no greater tragedy than that a man should escape from a stricken submarine and be lost on the surface. It has happened all too often but much is being done to lessen the risk today. Wherever compatible with a safe escape the timing is planned to give the greatest opportunity for surface craft to reach the area and to take place in daylight if possible.

The submarine escape immersion suit (Fig. 68) which can be inflated automatically when the surface is reached gives, with the inflated lifejacket, a high degree of insulation and comfort. Even in cold water many hours' survival can be expected. Attached to the life-jacket is a whistle and a light to aid location. One difficulty has been the problem of urination, often a necessity in cold climates, which is not easy to accomplish in the supine position and may, if achieved, cause considerable loss of insulation in the suits. Absorbent 'nappies' are now provided for wear under the suit.

That storage space is at a premium in the submarine must now be realized and therefore all escape equipment is designed to occupy the minimum volume. For this reason the inflatable life rafts which have proved so reliable in surface ships cannot be considered.

On the whole the submariner is well cared for by his escape planners for, as well as all the personnel techniques just described, great pains are taken to make sure that the loss of a submarine is immediately realized and a far reaching and efficient organization quickly comes into action. Submarines carry many devices to aid searching vessels to find them if necessary and behind all the safety precautions is the realization by constructors, as well as submariners, that the only true and valid requirement is that the disaster shall not occur.

As the sphere of operations and cruising depths of submarines increase so must the facilities for escape be developed, always however subservient to operational requirements. The physical difficulties increase and tax the skill of the physiologists and designers. Much is known about the problem and those who venture beneath the seas may rest assured that where their safety is concerned there is no complacency.

SUBMARINE ESCAPE TRAINING

The greatest importance is attached to training and both in this country and the United States special training tanks have been constructed. These consist of towers containing a 100-ft. high column of water below which is constructed the facsimile of a submarine's escape compartment and escape chamber (Fig. 64). (Smaller ones are also available in Sweden, the Argentine and Germany.) Men are thus trained under realistic conditions starting first from a chamber built into the side of the tank at 30 ft. (Crocker 1955). Next an ascent from 60 ft. is completed and finally one from the bottom.

Training is remarkably safe and before entering the water the technique is explained and demonstrated and the importance of complete relaxation and the free escape of air emphasized. Experienced instructors are in the water and should there be any evidence of lung damage a pressure chamber is always ready for immediate use at the top of the tower and the victim can be recompressed within seconds.

A total of 50,000 ascents were carried out in the British Training tank with only 25 accidents all of which responded to treatment and made a complete recovery. In 19 there was evidence of cerebral air embolism and in 4 there was mediastinal emphysema, one also having a severe pneumothorax. In addition two cases had no abnormality. There is no time for diagnosis before treatment and a medical officer follows the patient into the pressure chamber through the lock. A special chute is constructed to speed the entry of the casualty into the chamber.

The efficiency of the organization may be seen from the following example. A submariner on leaving the water bent down to rub a toe which he had stubbed on his way out of the bottom hatch. Before he had time to explain that he only wanted to rub his toe, instructors, thinking he was about to collapse, bundled him into the chamber and compressed him to 165 ft.

FREE ASCENT AND THE UNDERWATER SWIMMER

In the rare event of an underwater breathing apparatus failing under water it is essential that the user is able to abandon it and reach the surface. All sets should therefore be fitted with a quick release mechanism so that they can be abandoned without loss of time.

The technique is then exactly the same as that of ascent from a submarine with the advantage that the escaper is already in the water. If the set will allow it a final breath should be taken before abandoning (or 'ditching') it. If no air is available for this the lungs quickly fill as the ascent continues though the ascent may have to be assisted by swimming in the absence of added buoyancy.

During the ascent it is equally important to be completely relaxed and at all costs avoid panic which may result in pulmonary damage. The rarity of this event must be emphasized but when it does occur it can be dangerous. Underwater swimming organizations may practise the technique of ditching the set as part of their safety training programme. It is very doubtful whether it is justified to do this, except in swimming pools, unless the facilities of a pressure chamber are immediately to hand. Even an ascent from a shallow depth can result in a burst lung, for it is near the surface that the air in the lungs expands at the greatest rate.

The underwater swimmer who abandons his set is likely to be without additional buoyancy when he reaches the surface, unless he has an inflatable suit, or life-jacket, and for this reason it is desirable that he should be a good swimmer and also that he should not operate unless surface assistance is readily available.

READING AND REFERENCES

Crocker, W. E. (1955). 'Principles and Technique of Free Ascent in Submarine Escape.' *J. R.N. Med. Service. 41*, 133.

Davis, R. H. (1955). 'Escape from Sunken Submarines.' *Deep Diving*, p. 257. Siebe Gorman, London.

Elliott, D. H. (1966). 'Submarine Escape—The Hood Inflation System'. *J. Roy. Nav. Med. Service 52*, 120.

Schilling, C. W. and J. W. Kohl (1947). *History of Submarine Medicine in World War II*. U.S. Navy Submarine Base, New London.

Shelford, W. O. (1960). *Subsmash*. Harrap, London.

Taylor, H. J. (1953). 'Recent Research and Submarine Escape.' *M.R.C. (RNPRC) Report U.P.S.* 137.

A Condensed History of Submarine Escape in the Royal Navy (1959). Flag Officer, Submarines, Fort Blockhouse, Gosport.

CHAPTER XXI

Marine Animals

THERE is certainly very much more room for life in the sea than on land and although the fundamental dependence of animal life upon plants exists the picture is very different. Only in the shallowest waters do plants grow with any semblance of those on land and the majority of undersea 'growths', even though apparently rooted, stalked and branched, are animal.

Green plants are there in abundance and, though they bear no resemblance to their counterparts on land, they are essential to maintain the cycle of marine life.

Light is necessary and, because this does not penetrate far only the upper 150 ft. or so of the oceans can support vegetable life. The mineral and gaseous requirements of the plants are already dissolved in the water thus doing away with the need for supporting roots and branches. Plants however must float to be near the light and the most economical means of floating is to remain minute which also gives a greater surface-area-for-weight ratio than the complex multicellular structure of land vegetation.

The bulk of marine vegetation which is microscopic and invisible, consists of two types, the diatoms and flagellates known collectively as phyto-plankton. The distribution of phyto-plankton, depending on temperature changes in the sea and the activity of the currents, may, in some areas, be so dense as to discolour the sea. Generally speaking it is most abundant in the spring. It needs salts from the sea-bed to thrive and in winter the water, from which the salts have been exhausted by the previous season's phyto-plankton, is cooled and sinks. Warmer water rising from the sea-bed then brings the salts which are needed for further multiplication. Since almost all of the sea life is nourished by plankton its intensity waxes and wanes with the seasons as its essential mineral supplies arrive and are exhausted.

So small is this phyto-plankton that only the smallest units of animal life are able to eat it. The term plankton has a wider use and includes all living matter which drifts with the currents, the animal element of which is the zooplankton, the food of the larger whales. As a result the vast bulk of visible sea life is animal and carnivorous. The wastage of life is most extensive and eggs and offspring have to be produced in vast numbers if the species are to survive.

Flotation is an important problem becoming more difficult in the larger animals. Protoplasm is heavier than water and many ways are used to overcome this. If water is enclosed it will decrease the overall weight, and may be bound within a jelly to form a kind of structural skeleton. Some creatures are able to attain a degree of buoyancy by enclosing water containing less salt which is therefore lighter than sea water. One of the most valuable aids to buoyancy, fat, is used by many fishes and in the warm-blooded sea mammals serves also as insulation. Food reserves are stored in the form of oils rather than the heavier glycogen. In some bony fishes gas bladders may be used to give buoyancy. It is often difficult to find a compromise between speed and flotation for streamlining and heavy muscles lessen buoyancy. Gas bladders when present may also serve an additional function of depth gauge.

Strictly speaking only the upper layers which contain plant life are truly self-supporting. However not all the life in this area is consumed and a proportion of it dies to produce a continuous rain of organic debris through the depths. Although much of this falls to litter the sea-bed, a proportion is devoured by the inhabitants of the various layers and is essential for their survival. That which reaches the sea-bed provides food for a wide variety of fungi, bacteria and primitive scavenging animals.

The whole vast changing pattern of marine life provides a field for scientific investigation which is only just being explored. It is a delicately balanced cycle and when the time comes for man to control its rich harvest he will need to proceed with caution and understanding to prevent him from misusing and exhausting it. If he remembers some of the bitter lessons he has learnt on land he may escape the embarrassment of the results of thoughtless exploitation.

Little more can be done here than to try and tempt the reader with a few tit-bits in the hope that he will seek elsewhere for the knowledge which is already available on the very large subject of marine biology. The underwater swimmer may in time become an underwater farmer and he will need to know the habits of his flocks and requirements of his crops. There may be some trial and error but there is today better chance of a scientific approach.

Meanwhile in his attempt to perfect his underwater capabilities he may learn much from the aquatic mammals. He must also learn to know and combat those creatures which may become his enemies and rivals under water.

THE AQUATIC MAMMALS

The aquatic mammals are of particular interest to man in his study of the underwater environment for in their re-adaptation to the sea they took with them the lessons they had learnt on land. The whales and dolphins have made the most complete change, spending all their life in water, even mating and breeding. The seals are less adapted, retaining their fur and going ashore for breeding and basking.

All have taken with them a high degree of intelligence which is demonstrated by the ease with which these mammals can be trained to work

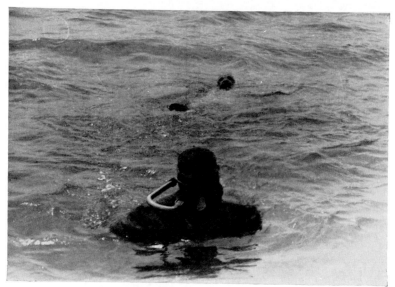

Fig. 69. Swimmer and towing seal

with man and perform tricks. They are said to be as intelligent as dogs and may well become the domestic animals of the underwater farms. The skills of dolphins, sea lions and seals are well known and if they work so well with man out of water they will most certainly work with him in water. Underwater swimmers interested in these possibilities have fitted seals with harnesses and been towed by them through the water (Fig. 69).

The vertebrate skeleton has become well adapted to streamlining which in the whale, where gills are unnecessary, has reached a very high degree of perfection. The neck has disappeared and lateral and dorsal fins are reduced in size to serve only for steering and stabilizing. The tail being the main propulsive unit has retained the up and down movements of the running land vertebrate, unlike that of fishes which is from side to side. This up and down movement is also a great advantage in the frequent rapid diving and surfacing so characteristic of these creatures.

Streamlining, powerful locomotion, and the small difference in specific gravity between body tissue and sea water have put no limit on size. As a result the largest animal that has ever lived, bigger even than the prehistoric monsters, is the whale which may have the bulk of fifty elephants. Locomotion is only really efficient when fully submerged for then the streamlining is most effective. To drive a 75-ft. whale on the surface at 15 knots ($17\frac{1}{4}$ m.p.h.) requires 1,775 h.p. and only 168 h.p. submerged (Barcroft, 1938). The actual efficiency of the whale's musculature is much the same as a fit animal or trained man but the whale scores over a rigid shape, such as a submarine, by the flexibility of its body which greatly reduces eddy formation and resistance.

In feeding habits a striking difference is found which divides the whales into two major groups, those which have teeth and those which do not. The toothed whales, the Odontoceti, which includes the killer whale, the sperm whale and the dolphins, feed on large fish and other sea mammals. The killer whale will attack other whales, enjoys seals and will eat man. It has a habit of tipping up ice flows on which seals are riding and would do the same with men. The teeth are not used for chewing and only with large animals such as other whales would they tear the flesh. Seals (and men) would be swallowed whole for most sea creatures are too slippery to chew and might easily be lost. How fortunate this practice was for Jonah!

The Whalebone-Whales, Mystotoceti, which include the rorquals and hump backs, grow very much bigger in spite of their diet of 'krill', small shrimp-like crustacea which are filtered from the sea water as it is drawn through the mouth.

DIVING AND RESPIRATION

Of great interest to the student of underwater medicine is the physiology of the diving mammal. This is believed to be similar in the whales, dolphins and seals though the first of these are not easy to study. Much more work needs to be done but there is general agreement as to how these animals are able to hold their breath for long periods and tolerate pressure changes. Since they must feed under water and since locomotion under water is so much more economical it is natural that a considerable proportion of these animals' life is spent in diving.

There is still much dispute as to the depth these creatures reach and the time they remain submerged. Many of the recorded times have been made with the animals under duress. The smaller dolphins and seals dive for about 10 minutes and the whales probably about 20 minutes with 4 minutes on the surface between-whiles. Hunted whales carrying a harpoon have been known to reach depths of 4,000 ft. or more (Gray, 1927) and remain submerged for an hour; when recovered however they appear far from well though no gas bubbles have been found in blood vessels or tissues.

Even though these very deep and prolonged dives are exceptional profound physiological adaptation is necessary to meet the normal underwater requirements. The main changes are in circulation, respiration and central sensitivity. Laurie (1933) investigated the problem in whales and made some interesting findings, the following of which throw some light on the process of adaptation.

(i) The basal metabolic rate of the whale is only one-fifteenth that of man in calories per kilogram of body weight and the blood will hold enough oxygen to maintain this for about 65 minutes.

(ii) A high concentration of haemoglobin in muscle will store sufficient oxygen to propel the whale at 5 knots for 25 minutes and it must be assumed that a further oxygen debt may be tolerated.

(iii) It is possible that the respiratory centre depends solely upon oxygen lack as a stimulant to breathing and not carbon dioxide excess. Very large quantities of carbon dioxide have been found dissolved in blood and other body fluids.

(iv) Micro-organisms found in the whale's blood have been shown to fix nitrogen enabling the blood to take up more of this gas than by simple solution. This gives some protection against decompression sickness.

(v) When submerged there is a profound slowing of the heart rate. In a seal recently studied, the rate fell from 120 per minute at the surface to 4 at 300 ft. The circulatory anatomy is such that large venous plexuses in the abdominal cavity are available for the pooling of considerable volumes of blood. When submerged only vital organs receive any blood. Furthermore blood supplied to the brain and spinal cord passes through a network of fine vessels, the 'retia mirabilia' which is believed to be a bubble trap so that in the event of the animal's activity leading to accidental bubble formation these may be held up without total blocking of essential circulation.

If these five possibilities are taken together they would seem to offer adequate explanation for the aquatic mammals' high degree of adaptation. Much more work is still to be done in this fascinating and promising field.

WATER BALANCE

Although spending its life in the sea the whale needs fresh water to maintain its fluid balance. It does not sweat but evaporation will take place from the respiratory passages. This may not be as great as might be thought as inspired air taken from immediately above the sea will be fairly well saturated itself. The fluid loss in urine however must be made good.

The salt concentration of the whale's body tissues though greater than man is still much less than that of sea water. The kidneys of the whale are relatively large and it is possible that they have the power of producing a urine more concentrated than body fluids.

If the air which the whale takes in is saturated with moisture, partial pressure of water will be increased as the animal dives and more will be absorbed. If by some physiological trick the loss of water vapour can be less on decompression it might be that the expired air was drier than inspired air. It would be most interesting to know if this actually happened.

OTHER AQUATIC ANIMALS

Many other animals exploit under water the potentialities though less completely. These include water rats, otters and beavers and the feats of diving birds are quite remarkable. Ducks have been widely studied and may remain submerged for as long as 20 minutes.

DANGEROUS MARINE ANIMALS

This heading is also the title of a recently published book by Halstead (1959) which gives a full and admirably illustrated account of the various creatures which the diver and swimmer may meet. A useful list of dangerous sharks and other marine hazards is also to be found in the *U.S. Navy Diving Manual* (1959). The most worthwhile information however can usually be obtained from local sources where the habits of the dangerous sea dwellers of the area will be well known and means of avoiding them practised.

The animal menaces of the ocean can be most conveniently divided into those which bite, those which sting and those which are dangerous to eat.

BITING FISHES

(i) *Sharks*

Sharks are possibly the most feared of sea creatures and many harrowing reports are available of their attacks on man. These attacks are usually confined to the warmer seas and rarely occur when the temperature of the water is less than 70° F. which conditions too are most attractive to man. Very roughly this means that sharks are dangerous all the year round between the latitudes of 30° N and 30° S extending in the northern summer to 40° N and in the southern summer to 40° S.

Not all sharks attack man, in fact only 6% of the known varieties do so. Some experience is however needed to recognize one species from another. It is wise therefore to regard any shark of over 4 ft. in length as potentially dangerous, especially if there is blood in the water. Normally the shark feeds in an orderly manner on anything from small marine organisms to seals or even man. They will feed from below and white arms carelessly trailing in the water or the unprotected legs of a swimmer are very tempting to them. It is generally believed that suited divers under water are safe from attack though they may invite some curiosity. The underwater swimmer confronted with a shark should remain still. If some form of weapon is carried it may be used to shove the shark away or failing this to hit it on the snout or gills. Underwater noises, especially explosions, tend to attract sharks.

On occasions when for some reason there is much food in the water as for example after a sea or air disaster or the dumping of offal sharks may become frenzied and slash indiscriminately at anything roundabout, even one another.

Coppleson (1958) describes three types of injury due to shark the first two of which are the results of playfulness. A shark may without malice buffet a diver producing widespread bruising or if the swimmer is unclothed its rough body may cause severe abrasions consisting of multiple parallel scratches. The bite itself is usually irregular with considerable tissue destruction, a tearing away of flesh rather than a clean bite. For this reason the shark bite has a high mortality possibly 80% due to massive haemorrhage and shock.

First-aid treatment consists of stopping the haemorrhage with packing and local pressure. Tourniquets may be difficult to apply and remembering that much blood may have been lost in the water, shock must be treated with intravenous plasma, blood or some equivalent. Antibiotic therapy and tetanus antitoxin should also be given.

To prevent shark attack there is no sure recommendation which can be given. Various repellents are available, a common one being copper acetate. It may be combined with a dye to hide the swimmer. Experiments have shown that the repellents rapidly become ineffective and ignored by the shark. They may however give sufficient protection to enable a survivor in the water to be picked up and without doubt they are good for morale. Work is progressing in various establishments to find some chemical which will irritate the shark's eyes, a relatively vulnerable site, and some success seems possible with the lachrimatory agents used in chemical warfare.

Where popular bathing beaches are menaced by sharks it is frequently possible by various netting techniques to keep them away and if required shark-proof enclosures can be also built. Look-outs from the cliffs or specially constructed towers are useful and in some areas even light aeroplanes or helicopters are used at the height of the bathing season.

Davies (1964) who had a vast experience of the shark menace on the South African beaches, recommends the establishment of 'first aid' stores at strategic points which contain, amongst the normal supplies, human blood plasma and equipment for its administration.

(ii) *Other Biting Fishes*

A close rival to the shark is the BARRACUDA which is fairly widely distributed in tropical and sub-tropical waters. In length it may reach eight feet. It has sharp teeth, is a swift attacker and makes a clean bite. Brightly coloured objects such as a fish on the end of a swimmer's spear, will attract it.

GROUPERS and MORAY EELS, though not normally in the habit of attacking man and tending to bask amongst rocks and caverns, will if disturbed produce a vicious bite. GIANT CLAMS, though they do not bite, may if a diver inadvertently steps into an open one, close upon and hold his leg. The knife which all divers should carry may then be used to sever the muscles which hold the two halves of the shell together.

SEA ANIMALS THAT STING

The power to sting is found both in the fishes and the invertebrates and all degrees of injury may occur from discomfort to rapid death.

(i) *Venomous Fishes and Sea Snakes*

Most important members of this group are the STING-RAYS which are usually found in shallow water often almost completely hidden in sand. They may be one or two feet in length and width and when stepped on strike the foot with the tail, the tip of which contains a sting-laden barb. Pain is the main feature with swelling surrounding a puncture wound. In rare cases there may be extreme toxic symptoms, vomiting, tachycardia, paralysis and even death.

In walking through sand suspected to contain sting-rays a shuffling gait rather than a stepping one should be used.

Other stinging fishes include the RAT FISH, CAT FISH, MORAY EEL, WEEVER FISH, SCORPION FISH, STONE FISH and many others.

The venom apparatus is usually contained in the tips of spines which make up the support of dorsal or pectoral fins. Others such as the SURGEON FISH have retractable spines for no other purpose than to sting.

In the TREATMENT of these stings the alleviation of pain is the prime concern and then neutralization of the venom. Many conventional methods are used including ligature, excision, hypertonic applications and compresses. More recently a method popular in the treatment of snake bite is being tried. This is 'cryotherapy' in which the injured area is immediately immersed in iced water. Finally the risk of secondary infection, which is great, must be met with active chemotherapy.

SEA SNAKES are not common but all are very poisonous. In appearance they resemble land snakes with the tail flattened from side to side to aid swimming. They likewise have venom fangs with which they promptly kill their prey, usually smaller fishes.

When a man is bitten there is little local pain but a gradual onset of general stiffness followed by paralysis. In severe intoxications there may be convulsions, loss of consciousness and death.

The treatment is identical with that of the land snake and should include the early intravenous injection of a polyvalent antivenin containing a 'krait' factor.

(ii) *Jelly Fishes and other Stinging Invertebrates*

Four groups usually described, are (i) Coelenterates, including Jelly fishes and Corals, (ii) Molluscs, shell-fish and octopuses, (iii) Stinging worms and (iv) Sea Urchins.

One of the most familiar stinging jelly fish is the Portuguese Man of War (strictly speaking this is not a true jelly fish but a 'Hydroid' found floating on the surface). From its balloon-like float hang trailing tentacles which may be many feet in length and contain the venom cells and stinging apparatus. The Portuguese Man of War (Physalia), sometimes called the Blue Bottle, has a world-wide distribution in temperate and tropical waters and is an occasional visitor to the British Isles. The stings are not dangerous but can be excruciatingly painful. The manifestation is an urticarial lesion on the skin and the victim may appear as if lashed by a whip.

Far more dangerous is the Sea Wasp (Chiropsalmus) which fortunately is localized to the North of Australia and the Indian Ocean. It is not unlike the Portuguese Man of War but is squatter with clusters of tentacles hanging from four corners of its base. It is without any doubt the most venomous creature in the sea and will kill a man in as little as three minutes. As with other stings there is local reddening, pain and swelling. In addition there are severe shock, cramps, paralysis, respiratory failure, convulsions and death.

The treatment of the Sea Wasp and Blue Bottle stings consists of relieving the pain for which morphia may be needed, neutralizing the effects of the poison and countering the shock. In less severe cases soothing lotions may help. Antihistamines and intravenous calcium gluconate have been used. Artificial respiration and cardiac stimulants may be needed in extreme cases but there is as yet no specific antidote. Australian marine biologists are working on the problem and some success is expected though in the case of the Sea Wasp the chances of injecting an antivenin in time are very slender.

Where these creatures are known to exist no chances should be taken. Furthermore, though the bodies of both the Sea Wasp and Blue Bottle may be seen and recognized on the surface, it should be remembered that their trailing tentacles may be as much as fifteen feet long. The underwater swimmer's suit gives complete protection except for any uncovered portion such as the hands.

CORAL stings are usually mild and unimportant but because of the razor sharp edges which commonly occur cuts from coral can readily be experienced. Such cuts, though superficial, are very slow to heal and often show a local toxic reaction which may lead to ulceration. Treatment for such cuts should be prompt and vigorous with magnesium sulphate or kaolin dressings. Antibiotics should also be given and antihistamine drugs may be helpful.

Well known among the stinging shell-fish are the CONE SHELLS of which there are many varieties all conical in shape and attractively marked. They are found in sand or under rocks and have a very effective venom apparatus including teeth which produce a bite into which the venom is pumped.

The sting of the Cone Shell produces a local redness, swelling and severe pain around the puncture wound. Numbness and tingling spread throughout the body and in severe cases death may follow respiratory paralysis and cardiac arrest.

It might have been thought that the evil-looking OCTOPUS would be one of the diver's most dangerous enemies but they and their kind are retiring animals content to lie hidden in the nooks and crannies of the ocean-bed. They do however possess a venom apparatus and can bite but this is only a real danger to man if they are thoughtlessly handled. Rarely are the bites serious and usually there is no more than a local wound and irritation.

There are also to be found under rocks the segmented ANNELID WORMS which, looking rather like legless millipedes, may have jaws to bite or bristles to sting. In both bite and sting there is a local reaction and the bristles may adhere to the skin.

The condition is not serious and little more than local soothing lotions are called for. Sticky tape will usually remove the bristles.

Lastly the SEA URCHINS, like curled-up hedgehogs with their vicious-looking spines may be found in crevices amongst the rocks. Their spines, tipped with venom cells, are long, sharp and brittle. They penetrate the skin deeply, break off and are difficult to remove. Invariably they produce the itching, redness and aching, so common in stings, which on occasions may be severe and fatal. Even if the poisoning is not severe the broken-off spines are very prone to produce a secondary infection. Care should be taken by divers to avoid contact with them and where they are handled gloves should be worn.

When all these dangerous marine animals are gathered together in a single chapter they may present a formidable picture but the sea is a vast expanse and these creatures are the least of the underwater swimmer's problems. It is important however that their existence is recognized and again it is emphasized that the best way to appreciate the risk is to make inquiries from the local experts before entering the water. It is even doubtful if the creatures of the sea are on the whole as dangerous as the creatures of the land.

SEA CREATURES DANGEROUS TO EAT

Many sea creatures are poisonous but this depends largely on what it eats. A fish may be poisonous in one part of the world but harmless elsewhere when on a different diet. Local information is here the best guide and Halstead, in his book, gives some useful advice and illustrations.

MAN—THE MARINE ANIMAL

It is not certain just what sort of animals the aquatic mammals were before they returned to the sea but there can be no doubt some instinct assured them that by doing so they would have a better chance of survival. Eminent zoologists have even suggested that man's ancestors made an attempt to do this, being forced to seek food in shallow waters. In so doing they lost their hair and learned to swim. Only in fiction however did any persist to become mermaids and mermen in Neptune's Kingdom.

Today science is coming to the aid of man, giving him the power to seek his fortune beneath the waves in the vast expanses of the sea and sea-bed. A great deal more imaginative and practical work is necessary. First, all the physiological and psychological functions of man must be completely studied in water and under pressure and secondly, the equipment designers must produce apparatus which will bring to man at any depth an environment within the limits required for normal behaviour and function. Breathing apparatus and clothing far in advance of what is available today will be needed. The first step towards this will be the design of a closed circuit breathing apparatus which will maintain a constant oxygen partial pressure irrespective of depth and activity. It must use a diluting gas of low density and low toxicity. Helium seems the best at present available though with care hydrogen might replace it. Ideally a gas which is also insoluble might be used if one exists.

A completely new approach to the problem of decompression is essential. Surface decompression procedures may be developed as an interim measure but the greatest promise would seem to be in man's adaptation to periods of prolonged high pressure. Weeks or months spent in sea-bed pressurized dwellings, breathing a safe and carefully controlled mixture, would enable frequent exploratory excursions into the surrounding water. Such a problem of maintaining a desired atmosphere is no more difficult than that facing submarine and space ship constructors.

FLUID BREATHING

Cousteau (1963) addressing the Second International Conference on Underwater Activities startled his audience by reference to 'homo aquaticus' whom he visualized as living underwater with his lungs and respiratory passages filled with a physiologically neutral salt solution to replace air spaces. Oxygen would be supplied to the tissues by diverting the blood flow from the circulation through a small oxygenating apparatus which obtained oxygen from hydrolysis of the sea water.

A much more practical and realistic approach is that of 'fluid breathing' proposed by Kylstra (1968). The breathing of gases must limit man's effective depth underwater but if the respiratory system were filled with fluid which could be breathed and supply oxygen his depth potential could be indefinitely increased subject of course to any direct effects of hydrostatic pressure.

23

Working first with mice and later with dogs, Kylstra has shown that a carefully balanced saline solution, in osmotic equilibrium with the blood, can be introduced into the lungs quite simply. If the experiments are conducted with the solution which has been, or is subjected to, high pressure oxygen sufficient of this may go into solution to oxygenate the tissues. With mice pressures of up to 30 ats. have been used. The animals have remained under water breathing the liquid for periods up to 18 hrs. without distress. When anaesthetized dogs were used the maximum period for survival was 45 minutes. The limiting factor in the technique is the elimination of carbon-dioxide. Fluid breathing produces considerable reduction in respiratory rate and carbon dioxide retention is inevitable. Before the technique became of practical value for man it would be necessary to find some fluid in which carbon dioxide would easily dissolve.

Meanwhile there is one possible compromise which might be of use to man. For example if divers accommodated under pressure in underwater chambers had their lungs filled with oxygenated fluids they might make short excursion dives to depths well beyond those attainable with gas breathing.

Fluid breathing however remains very much in the experimental stage but nevertheless shows great promise. It won't be long before human volunteers are breathing liquid under controlled laboratory conditions.

CONCLUSION

Man surely must extend his underwater activities to organized and profitable farming, mining, exploration and other occupations. In so doing it is absolutely inevitable that he will enrol the more advanced sea creatures, the mammals in particular, to aid him in his progress.

The potential such a future holds is beyond conception and assuredly once the significance of this is fully realized the great underwater adventure will proceed with gathering momentum. Many scientific disciplines will be involved, marine biology, oceanography, physiology and not the least underwater medicine.

Underwater medicine, as previous chapters must have shown, is very much in its infancy. Many gaps in knowledge must still be filled and much patient research remains to be done before the human race can enjoy, to the full, the fruits of the labours and triumphs of sub-aquatic man.

READING AND REFERENCES

Barcroft J. (1938). *Features in the Architecture of Physiological Function.* Cambridge University Press.

Coppleson, V. M. (1958). *Shark Attack.* Angus & Robertson Ltd., Sydney.

Cousteau, J. (1963). 'The Underwater Challenge.' The Palantype Organization, London.

Davies, H. D. (1964). 'About Sharks and Shark Attack.' Shuter & Shooter, South Africa.

Ewer, R. F. (1947). *New Biology 2.* Penguin Books, London.

Gray, R. W. (1927). 'The Depth to which Whales Descend.' *Nature.* *120*, 263.

Halstead, B. W. (1959). *Dangerous Marine Animals.* Cornell Maritime Press, Cambridge Md., U.S.A.

Kylstra, J. A. (1968). 'Experiments in Water Breathing.' *Scientific American 219*, 66.

Laurie, A. H. (1933). 'Some aspects of respiration in Blue and Fin Whales.' Discovery Report, Colonial Office, London.

U.S. Navy Diving Manual (1959). Navy Dept., Washington D.C.

INDEX

357